Vascular Surgery

Volume II
Peripheral Venous Diseases

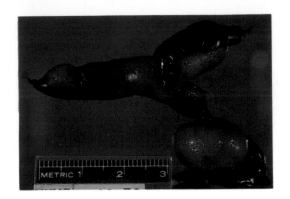

THROMBOGENESIS

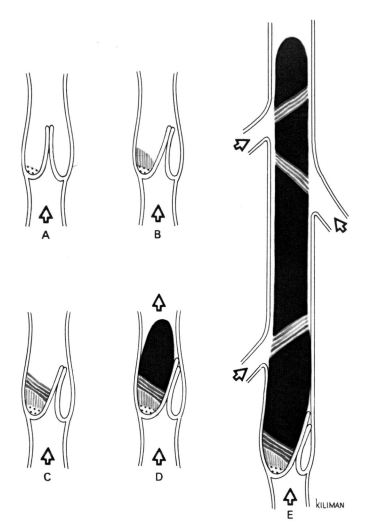

THROMBOGENESIS. (Redrawn in part from McLachlin, A. G., Venous Thrombosis and Pulmonary Embolism In Taylor, S. (ed.). *Recent Advances in Surgery.* London, Churchill, 1969, p. 341; and in part from a diagrammatic interpretation of thrombus propagation, p. 347, modified from Hadfield, G. Thrombosis. *Ann R Coll Surg* 6:219, 1950). (Courtesy of Dr. J. C. Parker, Lexington, Kentucky.)

Vascular Surgery

Volume II
Peripheral Venous Diseases

JOHN J. CRANLEY, M.D.

Director, Department of Surgery and Department of Medical Education, Good Samaritan Hospital, Cincinnati;

Director, Kachelmacher Memorial Varicose Vein Clinic, Logan; Kachelmacher Memorial Research Laboratory for Peripheral Venous Diseases, Good Samaritan Hospital, Cincinnati;

Assistant Clinical Professor of Surgery, University of Cincinnati College of Medicine, Cincinnati, Ohio

With Contributions by

CHARLES D. HAFNER, M.D.
RAYMOND J. KRAUSE, M.D.
ERNEST H. MEESE, M.D.

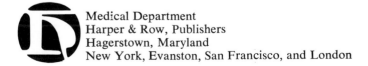

Medical Department
Harper & Row, Publishers
Hagerstown, Maryland
New York, Evanston, San Francisco, and London

Vascular Surgery

Volume II
Peripheral Venous Diseases

VASCULAR SURGERY:
  Volume II. Peripheral Venous Diseases

Copyright © 1975 by Harper & Row, Publishers, Inc.
All rights reserved. No part of this book may be used or reproduced in any
manner whatsoever without written permission except in the case of brief quo-
tations embodied in critical articles and reviews. Printed in the United States of
America. For information address Medical Department, Harper & Row, Publishers, Inc., 2350 Virginia Avenue, Hagerstown, Maryland 21740.

Library of Congress Cataloging in Publication Data

Cranley, John J.
  Peripheral venous diseases.

  (Vascular Surgery; v. 2)
  Includes bibliographical references and index.
  1. Peripheral vascular diseases.   2. Veins—
Diseases.   I. Title.   II. Series.
RD598.C73 vol. 2 [RC694] 617'.413'008s [617'.414]
ISBN 0-06-140666-X   75-6895

To
My Patient Wife, Helen

Contents

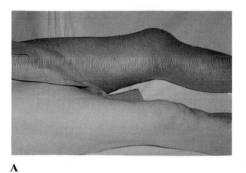

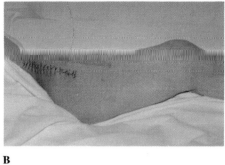

A

B

Figure A and B. "Benign" type of phlegmasia cerulea dolens with decrease in swelling and restoration of normal color of the skin a few hours following thrombectomy.

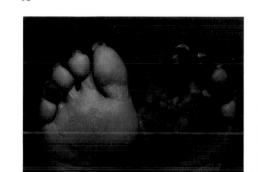

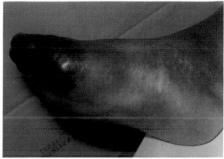

C

D

Figure C, D, E. and F. "Malignant" type of phlegmasia cerulea dolens. All occurred terminally.

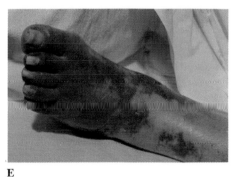

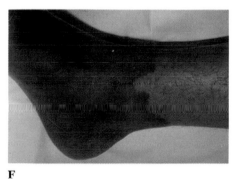

E

F

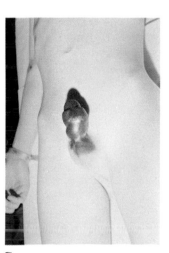

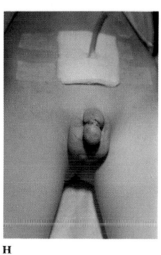

G

H

Figure G. Extensive venous thrombosis with apparent gangrene of the penis in a 10-year-old boy. Six hours prior to photograph, the penis was erect but with normal color. Condition was associated with disseminated intravascular coagulation, possibly due to a viral infection.

Figure H. Treatment consisted of surgical decompression and heparin therapy. The entire cast of the glans sloughed and separated. Normal functions restored, cystostomy tube removed the day of the photograph.

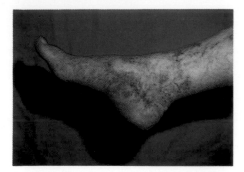

A

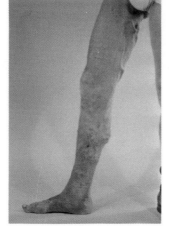

B

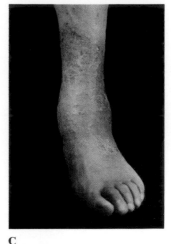

C

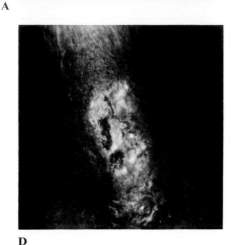

D

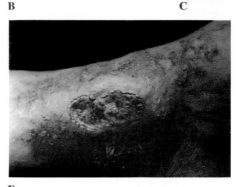

E

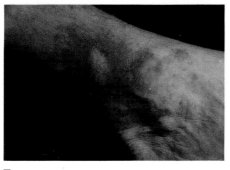

F

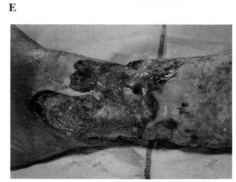

G

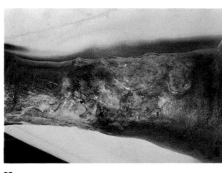

H

x

Figure A. The intracutaneous veins, greatly distended during pregnancy. They are frequently described by women as a "black" leg.

Figure B. Huge varicose veins associated with congenital arteriovenous fistulas. (See Case history; Figs. 9-14 A, B).

Figure C. Typical postphlebitic limb showing excoriation of skin and swelling centered around the malleoli.

Figure D. Postphlebitic ulcer nearly healed by application of pressure to demonstrate the brownish pigmentation of the skin as the ulcer heals. (See text under *Diagnosis*).

Figure E. Postphlebitic ulcer in a pregnant woman to demonstrate the bright red cellulitis frequently seen around such an ulcer. (See text under *Diagnosis*).

Figure F. A healed ulcer, to demonstrate the absence of reddish color and the presence of a brownish-tan color, indicating that the pathologic process is under control. (See text under *Diagnosis*).

Figure G. An extraordinarily dirty neglected postphlebitic ulcer. (See text).

Figure H. Postpartum phlebitis, 1929. Ulceration of the limb from 1938-55. The patient had had "successful" skin grafting procedures in 1953 and 1955. However, incompetent veins were not excised, and the limb was not treated with heavyweight elastic support after the patient left the hospital. (See *Technique, skin grafting*).

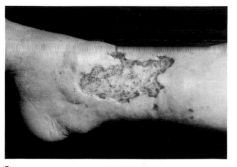

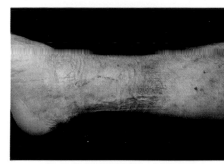

Figure I. Postphlebitic ulcer in an elderly woman.

Figure J. Treated by application of presure bandages. Healing required almost a year, but the patient carried on her housework while healing. (See text under *Pressure bandaging.*)

I

J

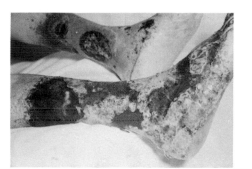

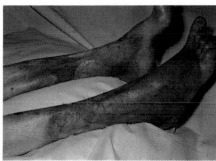

Figure K. Postphlebitic ulcers, neglected and aggravated by sitting in a rocking chair most of the time.

Figure L. Treated by bedrest and elevation, application of saline compresses changed 4 times daily for 1 month, followed by skin grafting, and afterward by use of heavyweight elastic support. (See text, under *Skin grafting.*)

K

L

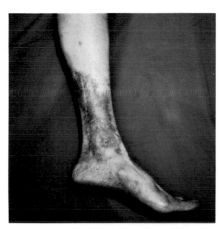

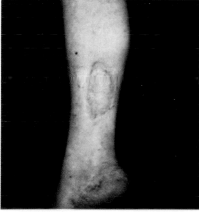

Figure M. 16-years post-Linton procedure for recurrent ulceration of the leg. Patient has worn heavyweight elastic support.

Figure N. 21-years post-Linton operation, followed by skin grafting for incisional slough. (See Case history No. 2.)

M

N

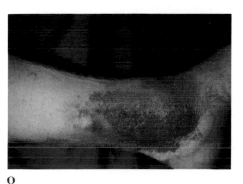

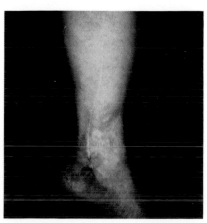

Figure O. (Case history No. 1) preoperatively.

O

Figure P. 21 years post-operative Linton operation. (See text, Case history No. 1.)

P

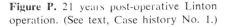

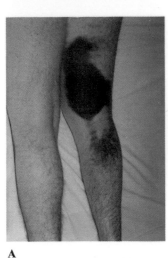

A

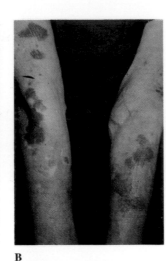

B

Figure A. Spontaneous hemorrhage of the leg. Before the ecchymosis appeared, patient was thought to have thrombophlebitis. This is one of the most common differential diagnoses encountered.

Figure B. Hemorrhagic blotching of the skin typical of patients receiving steroid therapy.

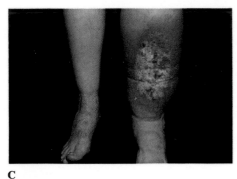

C

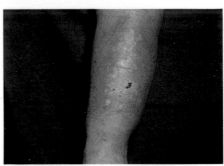

D

Figure C and D. Patient with lymphedema infection treated by bedrest, elevation, and continuous use of heavy-weight elastic support.

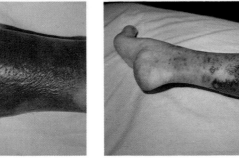

E

F

Figure E. Acute intradermal cellulitis associated with chills and fever, and in its less severe forms, mistaken for thrombophlebitis.

Figure F. A second patient with later phase of cellulitis which subsequently healed completely. This type of cellulitis is usually considered to be due to streptococcus.

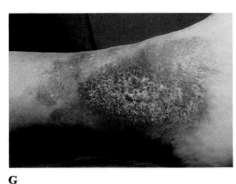

G

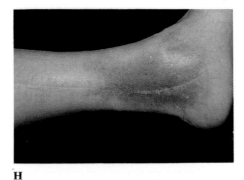

H

Figure G and H. Occasionally, atypical eczemas and ulcerations of the lower extremity are encountered, which cannot with certainty be ascribed to venous disease or to dermatologic disorders. If these lesions respond to pressure therapy, it is likely that a venous component is present, as is the case in this patient. He responded rapidly to pressure therapy and remained healed throughout a followup period of 3½ years after a Linton operation and the use of heavy-weight elastic stocking.

Contributors

CHARLES D. HAFNER, M.D., M.S., F.A.C.S.
Chief, Second Surgical Service, Good Samaritan Hospital; Chief, Vascular Surgery, Providence Hospital; Clinician, University of Cincinnati College of Medicine and Cincinnati General Hospital; Associate Attending Staff, St. Francis Hospital, Cincinnati, Ohio; Consulting Staff, Booth and St. Elizabeth's Hospitals, Covington, Kentucky; St. Luke's Hospital, Ft. Thomas, Kentucky.

Dr. Hafner prepared Chapter 10, "Portal Hypertension."

RAYMOND J. KRAUSE, M.D., F.A.C.S.
Attending Staff, Good Samaritan, St. Francis, St. George, and Providence Hospitals; Associate Attending Staff, Deaconess Hospital, Cincinnati, Ohio.

Dr. Krause collaborated on Chapter 6, "Operative Management of Acute Venous Thrombosis and Thrombophlebitis."

ERNEST H. MEESE, M.D., F.A.C.S., F.A.C.C., F.A.C.C.P.
Assistant Clinical Professor, Department of Surgery, Division of Cardiovascular and Thoracic Surgery, University of Cincinnati College of Medicine; Attending Surgeon, Division of Cardiovascular and Thoracic Surgery, Department of Surgery, Cincinnati General Hospital; Chief, Section of Thoracic Surgery, St. Francis Hospital; Attending Thoracic Surgeon, Good Samaritan and Providence Hospitals; Attending Thoracic Surgeon, St. George and Deaconess Hospitals, Cincinnati, Ohio; Consulting Thoracic Surgeon, St. Luke's Hospital, Ft. Thomas, Kentucky.

Dr. Meese prepared the section on syndromes of the superior vena cava in Chapter 7, "Special Syndromes," and the section on pulmonary embolectomy in Chapter 8, "Pulmonary Embolism."

Preface to Volume II

The intimate involvement of so many areas of medicine with the formation and pathologic consequences of venous thrombosis made the preparation of this volume far more complex than that of Volume I, Peripheral Arterial Diseases. It is impossible to discuss venous thrombosis comprehensively without at least touching on the mechanisms and abnormalities of coagulation, anticoagulation, and thrombolysis; nor can one deal with the diagnosis of venous thromboembolic disease without discussing electrocardiography, noninvasive and invasive radiography, and pulmonary physiology and pathology. To make these chapters as comprehensive and accurate as possible, we sought the counsel of many physician friends (see Acknowledgments) who contributed generously to our thinking. The result is, we believe, a compilation of the present state of knowledge of major venous problems encountered in clinical practice, with major emphasis placed on diagnosis and complete medical and surgical management.

The writing of Volume II, Peripheral Venous Diseases, coincided with the development in our research laboratory of the phleborheographic technique of diagnosing deep venous thrombosis, which is now a standard clinical test in our hospital. We believe this technique to be a major contribution to the diagnosis and differential diagnosis of acute and chronic venous thromboembolic disease, and it will also be useful in detecting concomitant obliterative arterial disease. We foresee phleborheography as the standard clinical test not only in hospitals but also in office practice, because of its great specificity and the ease with which it can be carried out.

As implied in the title, VASCULAR SURGERY stresses the operative *management of vascular problems. However, most patients with circulatory diseases are treated nonsurgically, and for this reason, the principles of medical and conservative therapy are equally stressed in this volume. As with Volume I, Peripheral Arterial Diseases, this second volume is addressed to internists as well as surgeons, to medical students, interns and residents, and to the physician in practice.*

Preface to Volume I

Prior to World War II, the field of vascular diseases was largely medical. Textbooks were usually written by internists and operative treatment consisted primarily of ligation of varicose veins, amputations, and an occasional lumbar sympathectomy. In the intervening 25 years, those of us in the field have participated in the birth and development of a new specialty. We have witnessed the development in rapid sequence of excisional therapy of arterial aneurysms, bypass grafting with homografts, several types of synthetic grafts, autogenous grafts, and even heterografts. We have learned to split the two layers of the media and to "thromboendarterectomize" the femoral artery, the iliac artery, the aorta, the renal arteries, and the carotid arteries. Some thrombi have been removed from veins; several types of portocaval shunts have effectively controlled portal hypertension. The heart has been entered, its valves replaced, aneurysms excised, its walls revascularized. These years can truly be called the Golden Age of Vascular Surgery.

A book written from the viewpoint of a participant in that creative period seems appropriate at this time. Even today there is a paucity of texts written by surgeons, and those available are quite often monographs on a particular subspecialty. This volume on arterial diseases and Volume II, on venous diseases, provides a succinct yet comprehensive commentary on the historical background of each topic with discussion of the important points of current diagnosis and management.

The surgeon will find this volume a comprehensive guide for the diagnosis and treatment of patients with vascular disease. Along with specific surgical procedures it includes detailed presentation of methods and techniques applicable to preoperative and postoperative examination and care. At the same time, the medical student, the intern and resident, and also the physician in other fields of practice will find in this text fundamental principles presented for his orientation.

Acknowledgments

A special debt of gratitude must be acknowledged to all my colleagues in a group practice that has grown since the publication of Peripheral Arterial Diseases *and that now includes: Raymond J. Krause, Edward S. Strasser, Charles D. Hafner, Ernest H. Meese, James J. Arbaugh, Rodolfo Q. Bruno, Ranjit Rath, and Richard E. Welling. All the materials herein presented are from our combined practice. Additionally, Dr. Hafner and Dr. Meese each contributed a chapter, and Dr. Krause joined me in preparing the chapter* Operative Management of Acute Venous Thrombosis and Thrombophlebitis. *Dr. Richard Mulvey worked with us in improving our phlebographic technique, and several of the photographs are his. In recent years Dr. Arbaugh and Dr. Bruno have performed most of our angiographic studies and many of their radiographs are used in this volume.*

Our thanks are given to Dr. Olga Dobrogorski for reviewing the pathology of pulmonary embolism; to Dr. J. C. Parker, Lexington, Kentucky, for lending us his superb photos, included in the frontispiece; to Dr. Donald Fischer for reviewing the section on cardiographic interpretation of pulmonary embolism; to Dr. Andrew Weiss for reviewing Chapters 2 and 8 and sections of Chapter 5, and for his valuable suggestions on coagulation in general; to Dr. Mohammad Atik for his generous help concerning dextran, and to Dr. Alec Haller, Baltimore, Maryland, for his detailed discussion of his work with dextran; to Dr. William Coon for consultation on the clinical aspects of pulmonary embolism; and to our British colleagues, Dr. N. M. Gibbs, for clarifying some details on the role of elevation in the discussion of prophylaxis of venous thrombosis and Dr. F. S. A. Doran and his associates for light they shed on galvanic stimulation of the calf muscle intraoperatively.

Our drawings were made by Gail Kiliman of the Good Samaritan Hospital Department of Medical Illustration, and by Carolyn Wehmann. Eric Soovere of our Department of Surgical Photography and Lewis O'Brien of the Cincinnati General Hospital Department of Surgical Photography provided our photographs.

The Herculean task of organization, preparation, and editing of the entire manuscript again was carried out by Rosamunde M. Preuninger, Ph.D., our Research Associate in Vascular Diseases and Supervisor of our Vascular Research Laboratory, who has been our statistician from the beginning of our practice.

Cincinnati, Ohio

J.J.C.

This work was supported in part by the Kachelmacher Memorial, Inc., Logan, Ohio

Vascular Surgery

Volume II
Peripheral Venous Diseases

1

The Venous System of the Lower Extremities

Man instinctively elevates his limbs for relief of tiredness and heaviness, thereby demonstrating the essentials of the anatomy, physiology, and pathology of the human peripheral venous system. This discussion is limited to the portions of these disciplines of interest to clinicians in their efforts to diagnose and treat venous insufficiency, particularly of the lower extremity. For detailed descriptions, textbooks on anatomy and physiology may be consulted.[1, 2] This treatise is based on our clinical experience spanning 25 years and on the treatment of approximately 10,000 patients seen in private practice, one third of whom had acute venous insufficiency and two-thirds with chronic venous incompetency. We are also able to draw on 13 years of experience with indigent patients in the vascular clinics at the Massachusetts General and Cincinnati General Hospitals. However, the statistical data that form the basis for this volume have been accumulated entirely from private practice.

ANATOMIC FACTORS OF CLINICAL SIGNIFICANCE

Five anatomic features are of significance to the surgeon: (1) The presence of venous valves, (2) the extensiveness of the normal venous network and the number of veins in the human body, (3) the connections between the superficial and deep venous systems in the lower extremities, (4) the potential points of compression of the major venous trunk, and (5) the soleal plexus of veins.

PRESENCE OF VENOUS VALVES

Although the *vis a tergo* (see section on Physiology) is the most important basic determinant for venous bloodflow back to the heart, unidirectional venous valves are necessary for maintaining a normal antigravity blood flow in the extremities, especially in the lower limbs.

When venous valves become incompetent due either to dilatation of the veins (varicose veins) or to destruction of the valves during recanalization of thrombosed veins the efficiency of the muscular pump or venous heart is reduced to the point of producing the pathologic changes typical of chronic venous insufficiency. The intensity of symptoms in patients with varicose veins and tissue destruction of the postphlebitic syndrome is believed to be directly related to the number of venous valves destroyed.

Extensiveness of the Normal Venous Network

Dissection of the veins of the body, particularly of the superficial system, is very difficult. For this reason, many anatomy textbooks depict the venous tree as being composed more or less of single veins which anastomose at various locations. Figure 1-1 indicates the extensiveness of the interconnections of the superficial veins of the lower extremities. The superficial veins are best thought of as an extensive network of innumerable interconnections, much

1

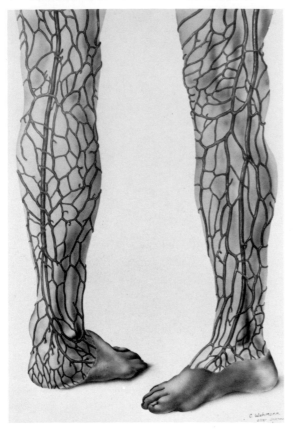

Figure 1-1. Anatomic diagram of extensive interconnections of superficial veins of the lower extremity. Posterior view, and anteromedial view. (*From Linton, R. R., Teaching collection. Original source unknown.*)

Figure 1-2. A. Patient with blockage of the deep major veins by thrombosis. Note extensiveness of collateral venous circulation in the thigh. **B.** Clot visible in vein just above the knee. Note extensiveness of collateral circulation in thigh.

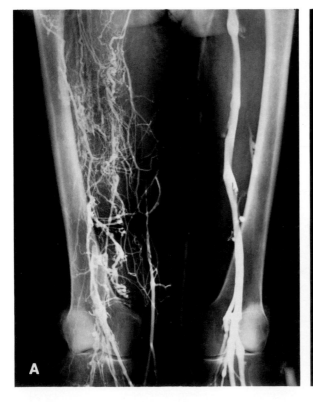

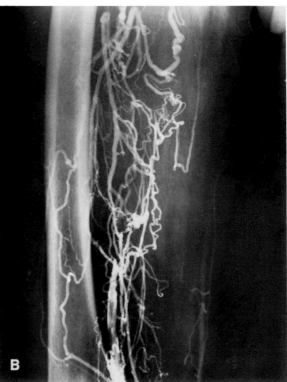

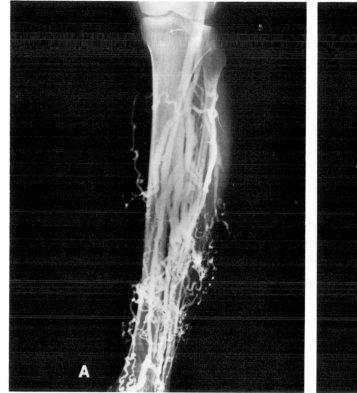
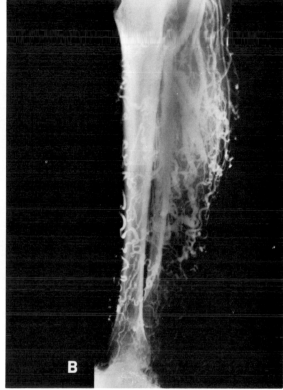

Figure 1-3. A. Phlebogram showing extensive duplication of major leg veins. **B.** Later phase of phlebogram, showing extensive venous circulation.

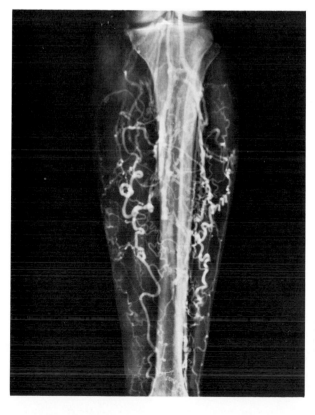

Figure 1-4. Phlebogram of leg following stripping of entire long and short saphenous veins, plus subfascial ligation of communicating veins, showing large number of incompetent veins remaining despite all efforts to eradicate them.

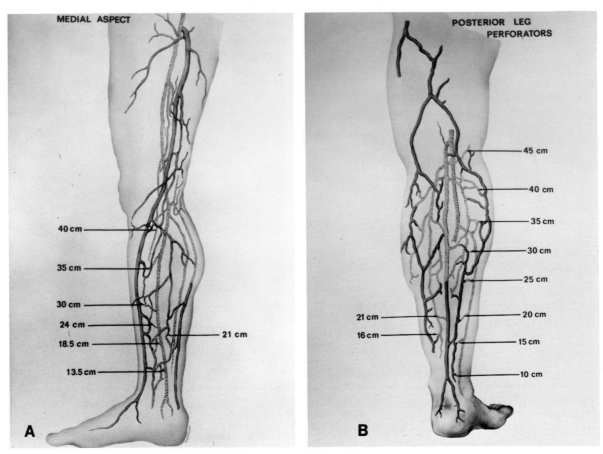

Figure 1-5. A and **B.** Anatomic location of the perforating (communicating) veins of the leg (after *Sherman*. Ann Surg 130:219, 1949.)

like the strands of a screen. Obviously, a radical surgical procedure is necessary for removal of all the incompetent veins in a patient with extensive varicosities. The phlebogram (Figs. 1-2 and 1-3), when performed on a patient with extensive venous thrombosis, strikingly demonstrates the tremendous number of deep veins that may exist in the extremity and which are not discovered by any other method of examination, not even during surgical procedures (Fig. 1-4). Of necessity, the veins greatly outnumber the arteries. The total venous return to the heart must at all times equal the total cardiac output; since the venous system is a low-pressure system, the large volume of blood can be handled only through channels larger and more numerous than the arteries. It is impossible to overstate the importance of the great number of veins. Surgeons experienced in peripheral vein surgery

who are aware of the intricate venous communications may ligate a single venous trunk for hemorrhage or for thrombosis without hesitation. If there is no secondary thrombosis, ligation of almost any vein in the extremities or the abdomen usually will not result in persistent swelling; however, if there is secondary thrombosis, the consequent obliteration of numerous venous channels may produce massive swelling. For this reason, anticoagulant therapy with heparin is of value following ligation of a major venous trunk.

Connections Between Superficial and Deep Venous Systems in the Lower Extremities

The connection of the superficial and deep veins via the communicating veins is an important anatomic concept that must be understood by the surgeon. Figure 1-5 is a reproduction of an anatomic dissection, showing the position of the communicating veins. Normally the flow of blood is from the superficial system to the deep system. When the communicators are incompetent, as in the postphlebitic syndrome, division and ligation of these veins is an essential portion of the operative treatment.

Points of Compression of a Major Venous Trunk

A vein can be compressed more easily than an artery. A superficial vein may be occluded by a tight belt or by tight garters. The gravid uterus may completely occlude the inferior vena cava during the late months of pregnancy,[3, 4] particularly when the patient is supine. A site of obstruction that is not widely recognized and that should be stressed is the point at which the right common iliac artery crosses the left iliac vein.[5] Fibrous stenosis of the iliac vein may occur at this point; in addition, retrograde thrombosis of the entire common iliac vein, a potential cause of swelling of the left lower extremity, may occur.

The normal vein is strong. In a normal person, rupture of a vein by increased internal pressure is very rare. In general, the veins are more resistant to pressure than the capillaries drained by them; with a rise in venous pressure, the capillaries filter at a progressively more rapid rate.[1] Toward the end of the nineteenth century, Gréhant and Quinquaud[6] concluded that the veins of an animal normally require a slightly higher internal pressure to rupture than the carotid arteries of the same animal. The bursting pressure of a normal carotid artery or iliac vein is between 7 and 8 atmospheres. It has now been proven that the normal saphenous vein is an almost perfect substitute for the femoral artery in direct arterial operative procedures. At times aneurysms have formed at the point of anastomosis of saphenous vein to femoral artery; however, an aneurysm of the vein itself is the rarest of complications.

The Soleal Plexus

The soleal plexus of large veins is probably designed to be the main peripheral venous heart. (See Chapter 2, Figs. 2-14 to 2-17.) These veins have not been extensively studied in the United States, but reports from abroad[7–10] indicate their great significance (Figs. 1-6 and 1-7). Note that the posterior tibial and peroneal are both paired veins.

Figure 1-6. **A.** Diagram of anatomy of deep veins. **P.V.** = popliteal vein. **P.T.V.** = posterior tibial. **Per.** = peroneal. **G** = gastrocnemial. **S** = soleal. **B.** Phlebogram of amputated limb injected with micropaque. **S** = soleal venous sinuses. (From *Cotton, L. T., & Clark, C.* Ann Roy Coll Surg Engl 36:*215, 1965.*)

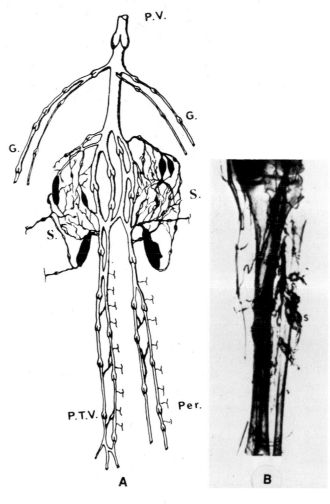

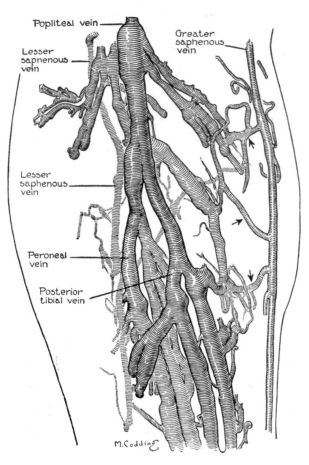

Popliteal vein

Greater saphenous vein

Lesser saphenous vein

Lesser saphenous vein

Peroneal vein

Posterior tibial vein

M.Codding

Figure 1-7. Anatomic sketch showing deep veins of the legs. Note duplication of major trunks and size of tributaries from the soleus muscle, constituting venous heart. Note that the posterior tibial and peroneal are paired veins. (*From Charles Rémy.* Traité des Varices, *Vigot Fréres, Paris, ca. 1905. Modified by Homans, J.* Circulatory Diseases of the Extremities. *New York, Macmillan, 1939.*)

PHYSIOLOGIC FACTORS OF CLINICAL SIGNIFICANCE

THE VIS A TERGO

The basic cause of flow in the venous system is the *vis a tergo* (the force from behind) of the heart. When a man is upright, his vascular system may be depicted as a U-tube, with the arteries forming the descending limb, the veins the ascending limb, and the capillaries the bottom of the tube. It is easy to see that little pressure is required to force the venous blood to return to the heart against gravity. Furthermore, the diameter of the venous system is enormous, making it truly a low-flow system that can transport large volumes of blood toward the heart under pressures that are scarcely measurable. It has been stated[2] that blood will flow upward from the extremity even in the absence of venous valves.

NEGATIVE PRESSURE WITHIN THE THORAX

The negative pressure in the chest is also a factor in augmenting the flow of venous blood toward the heart. This is particularly true when the body is recumbent. However, it is clear that some other factor is the critical one in patients with chronic venous insufficiency of the lower extremity. For example, it may be assumed that the forward propulsion of blood from the heart and the sucking action of the thorax in inspiration are equal in the patient with one normal extremity and one extremity with chronic venous insufficiency. Obviously, some inequality exists. The abnormal limb has symptoms such as tiredness, heaviness, aching pain, fullness, and nocturnal cramps; there is gradual abnormal hemosiderin pigmentation of the skin, atrophy, induration of the subcutaneous tissues, and eventual ulceration of the skin. A specific defect, i.e., a critical difference, exists between the extremities, viz., a loss of efficiency of the venous heart or muscular pump in the abnormal limb caused by damage to or destruction of the venous valves.

The Venous Heart

The venous heart is analogous to the thoracic heart. Contraction of the muscles of the limb thrusts the blood forward. Even without venous valves, the blood would be propelled toward the heart since there is less resistance to blood flowing proximally in the great veins than to blood flowing distally in the capillaries.

The Venous Valves

The efficiency of the venous pump or heart is enhanced by the one-way valves. These valves also protect the small venules and capillaries from the wave of pressure due to coughing, straining, lifting, and other exertions. In this regard, it is interesting that the valve in the jugular vein is unidirectional toward the heart despite the fact that the flow from the head is almost entirely gravitational.

The Veins as Blood Depots

The entire venous bed may be thought of as a variable blood depot that holds approximately 70 to 75 per cent of the circulating blood at any given moment.[11, 12] According to Brecher,[2] blood in this type of depot is not withdrawn from the active circulation. It merely circulates *slowly* when the venous channels are widened by prevailing parasympathetic tonus. Since the central veins constitute a considerable part of this "depot," blood is readily available for a sudden increase in right heart inflow and subsequent output as demand arises. A corresponding state prevails in the left side of the heart, as has been pointed out by Sjöstrand.[13] On the left side the pulmonary vascular bed represents a readily available large reservoir permitting a sudden increase of left-heart filling.[2]

EFFECT OF MUSCULAR CONTRACTION ON VENOUS PRESSURE

Carrier and Rehberg in 1923[14] showed that pressure in the superficial veins of the dependent leg could be reduced by muscular contraction. Further study by Walker and Longland,[15] Pollack *et al.,*[16] White and Warren,[17] and DeCamp *et al.*[18] has led to the formulation of the fundamental concept by means of which the physiology of the venous circulation of the lower extremities of man may be properly understood. Their findings can be summarized as follows:

If a needle (Fig. 1-8) is inserted at the ankle and connected to a manometer, the venous pressure can be measured when the patient is standing still or walking in place. When he is standing still, the pressure represents the weight of a column of blood from the needle to the left auricle. This pressure varies among individuals according to their height; however, it does not vary with the presence or absence of venous disease in the lower extremity unless there is an acute obstruction. In other words, the resting direct pressure is identical in both legs of a patient having one normal extremity and one extremity with varicose veins.[17] However, when the patient walks in place, the fall in pressure varies greatly and, if there is venous valvular incompetence, significantly. In the normal subject in the series of Pollack *et al.,*[16] the average fall in pressure was 64 mm Hg. When the subject stopped walking, it required an average of 31 seconds for the pressure to equilibrate at the initial level. In a subject with varicose veins (Fig. 1-9) and without evidence of deep venous insufficiency, the average fall in pressure in the same series was 37 mm Hg, and an average of only 2.8 seconds was required to regain the standing pressure. In the patient with the postphlebitic syndrome (Fig. 1-10), the average fall in pressure was only 11 mm Hg, and the resting level was reached again in 1 second. These findings are in close agreement with those of other investigators.[17, 18] In the patient with obstruction of the major veins (popliteal, femoral, or vena cava), the venous pressure became higher than the resting level after a period of walking.[15] Some difficulty was encountered in describing this phenomenon because in most patients with venous insufficiency caused by venous valvular incompetence, the pressure after walking, although higher than normal, is lower than the resting level. Therefore, "venous hypertension" could not be used and the term "ambulatory venous hypertension" was coined.

These studies conclusively demonstrate the following important clinical physiologic and pathologic points:

1. In a normal subject, the pressure in the superficial veins of the lower extremity is less when he is walking than when he is standing still. This explains why so many patients feel better when walking than when standing or sitting.

2. In a patient with primary varicose veins and without the postphlebitic syndrome, the pressure in the superficial veins is higher than normal when he is walking. This pressure can be restored to normal by removing the varicosities or by temporarily occluding them.[19] Our clinical experience corroborates this finding. Therefore, we have concluded that venous insufficiency is curable even when ulceration of the leg is present *if the insufficiency is secondary to varicose veins alone,* because after the ulcer is healed and the incompetent veins are removed, the patient has a normal lower extremity and does not need external support.

3. In the patient with the typical postphlebitic syndrome with venous valvular incompetence of the deep and superficial veins, there is a minimal drop in pressure when he is ambulatory. This pressure is not restored to normal by use of a tourniquet or by excision of the incompetent superficial veins. It is for this reason that ulcers of the leg that are secondary to deep venous valvular insufficiency are considered incurable, i.e., regardless of the operative treatment, the patient must wear external support for life. Furthermore, the external support must be sufficiently forceful to completely overcome the tendency to edema. In our opinion, venous pressure studies have significantly clarified our understanding of venous physiology and pathology of the lower extremity.

Figure 1-8. Venous return from lower extremity. Normal limb. See text for details.

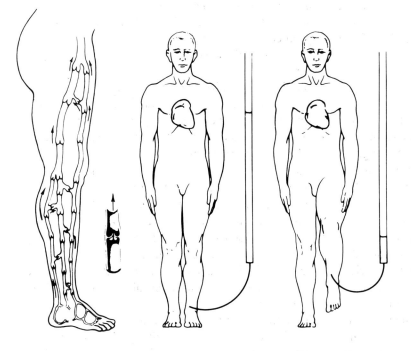

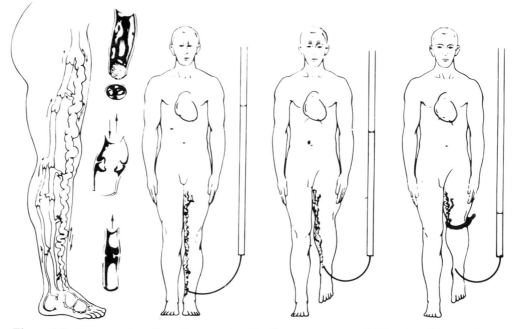

Figure 1-9. Venous return from lower extremity. Incompetent superficial veins. See text for details.

Figure 1-10. Venous return from lower extremity. Incompetent superficial, deep and communicating veins. See text for details.

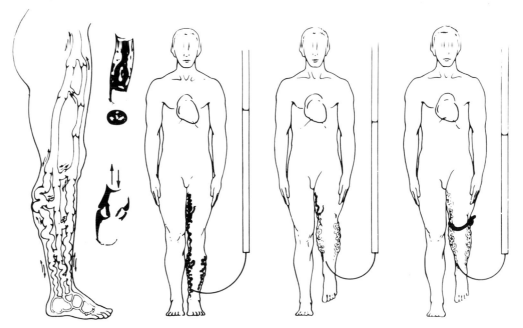

REFERENCES

1. Franklin, K. J. *A Monograph on Veins.* Springfield, IL., Thomas, 1937.
2. Brecher, G. A. *Venous Return.* New York, Grune & Stratton, 1956.
3. McRoberts, W. A. Postural shock in pregnancy. *Am J Obstet Gynecol 62:*627, 1951.
4. Howard B. K., Goodson, J. H., and Mengert, W. F. Supine hypotensive syndrome in late pregnancy. *Obstet Gynecol 1:*371, 1953.
5. Cockett, F. B., and Lea-Thomas, M. The iliac compression syndrome. *Br J Surg 52:*816, 1965.
6. Gréhant, N., and Quinquaud, H. Mesure de la pression nécessaire pour déterminer la rupture des vaisseaux sanguins. *J Anat Paris 21:*287, 1885.
7. Flanc, C., Kakkar, V. V., and Clarke, M. B. The detection of venous thrombosis of the legs using ^{125}I-labelled fibrinogen. *Br J Surg 55:*742, 1968.
8. Negus, D., Pinto, D. J., Le Quesne, L. P., Brown, N., and Chapman, M. ^{125}I-labelled fibrinogen in the diagnosis of deep vein thrombosis and its correlation with phlebography. *Br J Surg 55:*835, 1968.
9. Browse, Norman L. The ^{125}I-fibrinogen uptake test. *Arch Surg 104:*160, 1972.
10. Kakkar, V. V. The diagnosis of deep vein thrombosis using the ^{125}I-fibrinogen test. *Arch Surg 104:*152, 1972.
11. Green, H. D. Circulation: Physical principles. In Glasser, O. (ed.) *Medical Physics.* Chicago, Year Book, 1944, vol. 1, p. 208.
12. Landis, E. M., and Hortenstine, J. C. Functional significance of venous blood pressure. *Physiol Rev 30:*1, 1950.
13. Sjöstrand, T. Volume and distribution of blood and their significance in regulating circulation. *Annu Rev Physiol 33:*202, 1953.
14. Carrier, E. B., and Rehberg, P. B. Capillary and venous pressure in man. *Arch Physiol Skand 44:*20, 1923.
15. Walker, A. J., and Longland, C. J. Venous pressure measurements in the foot in exercise as an aid to investigation of venous disease in the leg. *Clin Sci 9:*101, 1950.
16. Pollack, A. A., Taylor, B. E., Myers, T. T., and Wood, E. H. The effect of exercise and body position on the venous pressure at the ankle in patients having venous valvular defects. *J Clin Invest 28:*559, 1949.
17. White, E., and Warren, R. The walking venous pressure test as a method of evaluation of varicose veins. *Surgery 26:*987, 1949.
18. DeCamp, P. T., Ward, J. A., and Ochsner, A. Ambulatory venous pressure studies in postphlebitic and other disease states. *Surgery 29:*365, 1951.
19. Lofgren, K. A. Measurement of ambulatory venous pressure in the lower extremity. *Surg Forum* pp. 163–168, 1954. Vol. 5, Saunders, Phila. 1955.

2

Venous Thrombosis and Thrombophlebitis

Venous thrombosis is the most precise term to describe intraluminal clotting in the deep venous system. At times the thrombus is attached to its point of origin; this may be a valve pocket, a site near the junction of two veins, or an area of dilatation or sacculation of a vein. The thrombus may be in contact with only a small portion of the vein wall; thus, its nonadherent tail floats freely in the venous bloodstream. This floating clot, which may produce minimal symptoms, is potentially the most lethal. Detachment of the clot, either complete or in part, converts a thrombus into an embolus which may then lodge in the pulmonary tree.

THROMBOPHLEBITIS

There is little evidence to suggest focal disease of the vein wall itself at the site of origin of a thrombus; nevertheless, it is generally accepted that if a thrombus becomes attached to the vein wall, by some unknown mechanism it initiates inflammation of the vein or *thrombophlebitis*. Such inflammation is secondary to the venous thrombosis. The clinical syndrome of thrombophlebitis is thus initiated. Depending on the degree of involvement of the vein wall and perivenous tissues, symptoms and signs may be absent, may include scarcely perceptible pain and tenderness, or may progress to include massive swelling of the entire extremity and severe pain. When the common femoral and external iliac veins are occluded, swelling is great. In the past, this type was termed milk leg or *phlegmasia alba dolens*. A better term is *iliofemoral thrombophlebitis*. Symptoms include swelling of the entire extremity to the groin, associated groin tenderness, pain in the calf and thigh, reddish-pink suffusion of the skin. Rarely, there is further spreading of the venous thrombosis into the smaller veins; obstruction then becomes so great that arterial inflow is significantly reduced. The limb turns a violaceous blue, then a deep blue (*phlegmasia cerulea dolens*), and finally blue-black as the limb becomes uniformly ischemic.

When intravenous thrombosis is initiated by injury to the vein wall, such as following the injection of a hypertonic or other irritating solution, or by infection secondary to venipuncture, or to an indwelling venous catheter, the term *thrombo-*

phlebitis seems most appropriate since the venous thrombosis is secondary to the inflammatory process in the vein wall.

PHLEBOTHROMBOSIS

The term "phlebothrombosis" was introduced by Ochsner and associates[1] in an attempt to distinguish between a freely floating thrombus with minimal symptoms but maximal danger and the more adherent type with maximal symptoms caused by extensive inflammation of the vein but with far less chance of detachment. This was an attractive concept and, in the ideal situation, meaningful. The clinical picture, however, is usually less clear cut. The patient with acute symptomatic thrombophlebitis may develop a soft clot or tail distal to the firmly adherent clot, so it is not safe to assume that the patient with maximal symptoms is in no danger of embolism. If embolization does not take place, a loose clot filling a vein may become attached to the wall in a very short time. Therefore, the period of "phlebothrombosis" is indeed brief and lacks real clinical significance. Actually, most clinicians recognize that pulmonary embolism does occur following deep thrombophlebitis,[2,3] however active and symptomatic it may be. "Phlebothrombosis" at best describes a transient distinction, one that compounds rather than clarifies the confusion surrounding the problem of venous thrombosis. Since it may give the physician a false sense of security, it has been well recommended that this controversial term be dropped from our vocabulary.

PULMONARY EMBOLISM

The subject of pulmonary embolism is covered in Chapter 8, and is the prime complication of thrombophlebitis. Without it, the disease would run a benign course and, in many instances would go undetected, since diagnosis is often made only after embolization has occurred. Obviously then, pulmonary embolism is intrinsic in any discussion of thromboembolic disease.

INCIDENCE

The incidence of thrombophlebitis is not only unknown, it has indeed been unknowable. The difficulty in establishing the incidence stems from the lack of firm evidence that the disease was diagnosed correctly in all cases so described and, conversely, that a significant number of cases have failed to be properly diagnosed as thrombophlebitis. While phlegmasia alba dolens or phlegmasia cerulea dolens and superficial thrombophlebitis may be recognized at a glance, other forms of the disease are difficult and sometimes impossible to diagnose on clinical examination. Until recently, the diagnostician had to rely largely on purely clinical findings. For this reason, past records are invalid for statistical use. Today, the availability of phlebography, techniques using the Doppler effect, impedance plethysmography, and phleborheography makes it possible for the physician to verify his clinical findings. The frequency of error is enough to cast doubt on the reliability of figures in the older reports. Our experience with phleborheography suggests that this technique offers the opportunity of making the correct diagnosis in almost all patients with thrombosis of the major veins, i.e., of the popliteal, femoral, iliac, or vena cava, and in the majority of patients with thrombosis in the posterior tibial or peroneal veins.[4] It is hoped that in the future, clinical records will furnish corroborative evidence of the correctness of the diagnosis. This in turn will permit a true basis for statistical studies. (See section on Incidence, Chapter 8.)

Our practice is centered around peripheral vascular diseases; therefore, our records on the incidence of the disease do not reflect the average regional or epidemiologic distribution. Still, certain observations and impressions have been inescapable.

1. *Superficial thrombophlebitis is a common and usually self-limited condition.* At least 70 per cent of the patients seen on an ambulatory basis have resolution of their symptoms and signs; this resolution is probably spontaneous, but it may possibly be influenced by prescribed conservative measures, i.e., use of supportive bandages or, occasionally, a day or two of bed rest. Occasionally in postpartum patients, completely spontaneous resolution of this type of thrombophlebitis has been noted within 24 to 48 hours. This indicates the ability of the normal physiologic processes to dissolve clots (Table 2-1).

2. *Deep thrombophlebitis is also very common* (Table 2-1). In our experience, it is approximately three times as common (excluding chemical phlebitis secondary to intravenous administration of solutions) as the superficial variety (Table 2-2) with which it shares basic similarities.[5] Based on a review of our patients, at least 70 per cent who have deep thrombophlebitis undergo spontaneous resolution without pulmonary embolism. This is supported by the large number of patients seen with the postphlebitic syndrome who either have no recollection of past thrombophlebitis or injury or recall having a painful, swollen limb that recovered without treatment.

3. *Pulmonary embolism is not a complication of superficial thrombophlebitis unless the process has extended into the deep venous system.*

4. *Few patients with thrombophlebitis of the deep and/or superficial venous systems die of pulmonary embolism. The majority of emboli to the lungs are small and cause minor symptoms or no symptoms at all.* When large enough for the diagnosis to be made (Table 2-3), pulmonary emboli are not fatal in the great majority of patients and cause few sequelae if treated with heparin and the prothrombin-depressant agents.

5. *The high annual mortality rate for patients with pulmonary embolism therefore indicates the far higher incidence of thrombophlebitis, the disease of which fatal embolism is a relatively uncommon complication.*

PATHOLOGY

Thrombophlebitis is a synthetic term of three Greek components. The two nouns, *phleb-,* meaning vein, and *thrombos,* a thickening (specifically, thickened blood or clot),[6] pose no difficulty in interpretation—they clearly mean a blood clot in a vein. The suffix *-itis,* which in medicine has come to mean "inflammation," makes the term "thrombophlebitis" unacceptable to those who dispute an inflammatory component. The inflammation in thrombophlebitis may be primary when caused by sepsis or chemical trauma or associated with blunt trauma; however, in most instances of deep venous thrombosis, inflammation is secondary to the thrombus.

Thrombus

The term *thrombus* was introduced into the medical literature by Virchow in 1846;[7] he commented that he did not deny the existence of phlebitis (i.e., inflammation of the vein wall), but at the same time he maintained that although the matter in clotted veins might *look* like pus, it was *not* pus. To describe this entity, he coined the word *thrombus* and defined "thrombosis" as "a real coagulation of

TABLE 2-1. Treatment of Acute Thrombophlebitis

	PATIENTS	%
Superficial		
Conservative treatment	717	79
Surgical treatment	195	21
Deep		
Conservative treatment	2384	89
Surgical treatment	307	11

TABLE 2-2. Acute Venous Thrombosis: 1952–1973

	NO. PATIENTS	%
Deep venous system only	2520	70.0
Deep and superficial	171	4.0
Phlegmasia cerulea dolens	48	1.3
Superficial system only	912	25.0

TABLE 2-3. Acute Deep Venous Thrombosis: 1952–1973

	NO. PATIENTS	%	DIAGNOSED PULMONARY EMBOLISM	%
Deep system alone	2520	91.5	323	12.8
Deep and superficial	171	6.0	14	8.2
Phlegmasia cerulea dolens	48	1.7	1	2.0

the blood at a certain fixed spot." He clearly stated that a thrombus is not necessarily associated with sepsis, is not necessarily adherent to the vein wall, and does not necessarily fill the vein. He further noted that a thrombus might liquefy with time, and/or the soft proximal clot might break loose and be carried to the lung; this process he described as "embolia."[8] He deduced that after lodging at the main bifurcation in the lung, the clot could subsequently break up into small pieces and be carried to the farthest recesses of the lung.

Welch[9] reviewed the literature in 1889 and further defined a thrombus as a solid mass of blood formed in the living heart or vessels from constituents of blood. He defined thrombosis as the act or process of thrombus formation or the condition characterized by its presence. Welch's definition is still valid. According to Hume et al.,[10] a thrombus is formed in flowing blood and is a layered structure containing varying amounts of red cells, groups of granular leukocytes, and condensed masses of platelets bound by fibrin. Depending on the rate of flow, i.e., on the degree of venous stasis, the venous clot will be more or less obviously layered. Changes in the clot with time tend to obscure the layering. The point of attachment, which may be minuscule and easily missed, may be white or red, depending on the extent of platelet involvement and the inflammatory component, i.e., the white blood cells. The tail of the venous clot is formed almost exclusively via coagulation and is red. Secondary points of attachment may have an inflammatory component. This is why it may be very difficult for a pathologist to differentiate a venous thrombus from a postmortem clot. Evidence of organization and chance sectioning showing points of attachment are among the few clues to identify the thrombus.

Exposure of the initial nidus on the vein wall to flowing blood permits the thrombus to grow by accretion until it occludes the vein wall. This layering stops when the flowing blood is halted by the occlusion and coagulation occurs in the quieted stream. The coagulation may proceed proximally and/or distally (Fig. 2-1). When this clot, growing by propagation, reaches another inflowing tributary, platelets adhere to it and new layering formation of a thrombus begins (see frontispiece). Thus, the eventual thrombus is a composite structure. The head and other areas where platelets have been de-

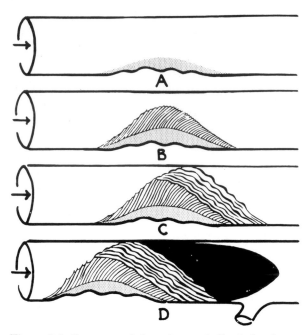

Figure 2-1. Sequence of thrombus and distal clot formation. (*From Hadfield, G.* Ann R Coll Surg Engl 6:224, 1950.)

posited are whitish in color; this is called a white thrombus. The areas composed of coagulated blood are red and are called red thrombus; this is composed mainly of red cells and fibrin. Grossly, the thrombus appears to be a firm, condensed, and relatively dry tubular structure, different from the moist, gelatin-like postmortem clot. Often, slightly granular, fine, circumferential lines known as the lines of Zahn,[11] are present (Fig. 2-2). They are considered to be external signs of lamination. Most venous thrombi are dark red from many red cells, but some are whitish or pink, depending on their leukocyte and platelet content. Lamination is always present in propagating thrombi and is also found in many retrograde extensions[10] (Fig. 2-3).

Arterial Thrombus

Arterial thrombosis differs distinctly from venous thrombosis. In arterial thrombosis, platelets adhere to exposed collagen or to broken or otherwise damaged intima, forming a platelet aggregate. Portions of this platelet aggregate may be swept away by the current, depending on the rapidity of the flow of the current. The swept-away platelet clumps may lyse, but new platelets adhere to the

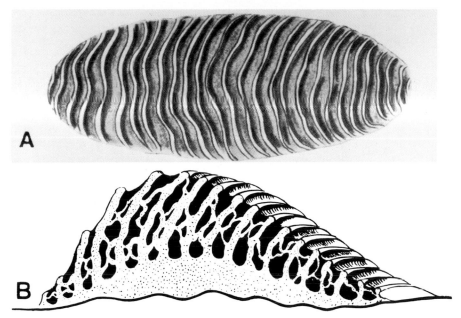

Figure 2-2. A. External appearance of thrombus. **B.** Cross section of thrombus. (*From Hadfield, G.* Ann R Coll Surg Engl 6:*225, 1950.*)

Figure 2-3. Basic thrombus structure. A coral-like framework of conglutinated platelets is covered by a condensed layer of fibrin containing leukocytes; the spaces between the framework are filled by blood clot. **A.** Longitudinal section. **B.** Transverse section. *Reproduced by kind permission from* General Pathology (*4th edition, 1970*), *edited by Lord Florey. London: Lloyd-Luke (Medical Books).*

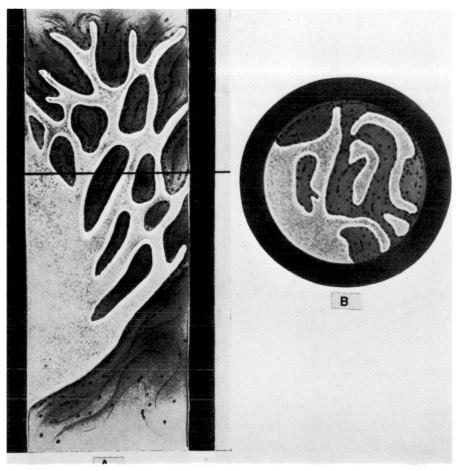

original clump, fibrin appears throughout the plug, and it then contracts. The fibrin itself initiates more platelet clumping; again a platelet mass forms by concretion and aggregation; again it is enmeshed in fibrin. This is the true building block of an intraluminal thrombus. The initial mass may appear on section to look something like a coral reef (see Figs. 2-2 and 2-3).

Postmortem Clot

A postmortem clot is similar to a blood clot that forms in a test tube. In each case, blood coagulation results in the formation of a fibrin mesh in which red cells, white cells, and platelets are trapped. This type of clot is red, gelatinous, and friable; it is called a red thrombus. The red and white cells and platelets in the fibrin mesh are scattered at random as they were in the liquid blood.

Collagen

Disruption of the vascular endothelium exposes the basement membrane and subendothelial collagen to the flowing blood. Collagen initiates clot

Figure 2-4. An artery injured by electric stimulus. Mass of platelets (**P**) is attached to wall at point (**arrows**) at which endothelium (**E**) has been destroyed (×3600). (*From French* et al. Br J Exp Path 45:467, 1964.)

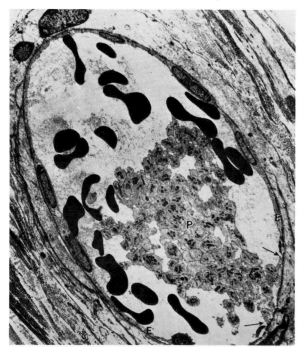

formation by two separate and distinct mechanisms: by induction of platelet aggregration and by activation of the Hageman factor (coagulation factor XII) to initiate the intrinsic clotting mechanism. The presence of a free amino group, especially the ε-amino group of lysine, specifically initiates platelet aggregation.[12] On the other hand, the negatively charged free hydroxyl groups of glutamic acid and aspartic acid in collagen are necessary for the activation of the Hageman factor.[12]

Platelet Aggregation

Within seconds after exposure of the blood to collagen, platelets can be observed adhering to the area of trauma and to each other (Figs. 2-4 and 2-5). More and more platelets are carried in the bloodstream to the site and stick to those which were initially deposited. This aggregation of platelets forms a loose hemostatic plug; this subsequently consolidates into a firm plug supported by a fibrin mesh. During this same time, the blood coagulation process is also activated and fibrin deposition is already evident, especially at the periphery of the hemostatic plug. Fibrin formation is the last event in primary hemostasis.

LYSIS OF PLATELETS

The intricacies of clotting are beyond the scope of this book. However, it must be recognized that the entire clotting mechanism, both platelet aggregation and coagulation, is balanced at all times by forces tending to lyse platelets and prevent coagulation. A slight shift in this equilibrium decides whether clotting occurs or bleeding becomes uncontrolled.

PATHOGENESIS OF THROMBOPHLEBITIS

It is convenient to study the pathogenesis of thrombophlebitis via the categories outlined in the famous triad of Virchow,[13] viz., changes in the vein wall, changes in the coagulability of blood, and changes in the velocity of bloodflow.

Changes in the Vein Wall

Until the mid-nineteenth century it was generally believed that the process of thrombophlebitis

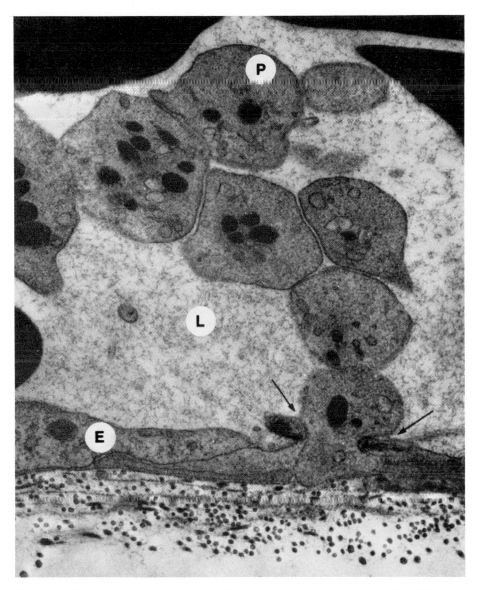

Figure 2-5. Part of wall of small vein in a hamster showing a group of platelets (**P**) in the lumen (**L**). One platelet occupies an intercellular gap (**arrows**) in the endothelium (**E**). (×26,000). (*From French* et al. Br J Exp Path *45:467, 1964.*)

started with inflammation of the vein wall. Virchow[14] was the first to raise doubts about this; since his time, more and more evidence has been accumulated that the pernicious type of deep venous thrombosis starts without any abnormality in the vein wall itself. There is no doubt, however, that injury to the vein wall can produce thrombosis, as originally shown by Eberth and Schimmelbusch in 1886.[15] In fact, in injection therapy for varicose veins, sclerosing solutions are used to produce venous thrombosis by irritating the vein wall.

TRAUMA

INJURY TO THE VEIN WALL. O'Neill in 1947[16] devised a method using silver nitrate solution whereby the entire endothelial surface of a vein could be studied. He was able to diagram (Fig. 2-6) the normal anatomy of the vein wall. He noted that the venules of the wall do not enter into the parent lumen; instead, venous capillaries form venules which emerge from the adventitia of the vein wall (usually as venae comites for entering arterioles) and then empty into the veins which run

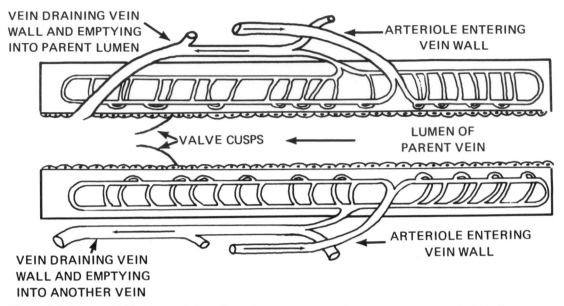

Figure 2-6. Pattern of blood vessels in vein wall. (*From O'Neill, J. F. Ann Surg 126:270, 1947.*)

Figure 2-7. Sequence of clotting in minimal injury. **A.** First phase: platelets depositing on the intercellular cement. **B.** Second phase: platelets form platelet thrombi. **C.** Third phase: fibrin deposits appear on platelet thrombi. **D.** Fourth phase: fibrin deposits spread along intercellular lines and over cell surface. (*From Samuels, P. B., and Webster, D. R. Ann Surg 136:428, 1952.*)

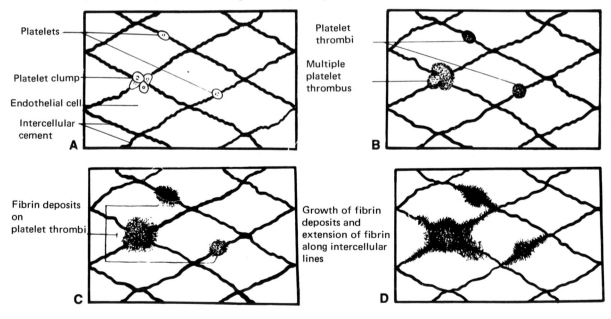

along the loose perivenous connective tissue. These veins in turn join others in the vicinity, and they finally empty as a true tributary into some other vein. (If it is in an extremity, the venules may empty into the parent vein at a more proximal site.) O'Neill's studies suggested that interruption of the vasa venarum could cause desquamation of the endothelium; thus, he hypothesized that this might be a cause of deep venous thrombosis, viz., interference with the arterial circulation of the vein wall.

Samuels and Webster[17] repeated O'Neill's studies, and although they agreed with all his observations, they reached the conclusion that this desquamation was an artifact due to the wrapping of the veins in a rubber dam for the experiment. These investigators observed that in minimal injury to a vein wall the sequence of clotting is as follows (Fig. 2-7): (1) the platelets, singly and in groups, adhere to the cement substance of the vein wall. (2) Adherent platelets metamorphose and coalesce to form platelet thrombi. (3) Fibrin deposits on the surface of the platelet thrombi. (4) Fibrin masses spread along the intercellular lines and across the cell bodies. Injury may stop at this stage; however, if the initial injury is severe or continued for a long period, the reaction progresses to the next stage, i.e., maximal reaction following injury to the vein wall. In this instance, the continuity of the endothelial surface is disrupted, and pathologic anatomic changes appear in the endothelial cells themselves. Large areas of the vein wall may desquamate, and fibrin is deposited on these desquamated areas. Samuels and Webster concluded that their results also indicated that heparinization of a normal dog and of dogs with experimentally injured veins prevents deposition of platelets on the intercellular cement in normal veins and limits (but does not prevent) local thrombosis on injured endothelium.

Today most forms of superficial thrombophlebitis begin by trauma to the endothelial lining of the vein. Most commonly, this results from intravenous injection of hypertonic solutions and from the insertion of intravenous catheters, with or without infection around the catheter. The injection of radiopaque media into veins during phlebography is another cause of thrombophlebitis.

DIRECT TRAUMA. Too many of our patients have insisted that superficial thrombophlebitis began with a blow to the area of their varicose veins for us to doubt that direct trauma may at times initiate the thrombophlebitic process. It is difficult to determine what part direct trauma plays in producing thrombophlebitis by damage to the vein wall in violent injuries. Certainly stretching a vein to the point of rupturing its intima causes thrombosis. This may be the mechanism of so-called effort thrombosis of the subclavian vein. Fracture of a vein by a spicule of bone or a crushing injury to a vein would be expected to cause venous thrombosis. Whether the trauma is mechanical, chemical, or thermal, disruption of the endothelial lining of the vein wall exposes subendothelial collagen, inducing platelet aggregation and/or coagulation. The release of tissue thromboplastin from injured cells directly initiates coagulation; in more extensive injuries, such as whole-body injuries, tissue thromboplastin from all the damaged tissues directly triggers coagulation.

Superficial thrombophlebitis resulting from trauma is almost invariably painful. The perivenous tissues are involved, and even the skin usually shows some redness over the thrombosed vein. The process extends proximally and distally but usually subsides before a major tributary is reached. Since it is an adherent type of thrombophlebitis, emboli do not break loose. However, if the thrombus extends into a major vein, e.g., the common femoral, then soft clot may form at its tip; this may indeed embolize. On a number of occasions we have teased soft clot out of the common femoral vein when dividing the saphenous vein at its termination for superficial thrombophlebitis.

SEPTIC THROMBOPHLEBITIS

The first clear cut medical history of septic thrombophlebitis was presented in a paper by John Hunter on February 6, 1784,[18] prior to the era of Lister, and in view of the fact that bacteria were still unknown, it is of interest to read some of Hunter's descriptive terms. In an arm after bleeding, he found the insides of veins to be "a seat of inflammation and abscesses" and found redness and inflammation. He observed that some wounds healed by "first intention" following a second bleeding of a person who developed inflammation of the opposite arm after the first bleeding. When a wound does not heal by first intention, it "festers or inflames then suppurates and ulcerates." He described a wound in the saphenous vein at the ankle as being inflamed all the way up the leg and thigh nearly to the groin, and he observed a string of abscesses along the entire course. He recalled having observed "inflammations of horses . . . [where] the jugular vein [is] inflamed through its whole length and all of the side of the head is considerably swelled. The inflammation carried along the vein quite into the chest. In these cases, there was always an abscess formed at the wound and often several along the vein, as in the human subject . . ."

Truly septic thrombophlebitis with abscesses in the veins as described by Hunter is rarely seen today. It has been seen only once in our experience. However, there is a definite possibility that some instances of superficial thrombophlebitis following intravenous catheterization are caused by infection.

L-FORM ORGANISMS. Altemeier et al.[19] introduced the concept that some forms of recurrent thrombophlebitis may be due to an obscure infection by an unusual organism of atypical morphology called an L-form of bacteroides. This organism is filterable and difficult to grow. It has been isolated in more than 50 patients with recurrent thrombophlebitis or pulmonary embolism.

Thrombosis Due to Decrease in Velocity of Bloodflow

The decrease in velocity of bloodflow or relative venous stasis is probably the most important factor in the pathogenesis of deep venous thrombosis. There is no doubt that rapidly flowing blood is less likely to clot than blood flowing slowly. Except in extreme dehydration, thrombosis rarely occurs in a normal artery. Arterial thromboses occur at sites of intimal injury by trauma or at arteriosclerotic plaques. On the contrary, deep venous thrombosis usually occurs in anatomically normal veins (Figs. 2-8 to 2-12). The frequency of venous thrombosis

and the rarity of arterial thrombosis in normal blood vessels may be explained in one of three ways: (1) there is a fault in the vein wall, (2) some fundamental change occurs in the character of blood each time it passes through the arterial tree and into the venous tree, or (3) the difference between the velocity of arterial and venous blood is a critical factor; the last is believed to be the most likely explanation. All vascular surgeons are very aware that a high velocity of bloodflow is essential for long-term patency of an endarterectomized or grafted artery and that the most common cause of

Figure 2-8. Beginning of platelet aggregation and thrombus formation in the valve of a vein. (**S** sinus; **E** fluid eddies at the cusp-free borders.)   (*From Cotton, L. T., and Clark, C. Ann R Coll Surg Engl 36:214, 1965.*)

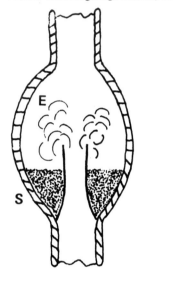

Figure 2-10. Clot located within a valve cusp and extend-► ing above it. (*From Paterson, J. C., and McLachlin, J. Surg Gynecol Obstet 98:101, 1954. By Permission of Surgery, Gynecology & Obstetrics.*)

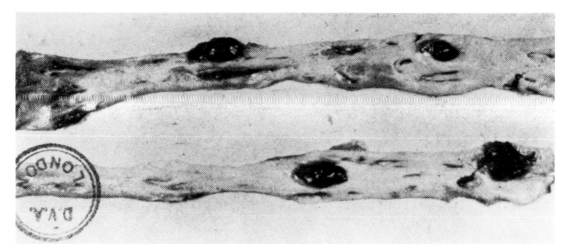

Figure 2-9. Gross clot found at autopsy in the valve cusps of femoral vein. (*From Paterson, J. C., and McLachlin, J. Surg Gynecol Obstet 98:100, 1954. By permission of Surgery, Gynecology & Obstetrics.*)

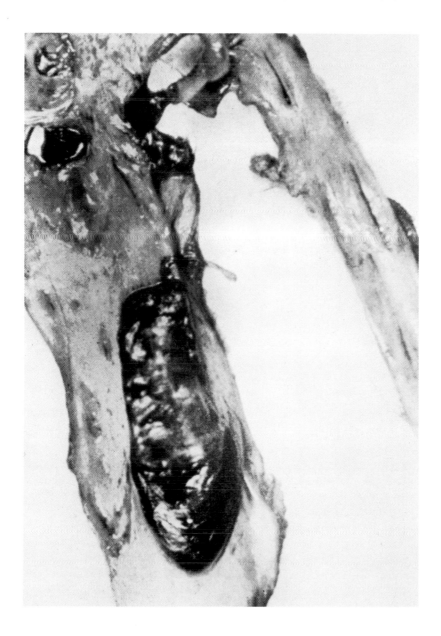

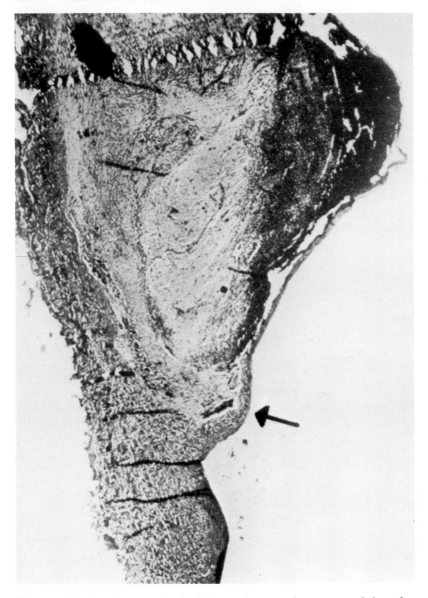

Figure 2-11. Thrombus contained within a valve cusp; lowest part of the valve pocket is primarily composed of platelets. In the large part of the valve, thrombus forms more proximally. (*From Paterson, J. C., and McLachlin, J. Surg Gynecol Obstet 98:99, 1954. By permission of Surgery, Gynecology & Obstetrics.*)

failure of arterial reconstructive surgery is slow bloodflow either into or out of the area of reconstruction. The decrease in velocity itself has certain definite effects. Platelets migrate from the axial stream to the wall of the vessel as the velocity decreases. With decreasing velocity, the viscosity of the blood increases. The decreased velocity also produces an increase in lateral pressure. This causes dilatation of the easily distensible veins, thus creating the type of cycle observed in arterial aneurysms, i.e., the greater the distention, the slower the velocity; the slower the velocity, the greater the lateral pressure, causing further increase in diameter. The high incidence of thrombosis of

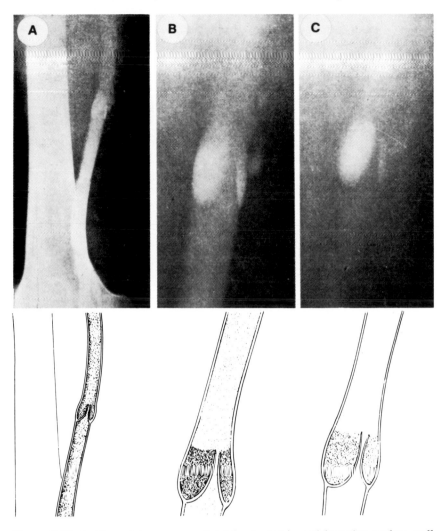

Figure 2-12. A. Normal human superficial femoral vein and its valve pockets well outlined 1 minute after injection of 50 per cent Hypaque into a dorsal vein of the foot. Tourniquet at the ankle has directed dye into the deep veins. **B.** Three minutes after the injection the vein is partially cleared, but there is poor emptying of the valve pockets. **C.** Five minutes after injection the main channel of the vein is barely visible, but stasis is again suggested by the good concentration of dye in the backwater of the valve pockets; at 12 minutes the valve pockets could still be seen. (*From McLachlin, A. D. Venous thrombosis and pulmonary embolism. In Taylor, S.* Recent Advances in Surgery. *London, Churchill, 1969, p. 12. Modified from Hadfield, G. Ann R Coll Surg Engl 6:219, 1950.*)

major veins with total arterial occlusion and the studies of Wessler *et al.*[20-23] demonstrating that serum causes thrombosis only in the veins in which bloodflow has been reduced all suggest that relative venous stasis plays a major part in venous thrombosis. A case in point is the postoperative patient whose venous flow is relatively sluggish; also the

incidence of venous thrombosis is markedly high after clipping procedures in prophylaxis for pulmonary embolism.[24, 25] Clinically, venous thrombosis is rare in an active person and exceptional in a child, but it is indeed common in adults who have been sitting for long periods. The likelihood of deep venous thrombosis increases with advancing age and debilitation. All of these predisposing factors are associated with decreased muscular activity and a consequent reduction in the velocity of venous bloodflow.

THE SOLEAL VEINS

Venous thrombosis does not occur haphazardly in the venous tree. The great majority of pulmonary emboli arise from the deep veins of the legs, thighs, and pelvis (Fig. 2-13). Much of our information regarding the sites of origin of deep vein thrombi stems from the few but extremely important studies in which the entire venous tree from the inferior vena cava to the ankle was exposed at autopsy.[26-29] These studies clearly indicate that valve pockets and the veins of the soleus muscle are the points of origin of many, if not most, venous thrombi. Other sites of origin are areas of dilatation or compression of a vein.

Of special importance is the peculiar anatomy and anatomic drainage of the soleal veins. The soleus muscle is the principal pump of the venous heart in the lower extremity. Some of its numerous veins may be considered as large sinuses measuring up to 1 cm in diameter and 4 to 5 cm in length. These veins have received little attention except from a few investigators.[30-32] Figures 2-14 to 2-17 show huge clots in the soleal sinuses. These sinuses lie outside the mainstream and do not fill on the ordinary phlebogram; however, they may be shown by a special technique which will be described later and by the technique recommended by Rabinov and Paulin.[31] When the patient is recumbent, the soleal veins drain directly ventrally, i.e., toward the ceiling. The soleal veins also drain indirectly into the popliteal vein, emptying first into the posterior tibial and peroneal veins, so that there is a slight bottleneck to the flow of blood.[32]

Figure 2-13. Sites of venous thrombosis in 133 dissected lower extremities. (*From Frykholm, R. Surg Gynecol Obstet 71:309, 1940. By Permission of Surgery, Gynecology & Obstetrics.*)

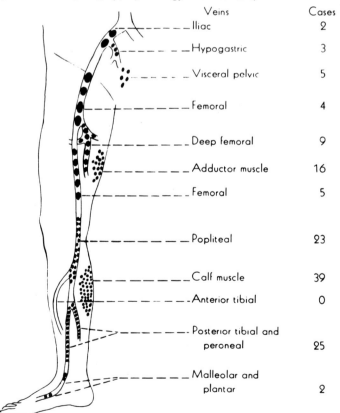

Veins	Cases
Iliac	2
Hypogastric	3
Visceral pelvic	5
Femoral	4
Deep femoral	9
Adductor muscle	16
Femoral	5
Popliteal	23
Calf muscle	39
Anterior tibial	0
Posterior tibial and peroneal	25
Malleolar and plantar	2

Figure 2-14. Transverse section through the soleus muscle showing thrombi in large soleal veins. (*From Dodd, H., and Cockett, F. B. The Pathology and Surgery of the Veins of the Lower Limb. Edinburgh, Livingstone, 1956, p. 297.*)

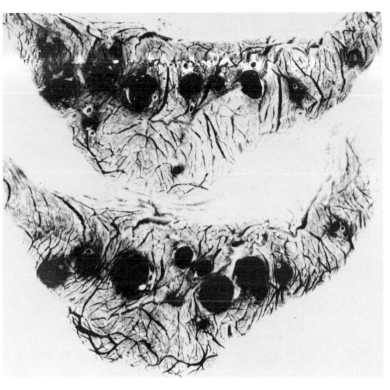

Figure 2-15. A. Phlebogram of isolated calf muscles. The size of a soleal sinus (**S**) is comparable to the size of a posterior tibial vein (**P.T.V.**). **B.** Corrosion cast of soleal veins. Relatively thin arborizing veins are seen above a soleal sinus (**S**) which connects with the posterior tibial veins. (*From Cotton, L. T., and Clark, C. Ann R Coll Surg Engl 36:216, 1965.*)

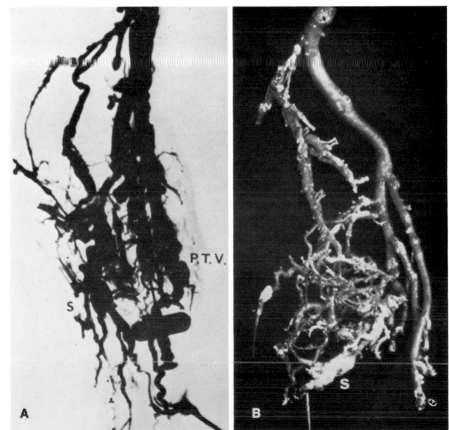

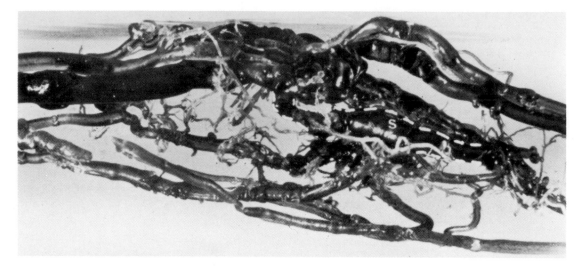

Figure 2-16. Corrosion cast of soleal veins. A typical soleal sinus (**S**) is outlined. It lies dependent in recumbency in the inferior part of the muscle. (*From Cotton, L. T., and Clark, C.* Ann R Coll Surg Engl 36:*216, 1965.*)

Figure 2-17. A. Corrosion cast showing thrombus in a soleal sinus (**S**). Only the sinus is affected. **B.** Corrosion cast showing thrombus in a soleal sinus (**S**) and in the posterior tibial vein (**P.T.V.**) near their junction. (*From Cotton, L. T., and Clark, C.* Ann R Coll Surg Engl 36:*216, 1965.*)

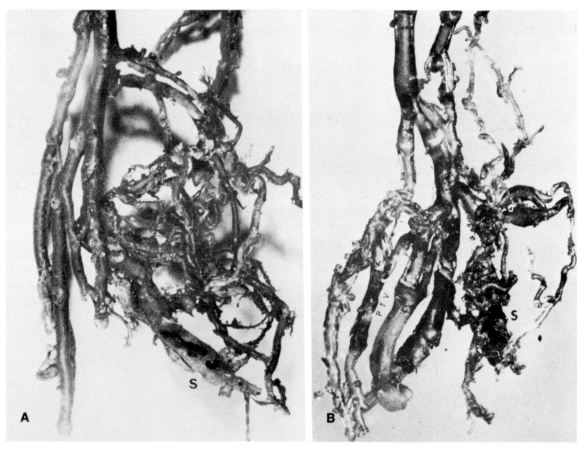

Prolonged bed rest results in relaxation and loss of tone of the leg muscles, more or less constant vasodilatation produced by blankets, decreased total velocity of bloodflow due to decreased cardiac output, increased viscosity caused by the slowing of bloodflow, and, lastly, further dilatation of the veins because of the slowed flow. All of these events contribute to thrombosis. Furthermore, the larger soleal veins are out of the mainstream; they are in the dependent position, frequently compressed by pillows; and they lie within a muscle that is used little when the patient is in bed. Evidence is accumulating that suggests that these large soleal veins are the most common source of deep venous thrombosis in bedridden patients.

Thrombosis Caused by a Defect in the Blood Itself

HYPERCOAGULABILITY OF BLOOD

Virchow logically deduced the possibility of hypercoagulability of blood as the cause of venous thrombosis,[13] but it has proved to be the most elusive of his three postulates to prove. The first question is, "Is it possible that a state of hypercoagulability of the blood can exist?" The answer to this is, "Yes." The strongest circumstantial evidence for this is found in the increased incidence of venous thrombosis in patients with cancer.[33] When associated with a neoplasm, thrombophlebitis tends to be migratory and appears in more than one extremity.[34] The association of venous and arterial thrombosis in patients with polycythemia vera is well recognized. It is not known whether it is caused by the hemoconcentration with increased viscosity, by the increased number of platelets, or by some specific factor.

The fundamental investigations of Wessler *et al.*[20-23] have demonstrated beyond doubt that a systemic infusion of serum injected at a distance from a site of venous stasis may produce massive thrombosis which closely resembles and is probably identical to the red thrombus or soft clot of a typical venous thrombosis. This thrombosis will not occur in the absence of venous stasis, nor will it occur in the presence of venous stasis without the injection of serum. This phenomenon is quantitatively related to the amount of serum infused and to the size of the vein. Thrombosis does not occur at the capillary level or in arteries or veins less than

50μ[35] in diameter, and it is produced less efficiently in smaller vessels than in large vessels.

Wright[36] reported that platelet adhesiveness may change and be greater, for example, in the postpartum and postoperative states. This work has been confirmed by Bennett.[37]

In recent years there has been a great increase in the knowledge of coagulation, so much so that a new specialty has emerged. Coagulationists are a valuable adjunct to pathology and hematology departments. It is beyond the scope of this book to discuss the intricacies of coagulation factors, inhibitors to natural coagulation, fibrinolysis, and the concept of continuous thrombin formation coincident with fibrinolysis. References made to these subjects in this chapter are admittedly of a general nature.

All three factors, i.e., intimal damage, decrease in the rate of bloodflow or relative stasis, and abnormal blood clotting, may coexist in the same patient. The debilitated or the postoperative patient may well have an increase in platelet adhesiveness plus some other factors as yet unknown that would increase hypercoagulability and at the same time cause pooling of blood in the soleal veins secondary to inactivity and debility. There also may be damage to the intima of the veins of the extremity from compression by pillows or sheets.

TESTS TO DETECT ABNORMALITIES OF CLOTTING MECHANISM IN PATIENTS WITH DEEP VENOUS THROMBOSIS

Perhaps the most ideal type of study to detect abnormal clotting factors in patients with deep venous thrombosis was conducted by Paterson and McLachlin[38] in 1952, involving 67 elderly veterans on the medical and surgical wards who were seriously ill. Blood tests were carried out almost daily for the duration of the serious illness, until the patients either recovered or died. At the death of a patient, the entire venous tree from the vena cava to the ankles was dissected out and a search made for thrombi; the presence or absence of thrombi was correlated with the *in vivo* tests. By this means they found that none of the following tests were of value in predicting the presence of venous thrombosis: plasma fibrinogen levels, fibrinogen D (which is "antithrombin"),[39] fibrinolytic activity, α-tocopherol, and probably the blood platelet count. Hume and Chan[40-42] have recently summarized the attempts of many workers to detect the test that would indicate the presence of venous thrombosis. At the present time there is no single blood test that indicates the presence of venous thrombosis. A high level of constituents of fibrin indicates that fibrin is being broken down somewhere in the body, but it does not necessarily indicate the presence of clinical thrombophlebitis.[41–43] Indeed, Wood et al.[44] found that a raised ratio of serum fibrin to fibrinogen degradation products (FDP) correlated more closely with infection and hemorrhage than with thrombosis. The depression of antithrombin III combined with acceleration of thrombin generation, as reported by von Kaulla et al.,[45, 46] gives promise of being an indicator of susceptibility to thromboembolism.

Predisposing Factors for Venous Thrombosis

The pathogenesis of venous thrombosis has been discussed under the headings of injury to the vein wall, decrease in velocity of bloodflow, and abnormality of bloodclotting.[13] Another way of looking at the problem is to consider the conditions regularly encountered in clinical practice that seem to predispose a patient to venous thrombosis. Most of these conditions probably produce their action through one or more of the mechanisms mentioned by Virchow[13] (see preceding section on pathogenesis).

AGE

Age must be considered as a predisposing factor.[47–49] Venous thrombosis and pulmonary embolism are rare in childhood and common in old age. Coon and Coller (Fig. 2-18) plotted the absolute incidence of pulmonary embolism by 10-year age groups in 4391 autopsies at the University of Michigan Hospital. These figures are absolute in that the incidence has been obtained by dividing the number of patients with pulmonary embolism in particular age groups by the total number of patients in the entire autopsy population that fall into that age group. The slight peak in the 10- to 19-year age group is thought to be due to the higher incidence of pulmonary embolism associated with the greater frequency of death due to physical trauma in males of this age. Daniel et al.[47] studied maternal deaths in England and Wales from 1961

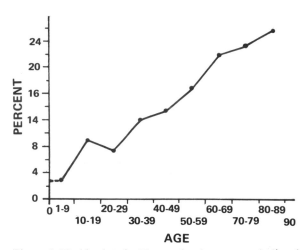

Figure 2-18. Absolute incidence of pulmonary embolism by 10-year age groups in 4391 autopsies at the University of Michigan Hospital. (*Redrawn from Coon, W. W., and, Coller, F. A.* Surg Gynecol Obstet 109:*489, 1959. By Permission of Surgery, Gynecology & Obstetrics.*)

to 1963; 41 per cent of the thromboembolic deaths occurred in mothers over 35 years of age, although that age group provided only 12 per cent of the registered births.

SEX

Coon and Coller[49] and Hunter et al.[48] found no significant difference in the incidence of venous thrombosis and thromboembolism in males and in females when the incidence was computed on an absolute basis and adjusted for age. Similarly, Sartwell and Anello[50] analyzed the mortality rates in the United States due to venous thrombosis and embolism for Caucasian males and females in five 10-year age groups covering the span from 15 to 65 years of age. During the period 1960 to 1966, there was an approximate logarithmic increase in mortality rate with advancing age over this age span. Although the rate rose somewhat more rapidly in males, there was no statistically significant difference between males and females.

THE ABO GROUP

Jick et al.[51–53] noted that among those patients being treated with anticoagulant therapy for venous thromboembolism, the number having blood group O was disproportionately small. This observation is supported by the findings of Preston and Barr[54] and Langman and Doll[55] who demonstrated that patients in blood group O are more likely to bleed as a complication of peptic ulcer than those in other blood groups. The reason for this difference has not yet been determined, but persons in blood group O have been found to have a slightly lower level of antihemophilic globulin (factor VIII) than people in group A. Following up their observations, Jick *et al.*[51–53] carried out a prospective study on groups of Caucasian women who developed thromboembolism while taking oral contraceptives, during pregnancy, or in the puerperium. These investigations were carried out in the United States, Sweden, and Britain. In each country, the group with thromboembolism showed a higher frequency of group A subjects and a lower frequency of group O subjects when compared with the controls. In two of the three series of pregnant or puerperal women and in each of the four series of patients using oral contraceptives, the deficit in group O patients was statistically significant.[51–53]

PREGNANCY

The incidence of thrombophlebitis during pregnancy is low. VillaSanta[56] found that the incidence given by various authors varied from 0.018 to 0.29/100 deliveries. The great variation is probably explained by the difficulty in diagnosis and by the fact that the figures for superficial thrombophlebitis and deep thrombophlebitis are not always reported separately. He analyzed 31 reports, covering the years 1904 to 1964, of patients with antepartum thromboembolic disease who were not treated with anticoagulant agents. Of 163 patients, 26 (15.9 per cent) developed a pulmonary embolus and 21 (12.8 per cent) died. He also collected 48 reports from the period 1945 to 1964 of patients with antepartum thromboembolic disease treated with anticoagulant agents. Of 134 patients, 26 (19.4 per cent) developed a pulmonary embolus but only 1 (0.7 per cent) patient died. Maternal complications were not common, most of them consisting of nonfatal hemorrhage. The incidence of fetal complications, however, was high. Of 92 pregnant women treated with warfarin sodium (Coumadin) derivatives alone or in conjunction with heparin, 14 delivered stillborn infants and 3 delivered infants who died in the neonatal period, a perinatal mortality of 18 per cent or almost 1 in 5 cases. In addition, 2 infants survived with congenital anomalies related to defects of coagulation.

MECHANISM INVOLVED. The veins of the lower extremities dilate during pregnancy, in fact, at a very early stage, much before the size of the uterus could have any effect on the venous outflow. Many of our patients have said that the first sign of pregnancy is dilatation of their leg veins. Goodrich and Wood[57] compared peripheral venous distensibility and the velocity of venous outflow in pregnant women and in women on contraceptive drugs with the distensibility and velocity in nonpregnant women not taking hormone therapy. Their results showed that the veins of the legs and forearms are more distensible in pregnant women and in women using oral contraceptives than in other women. Since distensibility increased in all four extremities, the cause for the increase could not be merely passive stretching of the veins secondary to pressure in the lower limbs. They also noted a decrease in linear velocity of venous bloodflow in the calf in such patients; in their view, this might be a contributing factor in the higher incidence of venous thrombosis in pregnancy and in women receiving oral contraceptive therapy.

THE PUERPERIUM

The incidence of thrombophlebitis during the puerperium is considerably higher than during pregnancy. Reporting from the Pennsylvania Hospital, Ullery[58] found the incidence 19 times higher post partum than ante partum. Aaro *et al.*[59, 60] reported the incidence at the Mayo Clinic as 0.18 per cent during pregnancy and 1.33 per cent during the puerperium. During pregnancy there is a gradual increase in the concentration of factors I, VII, VIII, IX, and X,[61] culminating during the puerperium in blood coagulation and fibrinolytic changes that reflect the dynamic changes in the hemostatic mechanism during this period. Such alterations may be presumed to be of importance as one of the etiologic factors in thrombus formation after delivery.

The absolute incidence of postpartum thromboembolic disease varies markedly from center to center, e.g., 0.34 per cent in Ullery's study[58] and 1.33 per cent in Aaro's report from the Mayo Clinic.[59, 60] The same is true of the absolute incidence of antepartum thrombophlebitis, 0.018 per cent vs. 0.18 per cent in these same reports. The disparity surely reflects a difference in diagnostic criteria and perhaps in the intensity of the investigation. However, despite the rather striking difference in the absolute incidence, the two studies agree that thrombophlebitis occurs much more frequently in the postpartum period than in the prepartum period.

ORAL CONTRACEPTIVES

As the use of synthetic estrogens and progesterones became popular for conception control, reports began to appear in the literature with increasing frequency suggesting the possible association of the use of such hormones and the development of deep venous thrombosis, thromboembolism, and arterial thromboses in the arteries of the brain, the heart, and the distal arterial tree. This discussion of necessity must be limited to venous thrombosis and thromboembolism.

In 1961, Jordan[62] presented the first report of a pulmonary embolism occurring in a woman on estrogen therapy. A year later at a special meeting called by the manufacturer of contraceptive pills, reports, some of them incomplete, were available of 118 cases of women of childbearing age in whom thromboembolic disease developed while they were taking the drug. Of these, 30 cases were associated with pulmonary embolism and 9 were fatal.[63] Within 3 months the number of reported cases more than doubled,[64] and in rapid sequence both abroad and in the United States[65-67] studies appeared implicating hormone therapy as a possible causative agent in venous thromboembolic disease.

Dugdale and Masi[68] recently collected and summarized the data of 41 investigators on approximately 1,000 patients receiving oral contraceptives. Of these, 412 were studied during the first three cycles (short-term group) and 530 for longer than 3 months. Their results showed that short-term use of oral contraceptives apparently has no effect on platelets except for altering their electrophoretic mobility; the physiologic significance has not been determined. Long-term use not only alters the electrophoretic mobility but also produces a rise in platelet count in two thirds of the users. There may be increased ability of the platelets to adhere to foreign surfaces. They also studied the effects of pregnancy, estrogens, and progestins on platelets. Some studies indicate increased aggregability of platelets in pregnancy. Estrogens, particularly the synthetic forms, increase the responsiveness of

platelets to aggregating agents. Progestins have no effect on platelet count or function. The investigations of von Kaulla et al.[45, 46] concerning antithrombin suggest that there is a decrease of this substance in the blood of patients receiving contraceptive therapy.[68]

The question arises whether the increased risk of venous thrombosis in the patient on contraceptive therapy is greater than the risk of pregnancy. The answer is not available at this time.

STATISTICAL ANALYSIS OF ORAL CONTRACEPTIVES AND THROMBOEMBOLIC DISEASE. The early reports from England tended to show a statistical relationship[69-73] between venous thromboembolic disease and the use of oral contraceptives; on the other hand, first reports from Drill et al. from the United States[74-76] failed to find causal evidence. More recently, however, both in Britain and America, an increased risk of thromboembolic disease attributable to the use of hormonal contraceptives has now been defined.[77-81]

Statistical analyses of this kind are open to criticism from many quarters. Perhaps the most fundamental problem has been pointed out by Hougie[82, 83] in 1969 and again in 1972: thromboembolic disease is underdiagnosed to a remarkable degree. The validity of the ninefold increase[71] of the disease in women taking contraceptive pills is not completely accepted. The higher incidence can easily be accounted for by an increase in the diagnosis of a disease that frequently goes unrecognized. When a woman is known to be receiving such therapy, special diagnostic procedures are more likely to be thought justifiable. In a recent prospective study of the association of oral contraceptives and thromboembolic disease carried out in Puerto Rico,[84] no correlation was found between the use of the drugs and the development of thrombophlebitis. Studies based on retrospective data have also come under attack from Drill[76] for failing to show cause-and-effect relationships. On the other hand, Sartwell[85] has criticized Drill and Calhoun[75, 76] for pooling heterogeneous material collected in different ways from multiple sources. Schrogie et al.[86] likewise found Drill's data not suitable for the analysis he undertook, because they can, to a limited extent, be interpreted as supportive of the results of the British reports.[87] Seltzer[88] objected to the data of Drill and Calhoun[75, 77] as being compilations from a large number of different investigators, using different sources, and posing problems of variable diagnosis and sampling. The difficulty of diagnosis of thromboembolic disease remains the crux of the problem. The pros and cons of methodology used in the compilation of various statistical analyses can be expected to be debated as long as the *diagnosis* of thromboembolic disease is such a variable factor.

Oral hormonal therapy has stirred the interest of physicians; however the controversy turns out, a far truer incidence of venous thrombosis and pulmonary embolism will be established than has heretofore been available. In 1967 Daniel *et al*[47] reported that in England pulmonary embolism was then second only to abortion as a cause of death in obstetrics patients. They studied the effect of suppression of lactation on the development of peripheral thromboembolism in 9324 women who delivered in Cardiff in the period 1965 to 1966. Of this group, 44 suffered attacks of thromboembolic disease. The incidence was influenced by the age and parity of the mother, "but even when allowance is made for these factors there was still a significantly higher incidence in the patients who had had lactation suppressed."[47] In the absence of other predisposing factors, the risk of developing deep vein thrombosis, pulmonary embolism, or cerebral thrombosis is increased approximately eight times by the use of oral contraceptives (Table 2-4).

In the United States, epidemiologic studies[89, 90] suggest that the risk of thromboembolism in a woman taking hormonal contraceptives is 4.4 times that in the nonuser.[81, 82] The studies showed that the excess risk did not persist after cessation of use and prolonged continuation of use did not enhance the risk. Quantitatively, the mortality from thromboembolic disorders attributable to oral contraceptive use is approximately 3/100,000 women per year.[81, 82] In 1973 the report of the Boston Collaborative Drug Surveillance Programme[81] confirmed the association between oral contraceptive use and venous thromboembolism. They estimated the incidence of idiopathic venous thrombosis to be 66 cases/100,000 users of contraceptive agents— approximately 1/1500 (this compares with Vessey and Doll's figure of 1/2000).[71] The incidence of idiopathic venous thrombosis in the Boston group is 11 times greater for women who were users of oral contraceptive agents.[81]

IMMOBILITY FOLLOWING TRAUMA

Immobility, combined with the liberation of tissue thromboplastins[20–23] and possibly other clotting factors in the bloodstream, probably largely accounts for the venous thrombosis that develops following major trauma. In violent wounds some of the veins may be directly traumatized; however, when such patients come to autopsy, thrombosis is a common finding in both lower extremities despite the absence of direct involvement of the limbs in the injury. Sevitt and Gallagher[29] dissected out the venous tree of the lower extremities of injured and burned patients at autopsy. They found an overall incidence of 65 per cent with intravenous thrombosis exclusive of patients with pulmonary embolism.

TABLE 2-4. Use of Oral Contraceptives in Women Suffering From "Idiopathic" Thromboembolic Disorders (Expected Numbers in Parentheses)

DISORDER	DATA SOURCE	NO. AFFECTED WOMEN WITH HISTORY OF ORAL CONTRACEPTIVE USE		NO. WOMEN STUDIED		RELATIVE RISK: USERS TO NONUSERS
		USED	NOT USED	AFFECTED	CONTROLS	
Deep-vein thrombosis or	Inpatients	26 (5.0)	32 (53.0)	58	116	8.6 to 1
pulmonary embolism	Deaths	16 (4.2)	10 (21.8)	26	998	8.3 to 1
Cerebral	Inpatients	5 (1.0)	4 (8.0)	9	116	10.0 to 1
thrombosis	Deaths	5 (1.5)	5 (8.5)	10	998	5.7 to 1
Coronary	Inpatients	0 (0.7)	13 (12.3)	13	116	
thrombosis	Deaths	18 (11.4)	66 (72.6)	84	998	1.7 to 1

From Doll, R. *Br Med J.* 2:69, 1969.

They believed, however, that the factors of patient age and the duration of bed rest were probably of greater importance in the development of thrombosis than the particular type of injury.

CANCER

The association of thrombophlebitis and carcinoma was first noted by Trousseau in 1877;[91] he observed that recurrent thrombophlebitis might be the first sign of an obscure cancer of a visceral organ, e.g., in patients with carcinoma of the stomach. (He later died of this same disease.) Gouget,[92] Osler and McCrae,[93] and Welch[94] confirmed this association of obscure visceral malignancy and venous thrombosis. In 1938 Sproul[95] reviewed 4258 consecutive necropsies and noted a significant relationship between cancer and thrombophlebitis. Of 16 patients with cancer of the body or tail of the pancreas, 9 (66 per cent) had venous thrombosis and 5 (31 per cent) *multiple* venous thromboses. This association was not limited to pancreatic carcinoma (Table 2-5); however, multiple thromboses were observed only with cancers of the pancreas, lung, and stomach.

Edwards[96] introduced the term "migrating thrombophlebitis." He reviewed the literature and discovered 23 cases in which a definite association of migrating thrombophlebitis and carcinoma was observed during life; to this group he added 6 cases of his own, a total of 29. In this series the primary site of cancer was the tail or body of the pancreas in 16 patients, the stomach in 4, the lung in 4, the gallbladder in 2, and undetermined in 3. Fisher et al.[97] presented 4 patients with cancer of the lung who were initially treated for thrombophlebitis which was resistant to anticoagulant therapy. Included in the 4 was a patient with a series of 10 attacks of thromboembolic phenomena involving all four extremities, including a pulmonary infarction. Two other patients also had multiple bouts. The fourth patient had a single attack and had no recurrence after removal of the carcinoma.

Hubay and Holden[98] reported 8 patients admitted to the hospital with thrombophlebitis and pulmonary embolism; in 7 of these, neoplasm was discovered. Tuberculosis was the associated disease in the eighth patient. The sites of the carcinoma were the colon, the cecum, the ovary, the lung, and the stomach, each with metastases. The uterus was the site of the neoplasm in 2 patients.

From the Mayo Clinic Barker[99] reported malignant lesions in 27 of 58 cases diagnosed clinically as venous thrombosis; in a follow-up report, Woolling and Shick[100] again called attention to the fact that thrombophlebitis is a clue to cryptic malignant lesions. Of 15 patients with thrombophlebitis seen

TABLE 2-5. Incidence of Thrombosis in Carcinoma of Various Organs

ORGAN IN WHICH TUMOR AROSE	TOTAL NO. CASES	CASES WITH THROMBOSIS		CASES WITH MULTIPLE THROMBOSES	
		NO. CASES	% OF TOTAL	NO. CASES	% OF TOTAL
Pancreas	47	14	29.7	8	17
Head of pancreas	31	5	16.1	3	9.7
Body or tail of pancreas	16	9	52.6	5	31.3
Lung	81	12	14.8	2	2.5
Liver	22	6	27.2	0	
Gallbladder	30	5	16.6	0	
Stomach	147	32	21.3	2	1.3
Duodenum	16	3	18.7	0	
Colon	94	15	15.9	0	
Kidney	27	7	25.9	0	
Prostate	43	7	16.3	0	
Uterus	27	6	22.2	0	
Ovary	17	4	23.5	0	

From Sproul, E. E. *Am J Cancer 34:*566, 1938.

at the Mayo Clinic between 1946 and 1952, 3 had associated cancer of the pancreas. Woolling and Shick believed that the thrombophlebitis was more extensive in this group than in other patients. The stomach, lung, ovary, and breast were the sites of the malignant lesions. The prostate was a probable site, and no site could be determined in 4 patients. Woolling and Shick[100] emphasized the point made earlier by Wilenski et al.,[97] i.e., a thorough and continuous study should be made to rule out developing carcinoma in any patient in whom at least two proven episodes of thrombophlebitis have occurred, provided there is no other convincing explanation for the thrombosis.

Lieberman et al.[34] reviewed 1400 case reports of patients with the diagnosis of venous thrombosis; in these they found 81 instances of associated cancer: 61 diagnosed clinically and 20 diagnosed at autopsy. They also noted the resistance of this group of patients to anticoagulant therapy[97] in the treatment of thrombophlebitis. The most frequent sites of the primary malignant lesion were the lungs, the female reproductive tract, and the pancreas.

Byrd et al.,[101] in a recent report from the Mayo Clinic, noted thromboembolism as an early complication in 37 patients with primary bronchogenic carcinoma. In 14 instances an attack of thrombophlebitis first called attention to the patient's disease. In their series, migrating thrombophlebitis involving unusual sites along with resistance to anticoagulant therapy often preceded recognition of the neoplasm by as long as 18 months.

The foregoing would suggest that one must always search for carcinoma in a patient presenting with thrombophlebitis. The relationship, however, is neither so constant nor so obvious. Autopsy studies show a high incidence of venous thrombosis in patients with malignancy of the abdominal viscera or of the lung. Also, a patient who presents with multiple or migrating instances of thrombophlebitis, especially if it is resistant to anticoagulant

TABLE 2-6. Patients Presenting With Carcinoma* and Deep Venous Thrombosis[†] of Lower Extremities

SITE OF MALIGNANCY	NO. PATIENTS		
	DEEP VENOUS THROMBOSIS	PHLEGMASIA CERULEA DOLENS	TOTAL
Brain	1		1
Lung		1	1
Splenic flexure (with metastases)	1		1
Liver	1		1
Pancreas (tail) (with metastases)	1		1
Vena cava obstructed by tumor	1	1	2
Colon	2		2
Bladder		2	2
Rectum	1		1
Prostate	3	1	4
Ovary	2		2
Endometrium	2		2
Cervix (with metastases)	2		2
Vulva	1		1
Melanoma (with metastases)	1		1
Lymphoma	1		1
Perihemangiocytoma of thigh		1	1
Site undetermined, metastatic	2	5	7
Total	22 (1%) of 2144 patients	11 (23%) of 48 patients	33 (1.5%) of 2192 patients

* 949 patients with carcinoma (3.4% with venous thrombosis)
† 2192 patients with deep venous thrombosis

therapy,[34, 97] certainly should have a thorough and complete study for hidden malignancy. Above all, involvement of the upper extremities in spontaneous phlebitis should immediately arouse suspicion. On the other hand, in our experience, if we consider only those patients presenting with superficial or deep thrombophlebitis of the lower extremities that is presumably idiopathic in origin, an exceedingly small percentage will be shown to have associated carcinoma. For instance, of 2144 patients seen between 1952 and 1972 with the diagnosis of deep venous thrombosis of the lower extremity, 22 (1 per cent) had associated carcinoma (Table 2-6). During this same period, however, 11 (23 per cent) of 48 patients seen with phlegmasia cerulea dolens also had malignant lesions: 2 in the bladder, 1 in the prostate, 1 obstructing the inferior vena cava, 1 perihemangiocytoma of the thigh, 1 in the lung, and 5 others for which the primary site could not be determined (Table 2-6). The overall total, then, of patients seen with venous thrombosis and a cancerous lesion still is only 32 (1.5 per cent). The total number of patients seen with carcinoma was 949 (Table 2-6); which indicates that the incidence of such patients with thrombophlebitis is still quite low, 3.4 per cent. The incidence of associated superficial venous thrombosis and neoplasm in the lower extremities was negligible, 2 of 712 patients (Table 2-7). In the upper extremities, however, the incidence was considerably higher, 2 of 17 patients or 11.6 per cent. One of these patients was seen for three attacks in his arms; the site of the carcinoma was the lung. In the other patient, the site was the larynx (Table 2-8).

It is our policy to study any patient who presents with three bouts of venous thrombosis for possible hidden malignancy. Table 2-9 presents the results of our 20-year experience with such patients. Since some of them had bouts of both deep and superficial thrombophlebitis and, at times, involvement of both deep and superficial systems simultaneously, the total number of patients studied was 45 (1.5 per cent of 3027 seen for any type of venous thrombosis with the exception of phlegmasia cerulea dolens). Despite the fact that some patients had as many as 14 bouts, no malignancy was found. On the other hand, Table 2-10 lists those patients whom we treated initially for venous thrombosis and who later developed carcinoma. The incidence is still quite low, i.e., 11 of 2144 patients or 0.5 per cent. The interval from treatment of thrombophlebitis until the diagnosis of carcinoma was established varied from 2 days (discovered at autopsy) to 5 years. Two additional patients were treated for superficial venous thrombosis; malignancy was found at exploration of the larynx (9 months later) and the breast (10 months later), respectively. The incidence for patients in whom superficial thrombophlebitis was the forerunner of carcinoma was 2 of 712 patients or 0.28 per cent (see Table 2-7).

THROMBOANGIITIS OBLITERANS AND THE COLLAGEN DISEASES

There are other disease states, such as thromboangiitis obliterans and some of the collagen diseases, in which there seems to be an increased incidence of thrombophlebitis. However, the mechanisms in these instances are obscure.

TABLE 2-7. Patients Presenting With Acute Superficial Venous Thrombosis of the Lower Extremities in Whom Cancer Was Diagnosed Later

PATIENT	NO. BOUTS	SITE OF CANCER	INTERVAL FROM FIRST BOUT TO DIAGNOSIS OF CANCER	METHOD OF DIAGNOSIS			
				PHYSICAL EXAMINATION	X-RAY	EXPLORA-TION	POST-MORTEM
1	2	Larynx with metastases	9 months			x	
2	3	Breast	10 months			x	

Total: 2 (0.28%) of 712 patients with acute superficial thrombophlebitis

TABLE 2-8. Patients With Carcinoma and Acute Venous Thrombosis of Upper Extremity

SITE OF MALIGNANCY	NO. PATIENTS	SUPERFICIAL VENOUS THROMBOSIS	DEEP VENOUS THROMBOSIS
Lung	1	1	0
Larynx	1	1	0
Total	2	2*	0†

* 11.6% of 17 patients with acute superficial venous thrombosis of upper extremity, 0.2% of 949 patients with malignancy
† None of 76 patients with deep venous thrombosis of upper extremity

TABLE 2-9. Patients With Multiple Bouts of Venous Thrombosis and No Cryptic Malignancy

NO. BOUTS	NO. PATIENTS DEEP VENOUS THROMBOSIS	NO. PATIENTS SUPERFICIAL VENOUS THROMBOSIS	TOTAL PATIENTS
3	20	2	22
4	8	0	8
5	7	0	7
6	0	0	0
7	2	0	2
8	2	0	2
More than 10			4*
Total			45†

* These had both superficial and deep bouts, with the highest number of bouts being 14.
† 1.5% of 3027 patients seen between 1952 and 1972.

TABLE 2-10. Patients Presenting With Acute Deep Venous Thrombosis of Lower Extremities In Whom Cancer Was Diagnosed Later

PATIENT	NO. BOUTS	SITE OF CANCER	INTERVAL FROM FIRST BOUT TO DIAGNOSIS OF CANCER	METHOD OF DIAGNOSIS PHYSICAL EXAMINATION	X RAY	EXPLORATION	POST-MORTEM
1	1	Gallbladder	2 days				x
2	1	Metastatic abdominal papillary carcinomatosis	3 weeks			x	
3	3	Cervix with metastases	2 mo			x	
4	3	Ovary with metastases	2 mo			x	
5	2	Prostate	5 mo	x		x	
6	2	Ureter, bladder	6 mo	x		x	
7	2	Lung	6 mo				x
8	1	Lung	11 mo		x		
9	2	Kidney	11 mo		x	x	
10	3	Breast	4 yr	x	x	x	
11	7	Lung	5 yr		x		

Total 11 (0.5%) of 2144 patients presenting with deep venous thrombosis of the lower extremities

CLINICAL PICTURE OF THROMBOPHLEBITIS

SUPERFICIAL THROMBOPHLEBITIS OF THE EXTREMITIES

Superficial thrombophlebitis is the most benign form of the disease and the easiest to detect; it can usually be diagnosed at a glance. There is a red globular enlargement of the vein that is tender to touch. The long saphenous vein or one of its tributaries is most frequently involved. The process may begin at the ankle and slowly and steadily progress all the way up to the saphenofemoral junction, or it may stop at any given point and subside.[34] It may begin near the middle of the leg and spread proximally, distally, or in both directions at the same time. The only condition simulating superficial thrombophlebitis is lymphangitis. In lymphangitis, the patient usually has lymphadenitis, leukocytosis, and fever; careful palpation reveals no large, clotted veins.

Treatment

The treatment rests on the fact that no patient (in our experience, at least) has been known to have a pulmonary embolism from superficial thrombophlebitis unless the thrombus has first propagated into the common femoral vein. Thus, the condition may be considered benign as long as it is within the saphenous system; however, it is potentially malignant and also the potential cause of the postphlebitic syndrome if the thrombus reaches the common femoral vein. Therefore, if a patient is encountered who has a thrombus of the saphenous vein at or near the common femoral vein, he should be admitted to the hospital immediately for heparin therapy or excision of the phlebitic veins.[102] On a number of occasions we have teased the head of the thrombus out of the common femoral vein. If the thrombus is not at the saphenofemoral junction or is not ascending rapidly, the disease can be controlled easily with bed rest, elevation of the extremities, and heparin therapy.

Less than a third of our patients with superficial thrombophlebitis have required hospitalization (see Table 2-1); the rest are treated as outpatients. The highest level of thrombus is marked on the skin with ink, and the patient is instructed that there is no need for alarm or hospitalization as long as the thrombus does not progress towards the groin. In most instances we simply recommend that the limb be wrapped with a rubberized bandage, and we encourage the patient to be normally active. If the pain is severe it may be relieved by bed rest with elevation of the extremities and (occasionally) by applications of moist heat. Aspirin or Empirin with codeine usually controls the pain. Enzymatic or anti-inflammatory agents have not been used.

UPPER EXTREMITY

Superficial thrombophlebitis of the upper extremity is so common that it is rarely recorded in our clinical charts. A very high percentage of patients who have been in the hospital for major surgical treatment and who have had intravenous therapy for any length of time complain of thromboses of the superficial veins of their arms where the intravenous needles and catheters were inserted. This is so commonplace that, after reassuring the patient, most surgeons dismiss it from their minds. Because of this, there is no way of relating the number of patients who occasionally are referred with extensive superficial thrombophlebitis of the upper extremity to the total number of occurrences. We have records of 11 patients referred to us with extensive idiopathic thrombophlebitis of the upper extremity for which no cause was apparent.

THROMBOPHLEBITIS OF THE CHEST WALL (MONDOR'S DISEASE)

Superficial thrombophlebitis of the chest wall (Mondor's disease) is a benign and relatively rare lesion. It presents as a painful, tender, cordlike (bowstring) lesion of the anterior chest wall, produced by thrombophlebitis of a superficial vein, usually the thoracoepigastric vein (Figs. 2-19 and 2-20). It is self-limited and unaffected by treatment. It is important because it is mistaken for lymphangitis and thus rouses apprehension that it connotes systemic disease or cancer; such fears are unfounded. Tenderness and pain persist for 1 to 6 weeks, and the palpable cord resolves in 1 to 7 months.[111]

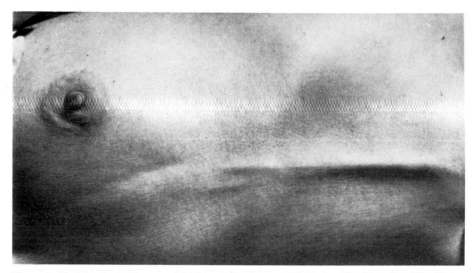

Figure 2-19. Mondor's disease: phlebitis of the thoracoepigastric vein. Note cordlike lesion in subcutaneous tissue of anterolateral chest wall and abdomen. (*From Thomford, N. R., and Holaday, W. J.* Ann Surg 170:*1036, 1969.*)

Figure 2-20. Marked fibrosis and scattered lymphocytes surrounding obliterated lumen of a subcutaneous vein in Mondor's disease. (*From Thomford, N. R., and Holaday, W. J.* Ann Surg 170:*1036, 1969.*)

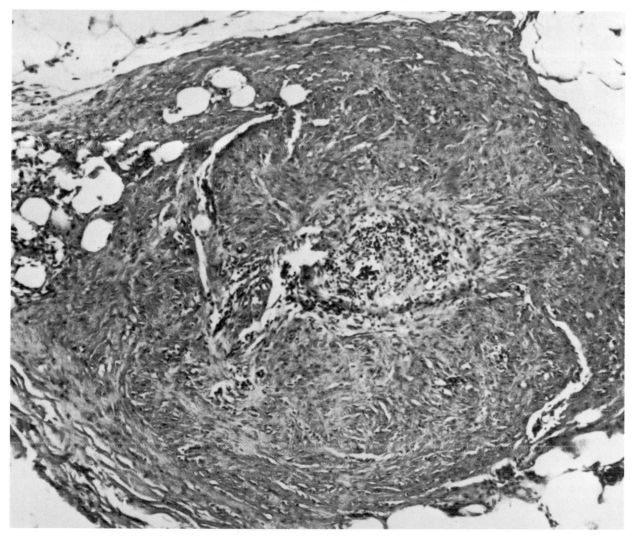

DEEP VENOUS THROMBOSIS OF THE LOWER EXTREMITY

Historically, thrombosis of the deep veins of the lower extremities has been linked with the use of the chair as a common household convenience.[113] The first documented case of venous thrombosis occurred in the thirteenth century.[114] Since then our society has become increasingly more sedentary, and deep venous thrombosis, once the rarest of disorders, is now one of the most common vascular diseases. Furthermore, it is the most pernicious form of thrombophlebitis in that the majority of the patients with pulmonary emboli have no prodromal symptoms or signs of venous thrombosis.

Clinical Diagnosis

HISTORY

A history of one of the above mentioned predisposing factors in deep venous thrombosis is exceedingly important. One rarely encounters a patient with deep venous thrombosis without one of the recognized predisposing factors.

A clinical history of a very sudden onset of chest pain associated with dyspnea, followed by pleuritic-type pain on breathing in a patient who also has a history of recent operation, injury, fracture, or pain in the lower extremity is so classic and so highly to be suspected that the physician should be led to make a tentative diagnosis of thrombophlebitis, until otherwise proven. In the absence of a pulmonary embolus, the onset of thrombophlebitis is likely to be gradual, as contrasted to the sudden onset of severe pain in the leg occurring with a ruptured tendon or muscle tear. The patient may experience pain that gradually intensifies over a period of several hours. The pain is definitely not as severe as with muscle hemorrhage or muscular cramps. In fact, in patients other than those with phlegmasia alba or cerulea dolens, the pain of thrombophlebitis is not excruciating; if the patient complains of pain of such a degree of severity, one should immediately suspect some other diagnosis. As the pain worsens, the patient himself may notice a sense of fullness or tightness or actual swelling of the extremity. In superficial phlebitis he notices the red streak in his leg. The pain of thrombophlebitis is usually relieved by elevation of the limb above heart level and is aggravated by sitting or standing.

PHYSICAL EXAMINATION

The medical initiate has difficulty accepting the fact that a patient may have extensive thrombophlebitis of the deep veins of the leg without any swelling. This was brought home to us early in our experience when we were asked to see a young woman who had been hospitalized with the presumptive diagnosis of small pulmonary emboli. Repeated examination of her extremities by several of us failed to reveal the slightest trace of swelling or even the feeling of fullness. (In the light of later experience, it is probable that this patient had an area of thrombosis localized to the groin.) Her lower extremities were entirely normal. However, the clinical picture was so suggestive of multiple pulmonary emboli that we elected to divide her superficial femoral veins. At operation she was found to have complete thrombosis of the entire left superficial and common femoral veins throughout the length of a rather large groin incision; the clots extended up into the pelvis. Had we not seen this ourselves, it would have been difficult to convince us that such extensive thrombosis could exist without any swelling. It is equally difficult for the clinician to believe that the patient may experience maximal swelling, pain, and tenderness of the limb without deep venous thrombosis of the major veins. Routine use of the phleborheograph or phlebography in patients suspected of having deep venous thrombosis demonstrates that this is not an uncommon occurrence. The degree of swelling is roughly quantitated and directly related to the extent of venous thrombosis and also to the number of hours in 24 that the limb is positioned above heart level. Thus, the patient with a small area of thrombosis may actually have no swelling while in bed, but if he were sitting or standing throughout the day, he would notice swelling. On the other hand, the patient with a large area of thrombosis, particularly if clots are present at the junction of the superficial femoral and saphenous veins, has massive swelling even though he is in bed. When there is unilateral swelling of the ankle, calf, and thigh, thrombophlebitis should immediately be suspected, since this is a cardinal sign of venous thrombosis. This swelling usually subsides in the night if the limb is elevated to above heart level.

In the mild form of thrombophlebitis there are no color changes in the skin; in the phlegmasia type, there is a reddish, suffused color which becomes bluish as the extent of thrombosis increases. The blueness is also related to the position of the limb in relation to the heart.

Venous distention, when present, is a most suggestive sign, especially if it is absent in the opposite extremity. Measurement of the maximal diameter of the calf and the minimal diameter of the ankle and thigh may reveal swelling that is not obvious on inspection.

Before palpating the extremity, the examiner should be certain that the patient is relaxed and supine and that the knees are flexed a few degrees to relax the gastrocnemius muscle. In extensive thrombosis the skin may be tight and the tissues tense. In the milder form, one can sometimes detect a slight tightness or doughy feeling in the muscles of one calf as compared with the other; in our experience this has been a most important sign. In palpating the calf, one should be certain that the tenderness is not in the skin only; one should palpate the calf muscles from front to back as well as from side to side to detect any localized areas of tenderness or induration, so often observed in patients with hemorrhages into the muscle. When tenderness is present either in the calf muscles or along the course of the veins in the thigh, it must be considered evidence of thrombophlebitis until proven otherwise. DeWeese and Rogoff[114] found that local tenderness was the most accurate sign of deep venous thrombosis, being present in 93 per cent of patients with iliofemoral involvement and in 81 per cent of patients with lower leg involvement, for all of whom phlebograms were also obtained.[114]

HOMANS' SIGN. When the knee is flexed, gentle dorsiflexion of the foot (Homans' sign)[115] may cause pain or discomfort in one calf but not in the other. In our experience, this sign has been suggestive of the diagnosis. However, the test is of no use if it is not carried out properly. Because the sign is not always present and because it is (obviously) not helpful in detecting deep venous thrombosis of the thigh or pelvis, its use in diagnosis is circumscribed.

THE LOWENBERG TEST. In the Lowenberg test,[116] a blood pressure cuff is placed around the normal extremity and inflated until discomfort causes the patient to say, "Stop." It is reinflated three times in order to accustom the patient to the test, which is then carried out on the limb thought to be involved. If pain is experienced at 20 to 30 mm Hg less on one side than on the other, it is suggestive of deep venous thrombosis. As a reliable diagnostic test, it has been found wanting by Barner and DeWeese[117] and in our own experience.

Despite the above well-known clinical signs and symptoms and the familiar clinical methods of detecting them, the ineffectiveness of clinical examination in establishing the presence of deep venous thrombosis has been repeatedly demonstrated by autopsy studies, phlebography, and, more recently, by other noninvasive laboratory instrumentation.

AUTOPSY STUDIES

When autopsy proof of venous thrombosis and/or pulmonary embolism is available, two questions may be raised: (1) In how many patients with such proof of thromboembolic disease was the diagnosis of thrombophlebitis of the lower extremity made prior to death? (2) If a retrospective search of the patients' charts were made, could the clinician have made or suspected the diagnosis of thrombophlebitis? Robertson[118] reported that only 4 per cent of 146 patients with fatal cases of pulmonary embolism presented warning signs of thrombophlebitis; Belt[119] found positive leg signs present in only 9 per cent of 56 cases of emboli, 19 of which were nonfatal. In Neuhof's study, 13 per cent of 88 cases of fatal pulmonary embolism had been diagnosed before death.[120] Crutcher and Daniel[121] reported 20 per cent of 55 fatal cases showing clinical evidence of deep venous thrombosis and 18 per cent having antemortem suggestions of pulmonary embolism. Ravdin and Kirby[122] studied 31 patients with fatal embolism proven by autopsy; in 74 per cent, the first striking clinical evidence of thromboembolic complications was massive pulmonary embolism; in the remaining 8 patients, there was definite evidence of thrombosis prior to embolization. In the largest series, 595 cases of autopsy-proven pulmonary emboli, Coon and Coller[49] found only 7.1 per cent with a clinical diagnosis of embolism; in this same series, only 10.6 per cent of patients had a clinical diagnosis of peripheral venous thrombosis during life.

In a carefully worked-out prospective study, McLachlin et al.[123] examined the lower extremities of seriously ill male patients twice weekly during the course of their illness. Those who subsequently died were autopsied with a complete venous dissection of the lower extremities. Table 2-11 is a summary of their true-positive and false-positive observations.

Retrospectively, Byrne and O'Neil[124] found definite evidence of venous thrombosis in 54 per cent of 130 patients with autopsy-proven fatal emboli. Leg signs were present prior to the embolus in 22 (58 per cent) of 38 cardiac patients, in 18 (56 per cent) of 32 surgical patients, and in 13 (60 per cent) of 22 hemiplegics; in each hemiplegic, the paralyzed extremity was the source of the lung clot. In the remaining 27 cases, the diagnosis was neoplasm in 11, ambulatory phlebitis in 8, and miscellaneous in 8. In over half, leg signs of thrombophlebitis were present prior to death. In retrospective examination of charts for possible symptoms and signs on which the clinical diagnosis of thromboembolic disease could have been based, the percentage of theoretic antemortem detection is not much more encouraging than when such prodromal signals are absent and not merely overlooked. For example, in a combined clinical and autopsy study of 100 patients with massive pulmonary embolism at Peter Bent Brigham Hospital, in 51 patients there was no mention of leg signs and symptoms. Retrospectively, however, Crane[125]

was able to find preliminary warning signs in approximately 80 per cent of the cases.

PHLEBOGRAPHY

Wesolowski et al.[126] reported a rate of diagnostic error on clinical grounds of 30 per cent proved by phlebography. Sanders and Glaser[127] divided their patients into those with "symptoms" and those with "minimal symptoms"; by phlebography, the rate of false-negative diagnosis was 53 per cent in patients with pulmonary embolism and asymptomatic legs. The rate of false-positive diagnosis was 38 per cent for patients with clinical "symptoms" and 80 per cent for those with "minimal" symptoms.

Approximately half of all patients referred to us for "deep vein thrombosis" and at least a quarter of those admitted to our hospital are found not to have thrombophlebitis. The experience of Hume et al.[128] parallels ours; in 54 per cent of their patients, the clinical impression was proved correct by phlebography. In Haeger's[129] retrospective analysis of 512 patients, all bearing the diagnosis of and undergoing treatment for deep venous thrombosis of the leg, subsequent phlebography proved that in 46 per cent the venous system was entirely normal. His second study[130] is of even greater significance. Surgeons with a particular interest in the diagnosis of deep venous thrombosis examined a group of patients for spontaneous calf pain, calf tenderness on palpation, temperature differences between the two legs, calf and ankle swelling, dilatation of superficial veins, Homans' sign,[115] and Lowenberg's sign.[116] If four or more of these signs were decidedly positive, the case was designated "highly suspected," bearing the marks of classic thrombosis. They believed that no experienced physician examining such patients would fail to make the

TABLE 2-11. True Positive and False Positive Clinical Observations

	TRUE-POSITIVE		FALSE-POSITIVE	
	INCIDENCE	%	INCIDENCE	%
Swelling at ankle	10/12	83	1/18	6
Local tenderness	5/12	41	2/18	11
Skin temperature changes	6/12	50	0/18	0
Homans' dorsiflexion sign	1/12	8	1/18	6
Venous dilatation	3/12	25	2/18	11

From McLachlin, J., Richards, T., and Paterson, J. C. *Arch Surg* 85:740, 1962.

diagnosis of deep venous thrombosis. If three of the signs were present, the patient was classified "suspected." In 40 patients with "classic venous thrombosis," the findings were positive by phlebography in only 22 (55 per cent). In the group of "suspected" patients, x-ray findings verified thrombosis in 11 (34 per cent). It is obvious from their findings (Table 2-12) that there is no significant difference between any sign or symptom in patients proven to have thrombosis and in patients with falsely diagnosed thrombosis. Even by splitting the data into two groups, i.e., "highly suspected" and "suspected," no difference could be established.

PHLEGMASIA CERULEA DOLENS

Phlegmasia cerulea dolens is a form of thrombophlebitis in which the venous outflow from the limb is sufficiently obstructed by venous thrombosis to cause cyanosis. In its mildest (benign) form, it differs from phlegmasia alba dolens in degree only. In its severest (malignant) form in which the venous obstruction becomes nearly total, the loss of fluid into the limb can be so great as to produce shock and death. If the patient survives long enough, the limb may become gangrenous due to the inability of arterial blood to enter the engorged limb.

Historical Review

Fabricius Hildanus[131–133] in 1593 recognized the possibility of gangrene of venous origin, and in the nineteenth century, several reports[134–137] suggested clear recognition of this entity. Godin,[134] in fact, declared the edema associated with gangrene to be of venous origin, he also stated that the venous occlusion causes the gangrene because once the blood reaches the distal parts, it cannot return. From then until 1938, investigators[138–141] published reports of gangrene in the presence of occluded veins and patent arteries of the extremities. The modern era of this subject can be said to begin in 1938, for in that year three significant articles appeared. Grégoire[141] published a case history and excellent clinical review under the title, "La phlébite bleue (phlegmatia caerulea dolens)" ("blue phlebitis"); in these two phrases he encompassed the distinguishing sign of this form of venous thrombosis. His name for the disease rapidly gained acceptance. In the same year, Tilley[142] in the United States and Pringle[143] in Scotland published the first case reports in English of the disease, the latter introducing the term "massive ischemic gangrene" in connection with venous thrombosis.

DeBakey and Ochsner[144] reviewed the subject in 1949 and concluded that blockage of the circulation by venous thrombosis afforded the most plausible explanation for the mechanism involved in the ischemia. In a series of excellent reports, Brockman and Vasko[145–148] have reviewed the subject again and added to our knowledge of the pathophysiology. Other terminology, such as "pseudoembolic thrombophlebitis," "arteriospasm due to venous thrombosis," and "fulminating deep

TABLE 2-12. Symptoms and Signs in True and False Thrombosis of the Leg

PRESENCE OF	TRUE THROMBOSIS		FALSE THROMBOSIS	
	%	n*	%	n*
Pain in the calf	90	33	97	39
Calf tenderness	84	33	74	39
Decrease of skin temperature	42	26	38	30
Unilateral ankle edema	76	33	76	39
Unilateral calf edema	42	32	32	36
Superficial venous dilation	33	27	18	34
Positive Homans' sign	33	33	21	37
Positive Lowenberg's sign	20	15	15	15

* The figures (*n*) indicate that all examinations were not performed in some cases.
From Haeger, K. *Angiology* 20:219, 1969.

venous thrombosis," has been proposed and abandoned. Läwen[149] and Veal et al.[150] suggested "acute massive venous occlusion"; although highly appropriate, this term has not become popular. Haimovici[133] recommended that the entire topic be included under the term "ischemic venous thrombosis" or "ischemic thrombophlebitis" and that the disease be subdivided into two clinical forms, viz., phlegmasia cerulea dolens (blue phlebitis) and venous gangrene. Phlegmasia cerulea dolens includes patients in whom the ischemic manifestations are reversible; in venous gangrene the ischemic manifestations are associated with a variable degree of tissue loss.

The term "phlegmasia cerulea dolens" remains in greatest usage.[146-148] Since it clearly describes the clinical picture, it should be retained; however, there are two clearly distinct clinical varieties, so they are referred to as "benign" and "malignant." The malignant type has been described by Haimovici[133] as "venous gangrene"; our reluctance to adopt his term arises from a distinct impression that the limb when first examined is not necessarily gangrenous. Therefore, if some new treatment is developed, e.g., effective enzyme therapy, some limbs may be salvageable.

Pathophysiology

The basic pathology in all instances of phlegmasia cerulea dolens is venous thrombosis. The pathophysiology, simply stated,[132] is that the arterial insufficiency is due to mechanical venous blockage. Brockman and Vasko[146-148] were able to produce typical examples of phlegmasia cerulea dolens in dogs; they created total venous occlusion by filling all veins of the lower extremity with inert barium sulfate solution following ligation of the entire iliofemoral system. In the untreated animals, swelling became apparent within 1 hour and increased rapidly within 3 hours; at the end of 4 to 6 hours, edema of the extremities was massive and marked tachycardia was present. In most animals the femoral pulse could not be palpated; however, the possibility that this might be due to edema was taken into consideration. Reaction to pinprick was negative. A sluggish or absent withdrawal reflex indicated impairment of motor power or sensation. At the end of 8 to 10 hours, profound shock was obvious. Death occurred in less than 24 hours in all

dogs. The average control hematocrit value increased 53 per cent; the average control blood volume decreased 52 per cent; the average control plasma volume decreased 57 per cent; the average red cell mass decreased 9 per cent. These data indicate that shock and hemoconcentration were caused by massive loss of plasma volume in the extremity. The administration of an amount of whole blood equal to the estimated blood volume (7 per cent of body weight in kilograms) and an equal amount of saline solution given over the first 12 hours resulted in 100 per cent survival.

Brockman and Vasko[146-148] demonstrated that venous ligation alone produced no effect on arterial blood pressure or flow; however, in the extremity in which there was massive venous occlusion, venous obstruction caused eventual collapse of the arterial tree. In further experiments they were able to demonstrate an excellent example of Burton's[151] concept of critical closing pressure. As the arterial pressure fell, the tissue pressure, normally close to 0, rose to between 25 and 48 mm Hg. Also, a point was reached at which the difference between tissue pressure and arterial pressure was less than the critical closing pressure (Fig. 2-21), estimated by Burton to be 20 mm Hg; at this point the arterial wall collapsed and all pulses disappeared. However, when the investigators restored the arterial pressure to above the critical closing pressure, the pulses promptly returned. This response was unaffected by sympathectomy produced either chemically or surgically. Brockman and Vasko[146-148] concluded that no evidence exists that "vasospasm" is involved in this pathologic process.

Clinical Features

PHLEGMASIA CERULEA DOLENS, BENIGN TYPE

The clinical feature that distinguishes this type of phlebitis from phlegmasia alba dolens or femoroiliac phlebitis is the presence or absence of cyanosis. Many patients with femoroiliac thrombophlebitis have a slight cyanotic hue to the skin of the limb when it is resting below heart level. After elevation of the limb, this hue disappears in minutes.

Figure 2-21. Mechanism of arterial occlusion as closing critical pressure is reached by increasing tissue pressure. (*From Brockman, S. K., and Vasko, J. S. Surgery 59:997, 1966.*)

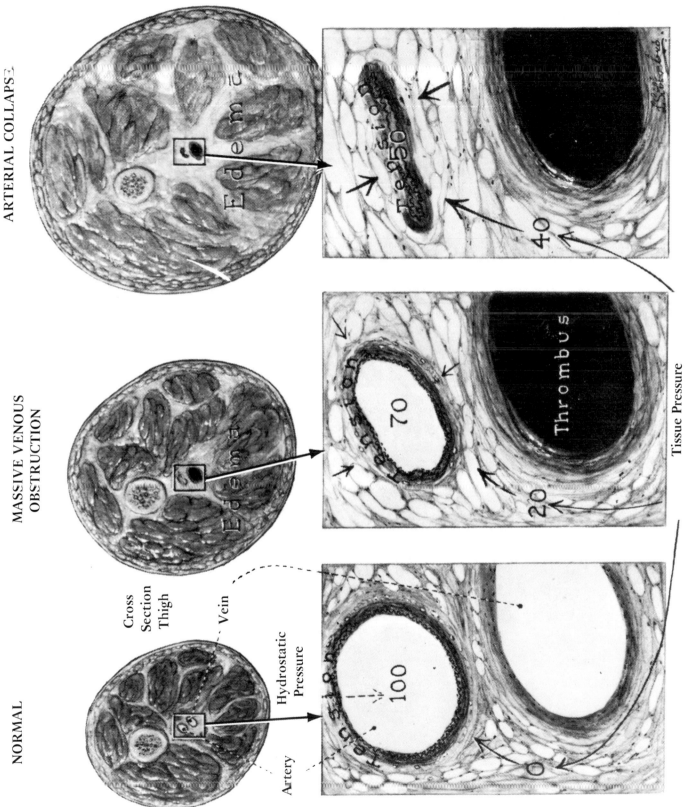

In another patient the cyanosis may be deeper and more pronounced, but nevertheless it subsides within a few hours of elevation of the limb. In some patients 12, 24, or even more hours may be necessary for the cyanotic hue to disappear. At times the cyanosis and swelling are of such intensity that it is feared the limb may soon become gangrenous. In such patients, thrombectomy of the femoroiliac veins causes a dramatic disappearance of the bluish discoloration with restoration of the normal pink color of the skin in a few minutes after operation.

It is difficult to believe that this type of the disease, which we have termed "benign," differs qualitatively from femoroiliac thrombophlebitis. As the limb becomes increasingly engorged with blood, due to increasing venous blockade, the amount of reduced hemoglobin continues to accumulate in the remaining blood, producing the typical bluish-purplish discoloration. In only a single instance in our series were we obliged to observe this process to its completion, viz., in a dying patient who had incipient signs of gangrene

Figure 2-22. A. Patient with phlegmasia cerulea dolens (benign type), treated conservatively. She developed superficial skin necrosis from the application of direct heat. Heat produces a burn more easily in such patients because of the inadequate heat dissipation due to inadequate venous outflow. **B.** Complete healing with scar formation.

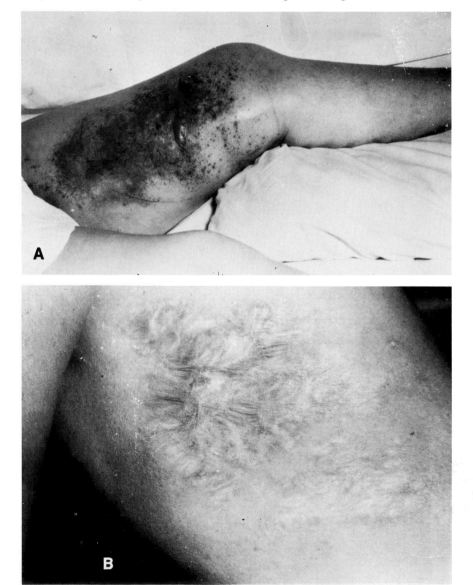

in the distal portion of his limb when he died. In all other instances it was possible to treat the extremity successfully, either by extreme pressure, elevation, and heparin therapy in our earliest experience (Fig. 2-22) or by thrombectomy in the last 20 years (Tables 2-13 and 2-14).

Thrombectomy

Thrombectomy is an excellent form of treatment for the patient with the benign form of phlegmasia cerulea dolens.[132] In the words of Brockman and Vasko,[147] "Venous thrombectomy is particularly applicable because it is based on the simple principle of mechanical intervention when a mechanical obstruction is the basic pathologic condition." Blood should be made available preoperatively, for not only are the patients in borderline shock due to loss of blood into their extremity but also they will hemorrhage extensively following thrombectomy because of engorgement of the vessels with blood, unless control is gained quickly. It has been our policy to ligate the vena cava before opening the groin in order to provide the utmost insurance against embolization of clot to the lung at operation or later. Brockman and Vasko[147] questioned the wisdom of this procedure, believing that there is little rationale in compromising this newly achieved unobstructed venous return by ligation of the major vein. On the other hand, Haller and Mays[152] experimentally demonstrated the extreme difficulty of producing edema in dogs by ligation of the entire iliac venous system. Clinically, it has been our impression also that ligation alone in the absence of thrombosis does not produce significant obstruction to venous bloodflow, because of the efficacy of the collateral circulation. It may not be necessary to provide protection to the patient undergoing thrombectomy; nevertheless, two deaths have been reported[153] from pulmonary embolism following thrombectomy with the cava unligated. Ligating or clipping the vena cava prior to thrombectomy continues to seem to be a reasonable precaution because there is no certainty that all clots have been removed (Figs. 2-23 to 2-26) or that new clots will not form in the immediate postoperative period.

TECHNIQUE

The Fogarty[154, 155] venous thrombectomy catheter has proved to be very efficacious in removing clots from the iliac system (Fig. 2-27). The saphenous vein or the femoral vein itself can be used for extracting thrombi. Using the catheter eliminates the extensive bleeding encountered sometimes when attempting evacuation of clots from the iliac system by other means. As a rule, the catheter is not easily passed into the femoral or popliteal vein due to the presence of venous valves. At times, however, large amounts of clot can be removed by massaging the femoral vein over the adductor canal with one's fist (Fig. 2-28).[156] Forcible dorsiflexion of the patient's foot by a member of the operating team may dislodge numerous thrombi. On one occasion,[156] this maneuver dislodged a clot that extended the entire length of the superficial femoral and possibly, the popliteal veins. It slithered out like a serpent, gathering velocity; as it left the vein it flew over the head of the anesthesiologist and struck the wall behind the operating table. This testifies to the tremendous force that may be exerted

TABLE 2-13. Phlegmasia Cerulea Dolens (Benign Type)

TREATMENT	NO. PATIENTS
Surgical treatment	21 (55%)
Vena cava ligation	13 (9 with thrombectomy)
Common iliac ligation	4
Common iliac thrombectomy only	2*
Common femoral vein and artery thrombectomies	1
Vena cava clipping	1
Anticoagulant therapy	17† (45%)

* One patient had prior vena cava ligation.
† One patient had vena cava ligation 14 years previously for femoroiliac thrombophlebitis of the opposite extremity.

TABLE 2-14. Hospital Deaths in Phlegmasia Cerulea Dolens (Benign Type)

TREATMENT	NO. DEATHS	CAUSE OF DEATH
Surgical	3 (total)*	
	1	Cardiac
	1	Diabetes plus renal insufficiency
	1	Carcinoma
Anticoagulants	1†	Cardiac

* 14% of 21 patients treated by surgery.
† 6% of 17 patients treated by anticoagulant therapy.

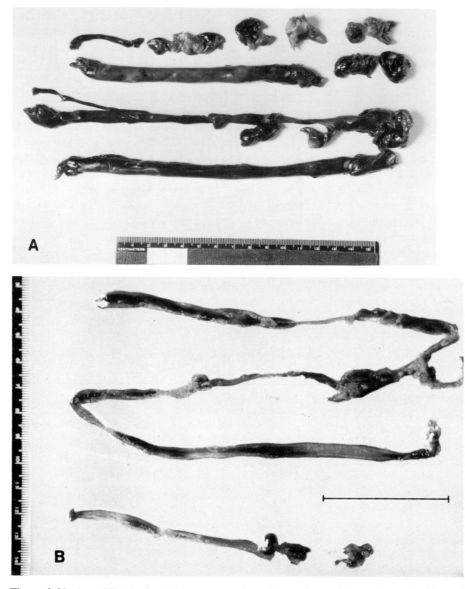

Figure 2-23. A and **B.** Typical clots removed from femoral and iliac veins at the time of thrombectomy for benign form of phlegmasia cerulea dolens.

by the soleal pump, especially if the limb is engorged. If the major portion of clots is successfully removed from the superficial femoral and popliteal veins as well as from the iliacs, the patient will make a dramatic recovery. The limb which had been so deeply violaceous will be of normal color and free of swelling within minutes or hours after thrombectomy. If heparin therapy is continued postoperatively, the end result may be an entirely normal limb. Such a result, however, is uncommon;

more often it is not possible to remove all clots and the patient is left with the postphlebitic swelling typical of one who has had femoropopliteal thrombophlebitis. Treatment in both instances is the same.

In some instances, it has been impossible to remove the thrombus from the superficial femoral vein. This indicates that the patient has had thrombosis of this vein for some time and that subsequently sudden thrombosis of the common femoral vein has occurred that also involves the mouth of the deep femoral, the saphenous, and the external iliac veins. Swelling which was minimal becomes massive. Removing the fresh clot from the sapheno-femoral junction and the iliac veins still produces a dramatic improvement in the color of the limb; however, despite the judicious use of heparin therapy postoperatively, all the residuals of deep venous thrombosis of the femoropopliteal vessels will be present in the lower extremity.

PHLEGMASIA CERULEA DOLENS, MALIGNANT TYPE

Haimovici[133] refers to this type of the disease as "venous gangrene." This must be separated from the benign type if there is to be any hope of delineating patients sufficiently to permit evaluation of different forms of therapy. The term "malignant type" seems preferable because it avoids abolishing any ray of hope for treatment that might be implied by "venous gangrene" (death of tissue.)

The malignant type of cyanotic thrombophlebitis (See Color Plate I. *D* to *H*) differs, in our opinion, from the benign type to a far more significant degree than does the benign type from femoroiliac thrombophlebitis (phlegmasia alba dolens). The malignant form has been encountered rarely in our practice; in most instances, the bluish discoloration has been noted to start in the toes and spread proximally to include the whole foot and distal limb (see Color Plate I. *D*). The progression of the process has been unremitting and uninfluenced by any attempts at treatment, i.e., intravenous heparin in as large a dose as deemed safe combined with steep elevation of the limb. Four patients have survived long enough to undergo thigh amputation,

Figure 2-24. Thrombectomy. The ideal location of thrombus for thrombectomy.

Figure 2-25. Area of thrombus frequently found in patients with femoroiliac thrombophlebitis. Clots can be easily removed from the iliac portion but only with great difficulty from the femoral portion.

Figure 2-26. With very extensive thrombosis, removal of the portion in the common femoral and iliac veins may give marked relief even though the surgeon is unable to extract all the clots from the deep system of the thigh and leg.

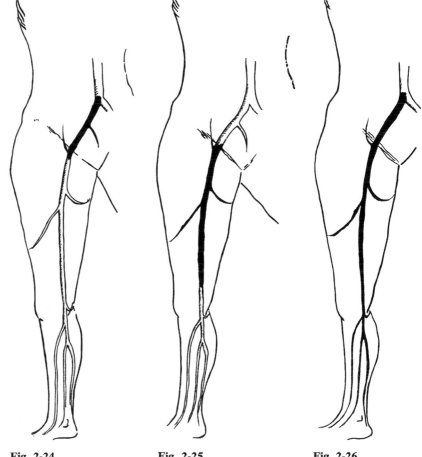

Fig. 2-24.   Fig. 2-25.   Fig. 2-26.

Figure 2-27. Thrombectomy using Fogarty venous catheter. (*From Hafner, C. D., et al. Ann Surg 161:411, 1965.*)

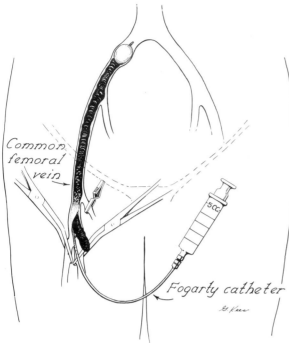

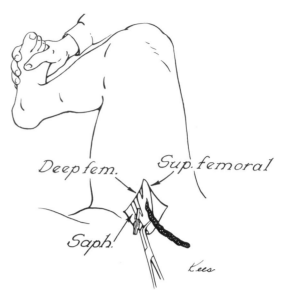

Figure 2-28. Maneuver sometimes of help in extracting clot from the superficial femoral vein. The foot is forcibly dorsiflexed, stretching the soleal muscle and thus pumping the clot proximally. (*From Hafner, C. D., et al. Ann Surg 161:411, 1965.*)

2 bilaterally; of the 11 patients seen, 10 have died while hospitalized (Table 2-15). A recent patient (see Case Report 2-2), having undergone a thigh amputation, died 6 weeks after leaving the hospital; the cause of death was carcinoma of the lung.

Case Report 2-1

R. T., a 47-year-old male Caucasian, a spray painter, was seen on the third day of hospitalization in January, 1963. His present illness had begun 11 days earlier when he noted blistering of his right foot which he attributed to wearing shoes heavily coated with paint. Gradually pain and swelling of his right foot developed, and with this, he was admitted. Examination by the intern showed no discoloration of

the feet bilaterally but redness and swelling of the right foot, ankle, and calf. Treatment consisted of heparin, phenylbutazone (Butazolidin), and penicillin. Initial WBC was 10,385, with 35 per cent neutrophiles, 29 per cent lymphocytes, 5 monocytes, 1 basophile, and 4 eosinophiles, with 2 juvenile myelocytes. Chest x ray showed no acute pulmonary pathologic changes, although fluid was present in both bases. In the opinion of the radiologist, the densities in the lung fields represented metastatic disease. On the day after admission, cyanosis developed on the dorsum of the right foot; within 12 hours, the entire foot was purplish-blue. In the next 12 hours, discoloration developed in the left foot. Temperature was elevated to 101 F.

On our examination, total blue-black discoloration of the entire right foot up to the ankle was noted,

TABLE 2-15. Malignant Form of Phlegmasia Cerulens Dolens

	NO. PATIENTS	ABOVE-KNEE AMPUTATION	IN-HOSPITAL DEATHS
Anticoagulant therapy	5	2 (Unilateral)	4*
No specific treatment	6	2 (Bilateral)	6
Total	11 patients with 14 involved extremities		

* One additional patient died 6 weeks after discharge from the hospital.

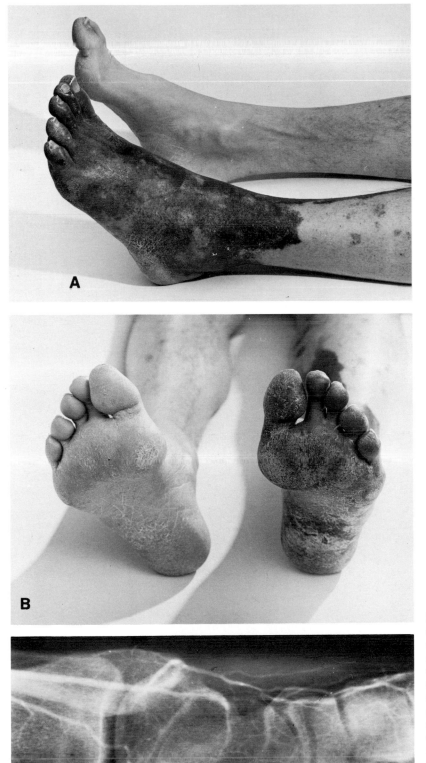

Figure 2-29. A. Lateral view of left limb within 48 hours of first appearance of violaceous discoloration of toes and dorsum of foot. At this time the family was told that this was the malignant type of phlegmasia cerulea dolens and that the patient probably had a malignancy and would not recover. **B.** Plantar aspect of foot. Color was bluish-black. **C.** Arteriogram taken on the day prior to amputation, showing the anterior tibial and dorsalis pedis arteries both patent.

(continued)

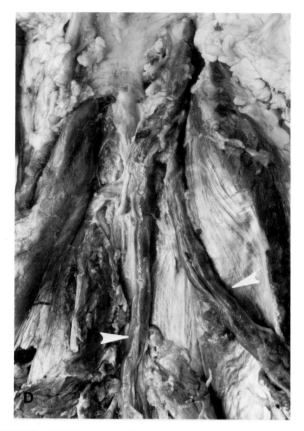

Figure 2-29 D. At operation (above-knee amputation), every major vein encountered was found to be thrombosed, including the superficial and deep femorals. It was not possible to extract this clot with the Fogarty venous catheter. The amputated specimen similarly showed thrombosis of all visible veins. Paired posterior tibial and peroneal veins are shown to be solidly thrombosed; the anterior tibial and soleal veins were similarly thrombosed. **E.** Microscopic photo through area of bluish black discoloration, showing all veins to be thrombosed. (Patient was found to have carcinoma of the lung and died at home of cerebral metastases within 6 weeks of admission to this hospital.)

i.e., the purplish discoloration usually observed with phlegmasia cerulea dolens or gangrene of the skin. The right leg was swollen, red, and tender. Discoloration similar to that of the right foot was noted on the dorsum of the left foot. The left foot was not swollen, and the calf muscles were not tender. Femoral pulses were palpable bilaterally, but pulsations were absent below that point. There was tenderness of both popliteal spaces.

It was our impression that this patient presented with the malignant form of phlegmasia cerulea dolens, that he was moribund, and, in the event that he survived, that bilateral amputation would be necessary. No surgical treatment was recommended.

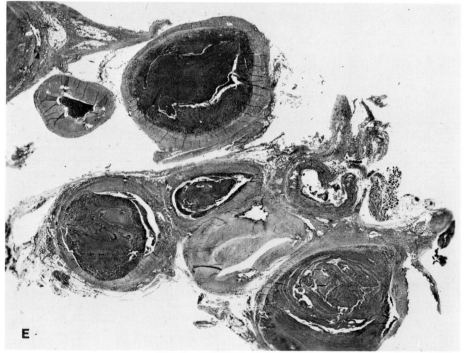

A second vascular consultation was sought later; by this time, x-ray evidence was present to suggest infarction of the lungs, and the vena cava was ligated by the second surgeon. The patient continued to deteriorate and died 17 days after admission.

At autopsy there was gangrene of both feet and legs, with thrombosis of all veins that were examined in the limbs and of several of the arteries, including the internal iliacs, deep femorals, and popliteals bilaterally. All veins examined were thrombosed from the site of ligature of the vena cava down. No thrombi were present above the vena caval ligation. Findings also included large mural thrombi of the right and left ventricles, infarcts of the lung, spleen, and kidneys, replacement of the thymus by a tumor, and lymphocytic infiltration of almost all of the abdominal viscera.

Final diagnosis was considered to be lymphocytic lymphoma, involving the abdominal and mediastinal nodes, intestines, thymus, pancreas, kidneys, and prostate gland.

Case Report 2-2

J.M., a 61-year-old male Caucasian, was under treatment at another hospital for superficial thrombophlebitis of the left lower extremity. On the evening of January 18, 1974, the patient, the family, and their physician stated that the limb appeared to be normal. At 3 AM on the morning of January 19, the patient felt a stinging pain in his foot; at 9 AM the physician noticed that the patient had a slight bluish discoloration of his toes. He was transferred to Good Samaritan Hospital. On examination at 7 PM, all toes were blue and there was a bluish-purplish discoloration of the dorsum of the foot (Fig. 2-29*A, B*). He could move his toes but there was hypesthesia. The diagnosis of the malignant type of phlegmasia cerulea dolens was made by inspection. Despite the fact that he was given 31,000 units of heparin intravenously over the next 8 hours, the bluish-black discoloration was present within 15 hours of entering the hospital and within 24 hours after the first slight bluish discoloration was noted. Although he had obliterative arterial disease, an arteriogram at this time showed the anterior tibial and dorsalis pedis arteries still patent (Fig. 2-29*C*). At amputation every visible vein in the thigh was thrombosed. A Fogarty venous catheter was inserted up the superficial femoral vein to the area of the iliac vein, and although much clot was removed, it was obvious that it was not all removed. Dissection of the amputated limb (Fig. 2-29*D*) showed every visible vein clotted, including the paired named veins, com-

Figure 2-30. Malignant type of venous gangrene. The color which appears to be black in the photo was actually blue-black and not the brownish discoloration of arterial gangrene. Patient died of metastatic carcinoma within 10 days after this photo. **A.** Toes. **B.** Sole of foot.

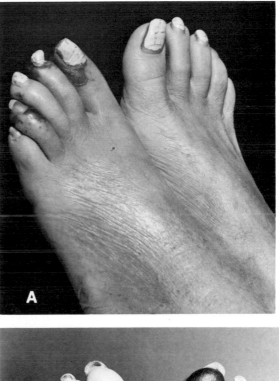

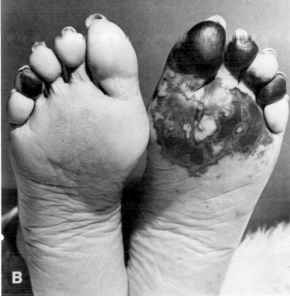

municating veins, soleal veins, and every vein large enough to be seen. Microscopic section (Fig. 2-29*E*) showed thrombosis of all veins apparent on every section. While the patient was being treated, complete work-up at the hospital showed carcinoma of the right lung, proven by brush biopsy and resected in the hope that similar episodes might be prevented in the right lower extremity. Despite the fact that the patient looked and felt well following amputation, he died within 6 weeks after discharge from the hospital. His right limb was slightly cyanotic but had not become gangrenous.

In Haimovici's review[133] of all reported cases of venous gangrene, not all were fatal. It may be that we have witnessed a group of particularly virulent examples of the malignant type (Figs. 2-30 and 2-31), or it may be that in the collected series other entities have been included. It can be gleaned from some of the reports that the term "venous gangrene" may be erroneously used in a patient with gangrene of the toes in the presence of patent major arteries. This condition, far from rare, should be considered to represent arteriolar thrombosis. (See Volume I, *Peripheral Arterial Diseases,* Chapter 1, Fig. 1-10*A,* p. 13.[157])

Figure 2-31. Gangrene of venous origin in a moribund patient. **A.** Toes, dorsal aspect. **B.** Plantar aspect of toes. **C.** Lateral view of left limb.

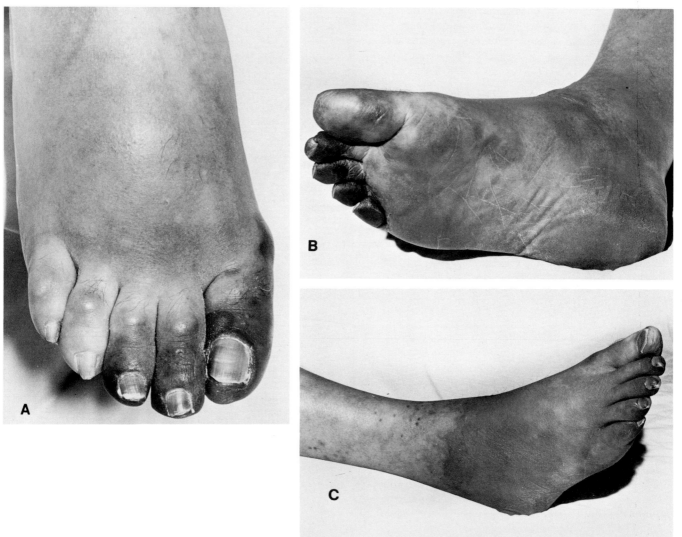

REFERENCES

1. Ochsner, A. Venous thrombosis. *Surgery 24:*445, 1940.

2. Allen, E. V., Barker, N. W., and Hines, E. A. Jr. Peripheral Vascular Diseases, ed 3. Philadelphia, Saunders, 1962.

3. McLachlin, J., and Paterson, J. C. Some basic observations on venous thrombosis and pulmonary embolism. *Surg Gynecol Obstet 93:*1, 1951.

4. Cranley, J. J., Gay, A. Y., Grass, A. M., and Simeone, F. A. A plethysmographic technique for the diagnosis of deep venous thrombosis of the lower extremities. *Surg Gynecol Obstet 136:*385, 1973.

5. Hume, M. Blood coagulation in deep and superficial thrombophlebitis. *Arch Surg 92:*934, 1966.

6. Liddell, H. G., and Scott, R. A Greek-English Lexikon, ed 9. Oxford, Clarendon, 1953, p 807.

7. Virchow, R. I. Ueber die Verstopfung der Lungenarterie. *Froriep's Notizen Nr 794,* 1846.

7a. Virchow, R. II. Weitere Untersuchungen über die Verstopfung der Lungenarterie und ihre Folgen. *Traube's Beitr z exper Path u Physiol Heft 2,* Berlin, 1846.

8. Virchow, R. Neuer Fall von tödlicher Embolie der Lungenarterie. *Arch Path Anat 10:*225, 1856.

9. Welch, W. H. Thrombosis and embolism. In Albutt, T. C. (ed.) *A System of Medicine.* London, Macmillan, 1889, vol. 6, p 155.

10. Hume, H., Sevitt, S., and Thomas, D. P. Venous thrombosis and pulmonary embolism. Cambridge, Harvard University Press, 1970, p 3.

10a. Hadfield, G. Thrombosis. *Ann R Coll Surg Engl* 1 1 1 1, 1 9 0 0.

11. Zahn, W. Untersuchungen über Thrombose: Bildung der Thromben. *Virchows Arch [Pathol Anat] 62:*81, 1875.

11a. Florey, H. W. (ed.) *General Pathology,* ed 4. Philadelphia, Saunders, 1970.

12. Marcus, A. J. Platelet Function. *N Engl J Med 280:* 1213, 1278, 1330, 1969.

12a. French, J. E. MacFarlane, R. G., and Sanders, A. G. The structure of haemostatic plugs and experimental thrombi in small arteries. *Br J Exp Path 45:*467, 1964.

13. Virchow, R. Cellular pathology as based upon physiological, pathological histology. New York, DeWitt, 1860.

14. Virchow, R. IV. Thrombose und Embolie. Gefässentzündung und septische Infection. In *Gesammelte Abhandlungen zur Wissenschaftlichen Medicin.* Frankfurt, Meidinger Sohn, 1856.

15. Eberth, J. C., and Schimmelbusch, C. Die Thrombose nach Versuchen und Leichenbefunden. Stuttgart, Ferd. Enke, 1888.

16. O'Neill, J. F. The effects on venous endothelium of alterations in blood flow through the vessels in vein walls, and the possible relation to thrombosis. *Ann Surg 126:*270, 1947.

17. Samuels, P. B., and Webster, D. R. The role of venous endothelium in the inception of thrombosis. *Ann Surg 136:*422, 1952.

18. Hunter, J. Observations on the inflammation of the internal coats of veins. In Palmer, J. F. *The Works of John Hunter, F.R.S.,* ed 3. London, Longman, 1857, p 581.

19. Altemeier, W. A., Hill, E. P., and Fullen, W. D. Acute and recurrent thromboembolic disease: A new concept of etiology. *Ann Surg 170:*547, 1969.

19a. Cotton, L. T., and Clark, C. Anatomical localization of venous thrombosis. *Ann R Coll Surg Engl 36:*214, 1965.

19b. McLachlin, A. D. Venous thrombosis and pulmonary embolism. In Taylor, S. *Recent Advances in Surgery.* London, Churchill, 1969, p 12.

20. Wessler, S., Reiner, L., Freiman, D. G., Reimer, S. M., and Lertzman, M. Serum-induced thrombosis: Studies of its induction and evolution under controlled conditions in vivo. *Circulation 20:*864, 1959.

21. Wessler, S. Studies in intravascular coagulation: III. The pathogenesis of serum-induced venous thrombosis. *J Clin Invest 34:*647, 1955.

22. Wessler, S., Reimer, S. M., and Sheps, M. C. Biologic assay of a thrombosis-inducing activity in human serum. *J Appl Physiol 14:*943, 1959.

23. Wessler, S., and Reimer, S. M. The role of human coagulation factors in serum-induced thrombosis. *J Clin Invest 39:*262, 1960.

24. Craven, J. L. Panel Discussion on Pulmonary Embolism, University of Kentucky, Lexington, Ky, April 18–21, 1973.

25. Crane, C. Panel Discussion on Thromboembolism, American College of Surgeons, Western New York Chapter, State University of New York, Buffalo, NY, May 3, 1973.

25a. Frykholm, R. Pathogenesis and mechanical prophylaxis of venous thrombosis. *Surg Gynecol Obstet 71:*309, 1940.

26. McLachlin, J., and Paterson, J. C. Some basic observations on venous thrombosis and pulmonary embolism. *Surg Gynecol Obstet 93:*1, 1951.

27. Paterson, J. C., and McLachlin, J. Precipitating factors in venous thrombosis. *Surg Gynecol Obstet 98:*96, 1954.

28. Gibbs, N. M. Venous thrombosis of the lower limbs with particular reference to bed rest. *Br J Surg 45:*209, 1957.

29. Sevitt, S., and Gallagher, N. G. Venous thrombosis and pulmonary embolism: A clinico-pathological study in injured and burned patients. *Br J Surg 48:*475, 1961.

30. Dodd, H., and Cockett, F. B. *The Pathology and*

Surgery of the Veins of the Lower Limb. Edinburgh, Livingstone, 1956, p 297.

31. Rabinov, K., and Paulin, S. Roentgen diagnosis of venous thrombosis of the leg. *Arch Surg 104:*134, 1972.

32. Homans, J. Thrombosis of the deep veins of the lower leg, causing pulmonary embolism. *N Engl J Med 211:*993, 1934.

33. Sise, H. S., Moschos, C. B., and Becker, R. On the nature of hypercoagulability. *Am J Med 33:*667, 1962.

34. Lieberman, J. S., Borrero, J., Urdaneta, E., and Wright, I. S. Thrombophlebitis and cancer. *JAMA 177:*542, 1961.

35. Ashford, T. P., Freiman, D. H., and Weinstein, M. C. The role of the intrinsic fibrinolytic system in the prevention of stasis thrombosis in small veins. *Am J Path 52:*1117, 1968.

36. Wright, H. P. Changes in the adhesiveness of blood platelets following parturition and surgical operations. *J Path Bact 34:*461, 1942.

37. Bennett, P. N. Postoperative changes in platelet adhesiveness. *J Clin Path: 20:*708, 1967.

38. Paterson, J. C., and McLachlin, J. A critical evaluation of the anti-thrombin test for venous thrombosis. *Surg Gynecol Obstet 94:*297, 1952.

39. Kay, J. H., Hutton, S. B., Weiss, G. N., and Ochsner A. Studies on antithrombin-III, a plasma antithrombin test for the prediction of intravascular clotting. *Surgery 28:*24, 1950.

40. Hume, M. Platelet adhesiveness and other coagulation factors in thrombophlebitis. *Surgery 59:*110, 1966.

41. Hume, M. Platelet entrapment in glass spheres: Clinical and experimental application. *Ann Surg 166:*569, 1967.

42. Hume, M., and Chan, Y.-K. Examination of the blood in the presence of venous thrombosis. *JAMA 200:*747, 1967.

43. Gurewich, V., and Hutchinson, E. Detection of intravascular coagulation by a serial-dilution protamine sulfate test. *Ann Int Med 75:*895, 1971.

44. Wood, E. H., Prentice, C. R., and McNicol, G. P. Association of fibrinogen-fibrin-related antigen (F.R.-antigen) with postoperative deep-vein thrombosis and systemic complications. *Lancet 1:*166, 1972.

45. von Kaulla, E., Droegemueller, W., Aokl, N., and von Kaulla, K. N. Antithrombin III depression and thrombin generation in women taking oral contraceptives. *Am J Obstet Gynecol 109:*868, 1971.

46. von Kaulla, E., and von Kaulla, K. N. Antithrombin III and diseases. *Am J Clin Path 48:*69, 1967.

47. Daniel, D. G., Campbell, H., and Turnbull, A. C. Puerperal thromboembolism and suppression of lactation. *Lancet 2:*287, 1967.

48. Hunter, W. C., Sneeden, V. D., Robertson, T. D., and Snyfer, G. A. C. Thrombosis of the deep veins of the leg: Its clinical significance as exemplified in 351 autopsies. *Arch Int Med 68:*1, 1941.

49. Coon, W. W., and Coller, F. A. Some epidemiologic considerations of thromboembolism. *Surg Gynecol Obstet 109:*487, 1959.

50. Sartwell, P., and Anello, C. Trends in mortality from thromboembolic disorders. In Advisory Committee on Obstetrics and Gynecology, Food and Drug Administration. *Second Report on the Oral Contraceptives.* US Government Printing Office, August 1, 1969, pp 37–40.

51. Jick, H., Slone, D., Westerholm, B., Inman, W. H. W., Vessey, M. P., Shapiro, S., Lewis, G., and Worcester J. Venous thromboembolic disease and ABO blood type. *Lancet 1:*539, 1969.

52. Slone, D., Jick, H., Borda, I., Chalmers, T. C., Feinleib, M., Muench, H., Lipworth, L., Bellotti, C., and Gilman, B. Drug surveillance utilizing nurse monitors. *Lancet 2:*901, 1966.

53. Borda, I., Slone, D., and Jick H. Assessment of adverse reactions within a drug surveillance program. *JAMA 205:*645, 1968.

54. Preston, A. E., and Barr, A. The plasma concentration of Factor VIII in the normal population: II. The effects of age, sex and blood group. *Br J Haemat 10:*238, 1964.

55. Langman, M. J. S., and Doll, R. ABO blood group and secretor status in relation to clinical characteristics of peptic ulcer. *Gut 6:*270, 1965.

56. VillaSanta, U. Thromboembolic disease in pregnancy. *Am J Obstet Gynecol 93:*142, 1965.

57. Goodrich, S. M., and Wood, J. E. Peripheral distensibility and velocity of venous blood flow during pregnancy or during oral contraceptive therapy. *Am J Obstet Gynecol 90:*740, 1964.

58. Ullery, J. C. Thromboembolic disease complicating pregnancy and the puerperium. *Am J Obstet Gynecol 68:*1243, 1954.

59. Aaro, L. A., Johnson, T. R., and Juergens, J. L. Acute deep venous thrombosis associated with pregnancy. *Obstet Gynecol 28:*553, 1966.

60. Aaro, L. A., Johnson, T. R., and Juergens, J. L. Acute superficial thrombophlebitis associated with pregnancy. *Am J Obstet Gynecol 97:*514, 1967.

61. Ygge, J. Changes in blood coagulation and fibrinolysis during the puerperium. *Am J Obstet Gynecol 104:*2, 1969.

62. Jordan, W. M. Pulmonary embolism. *Lancet 2:*1146, 1967.

63. *Thromboembolic Phenomena in Women,* Proceedings of a Conference, Chicago, September 10, 1962. Chicago, G. D. Searle.

64. Tyler, E. T. Oral contraceptives and venous thrombosis. *JAMA 185:*131, 1963.

65. Schatz, I. J., Smith, R. F., Breneman, G. M., and Bower, G. C. Thromboembolic disease associated with norethylnodrel: Report of 6 cases. *JAMA 188:*493, 1964.

66. Nevin, N. C., Elmes, P. C., and Weaver, J. A. Three cases of intravascular thrombosis occurring in patients receiving oral contraceptives. *Br Med J 1:* 1586, 1965.

67. Ballar, J. C. Thromboembolism and oestrogen therapy. *Lancet 2:*560, 1967.

68. Dugdale, M., and Masi, A. T. Effects of the oral contraceptives on blood clotting. In Advisory Committee on Obstetrics and Gynecology, Food and Drug Administration. *Second Report on the Oral Contraceptives.* US Government Printing Office, August 1, 1969, p 43.

69. Inman, W. H. W., and Vessey, M. P. Investigation of deaths from pulmonary, coronary, and cerebral thrombosis and embolism in women of child-bearing age. *Br Med J 2:*193, 1968.

70. Vessey, M. P., and Weatherall, J. A. C. Venous thromboembolic disease and the use of oral contraceptives. *Lancet 2:*94, 1968.

71. Vessey, M. P., and Doll, R. Investigation of relation between use of oral contraceptives and thromboembolic disease: A further report. *Br Med J 2:*651, 1969.

72. Doll, R., Inman, W. H. W., and Vessey, M. P. Concerning the British data: Letter to the editor. *JAMA 207:*1150, 1969.

73. British Medical Research Council. Risk of thromboembolic disease in women taking oral contraceptives. *Br Med J 2:*355, 1967.

74. Drill, V. A., and Calhoun, D. W. Oral contraceptives and thromboembolic disease. *JAMA 206:*77, 1968.

75. Drill, V. A. Response to Letter to the Editor concerning British data. (Ref. 72) *JAMA 207:*1151, 1969.

76. Drill, V. A., and Calhoun, D. W. Oral contraceptives and thromboembolic disease: I. Prospective and retrospective studies. *JAMA 219:*583, 1972.

77. Drill, V. A., and Calhoun, D. W. Oral contraceptives and thromboembolic disease: II. Estrogen content of oral contraceptives. *JAMA 219:*593, 1972.

78. Markush, R. E., and Seigel, D. G. Oral contraceptives and mortality trends from thromboembolism in the United States. *Am J Pub Health 59:*418, 1969.

79. Advisory Committee on Obstetrics and Gynecology, Food and Drug Administration. *Second Report on the Oral Contraceptives.* US Government Printing Office, August 1, 1969.

80. Preston, S. N. The oral contraceptive controversy. *Am J Obstet Gynecol 111:*994, 1971.

81. Boston Collaborative Drug Surveillance Programme. Oral contraceptives and venous thromboembolic disease, surgically confirmed gallbladder disease, and breast tumors. *Lancet 1:*1399, 1973.

82. Hougie, C. Thromboembolic disorders and oral contraceptives: Letter to editor. *JAMA 208:*865, 1969.

83. Hougie, C. Oral contraceptives and thromboembolic disease: Letter to editor. *JAMA 221:*194, 1972.

84. Fuertes-de la Haba, A., Curet, J. O., Pelegrina, I., and Bangdiwala, I. Thrombophlebitis among oral and nonoral contraceptive users. *Obstet Gynecol 38:*259, 1971.

85. Sartwell, P. E. Oral contraceptives and thromboembolic disease: Letter to editor. *JAMA 220:*416, 1972.

86. Schrogie, J. J., Seigel, D., Corfman, P. A. Oral contraceptives and thromboembolic disease: Letter to editor. *JAMA 220:*416, 1972.

87. Doll, R., and Vessey, M. Oral contraceptives and thromboembolic disease: Letter to editor. *JAMA 220:*417, 1972.

88. Seltzer, C. C. An editorial viewpoint. *JAMA 207:* 1152, 1969.

88a. Doll, R. Recognition of unwanted drug effects. *Br Med J 2:*69, 1969.

89. Hellman, L. M. Chairman's summary. In Advisory Committee on Obstetrics and Gynecology, Food and Drug Administration. *Second Report on the Oral Contraceptives.* US Government Printing Office, August 1, 1969, p 5.

90. Sartwell, P. E., Masi, A. T., Arthes, F. G., Greene, G. R., and Smith, H. E. Thromboembolism and oral contraceptives: An epidemiological case-control study. In Advisory Committee on Obstetrics and Gynecology, Food and Drug Administration. *Second Report on the Oral Contraceptives.* US Government Printing Office, August 1, 1969, p 21.

91. Trousseau, A. Clinique médicale de l'Hôtel-dieu de Paris, ed 5. Paris, Ballière, 1877, vol. 3, p 94.

92. Gouget, W. *Bull Soc Anat 13:*203, 1894. Cited by Welch, W. H. Thrombosis. In Albutt, T. C., and Rollston, H. D. (eds.) *A System of Medicine.* London, Macmillan, 1909, vol. 6, p 691.

93. Osler, W., and McCrae, T. Cancer of the stomach: A clinical study. Philadelphia, Blakiston, 1900, vol. 57, p 204.

94. Welch, W. H. Thrombosis. In Albutt, T. C., and Rolleston, H. D. (eds.) *A System of Medicine.* London, Macmillan, 1909, vol. 6, p 691.

95. Sproul, E. E. Carcinoma and venous thrombosis: The frequency of association of carcinoma in the body or tail of the pancreas with multiple venous thrombosis. *Am J Cancer 34:*566, 1938.

96. Edwards, E. A. Migrating thrombophlebitis associated with carcinoma. *N Engl J Med 240:*1031, 1949.

97. Fisher, M. M., Hochberg, L. A., and Wilenski, N. D. Recurrent thrombophlebitis in obscure malignant tumor of the lung: Report of 4 cases. *JAMA 147:* 1213, 1951.

98. Hubay, C. A., and Holden, W. D. Venous thrombosis, necrosis and neoplasia. *Surg Gynecol Obstet 98:*309, 1954.

99. Barker, N. W. Thrombophlebitis complicating infectious and systemic diseases. *Proc Staff Meet Mayo Clin 11:*513, 1936.

100. Woolling, K. R., and Shick, R. M. Thrombophlebitis: A possible clue to cryptic malignant lesions. *Proc Staff Meet Mayo Clin 31:*227, 1956.

101. Byrd, R. B., Divertie, M. B., and Spittell, J. A. Bronchogenic carcinoma and thromboembolic disease. *JAMA 202:*1019, 1967.

102. Hafner, C. D., Cranley, J. J., Krause, R. J., and Strasser, E. S. A method of managing superficial thrombophlebitis. *Surgery 55:*201, 1964.

103. Mondor, H. Tronculite sous-cutanée subaigue de la paroi thoracique antéro-latérale. *Mem Acad Chir 65:*1271, 1939.

104. Mondor, H., and Bertand, I. Thrombo-Phlébites et periphlébites de la paroi thoracique antérieure. *Presse Med 59:*1533, 1951.

105. Farrow, J. H. Thrombophlebitis of superficial veins of breast and anterior chest wall (Mondor's disease). *Surg Gynecol Obstet 101:*63, 1955.

106. Karlan, M., and Traphagen, D. Superficial phlebitis of breast. *Am J Surg 94:*981, 1957.

107. Miano, B. D. Mondor's disease. *Calif Med 89:*221, 1958.

108. Kaufman, P. A. Subcutaneous phlebitis of breast and chest wall. *Ann Surg 144:*5, 1956.

109. Honig, C., and Rado, R. Mondor's disease—superficial phlebitis of the chest wall: A review of seven cases. *Ann Surg 153:*589, 1961.

110. Johnson, W. C., Wallrich, R., and Helwig, E. B. Superficial thrombophlebitis of the chest wall. *JAMA 180:*103, 1962.

111. Castleton, K. B., Cloud, R. S., and Ward, J. R. Anterior chest wall-superficial thrombophlebitis: Mondor's disease. *Arch Surg 88:*1010, 1964.

112. Thomford, N. R., and Holaday, W. J. Mondor's disease (phlebitis of the thoracoepigastric vein). *Ann Surg 170:*1035, 1969.

113. Dexter, L. The chair and venous thrombosis. *Trans Am Clin Climat Assoc 84:*1, 1972.

113a. Dexter, L., and Polch-Pi, W. Venous thrombosis. An account of the first documented case. *JAMA 228:*195, 1974.

114. DeWeese, J. A., and Rogoff, S. M. Functional ascending phlebography of the lower extremity by serial long film technique. *Amer J Roentgen 81:*841, 1959.

115. Homans, J. Thrombosis as a complication of venography. *JAMA 119:*136, 1942.

116. Lowenberg, R. I. Early diagnosis of phlebothrombosis with aid of a new clinical test. *JAMA 155:*1566, 1954.

117. Barner, H. B., and DeWeese, J. A. An evaluation of the sphygmomanometer cuff pain test in venous thrombosis. *Surgery 48:*915, 1960.

118. Robertson, H. Clinical study of pulmonary embolism: Analysis of 146 fatal cases. *Am J Surg 41:*3, 1938.

119. Belt, T. H. Thrombosis and pulmonary embolism. *Am J Path 10:*129, 1934.

120. Neuhof, H. Venous thrombosis and pulmonary embolism. New York, Grune & Stratton, 1948.

121. Crutcher, R. R., and Daniel, R. A. Pulmonary embolism: Correlation of clinical and autopsy studies. *Surgery 23:*47, 1948.

122. Ravdin, I. S., and Kirby, C. K. Experiences with ligation and heparin in thromboembolic disease. *Surgery 29:*334, 1950.

123. McLachlin, J., Richards, T., and Paterson, J. C. An evaluation of clinical signs in the diagnosis of venous thrombosis. *Arch Surg 85:*738, 1962.

124. Byrne, J. J., and O'Neil, E. E. Fatal pulmonary emboli: Study of 130 autopsy-proven fatal emboli. *Am J Surg 83:*47, 1952.

125. Crane, C. Deep venous thrombosis and pulmonary embolism. *N Engl J Med 257:*147, 1957.

126. Wesolowski, S. A., Greenfield, H., Sawyer, P. N., Fries, C. C., Schaefer, H. C., and Martinez, A. Diagnostic value of phlebography in venous disorders of the lower extremity. *J Cardiov Surg (suppl) 133*–151:16–18 (Sept) 1965.

127. Sanders, R. J., and Glaser, J. L. Clinical uses of venography. *Angiology 20:*388, 1969.

128. Hume, M., Glancy, J. J., and Chan, Y.-K. Blood tests and Doppler flowmeter examination: Compared with phlebograms in venous thrombosis. *Arch Surg 97:*894, 1968.

129. Haeger, K. Problems of acute deep venous thrombosis: I. The interpretation of signs and symptoms. *Angiology 20:*219, 1969.

130. Haeger, K. Den kliniska trombosdiagnosens (o)tillförtlitlighet. *Lakartidn 62:*1067, 1965.

131. Fabricius Hildanus, G. De gangraena et sphacelo. Cologne, 1593.

132. Fogarty, T. J., Cranley, J. J., Krause, R. J., Strasser, E. S., and Hafner, C. D. Surgical management of phlegmasia cerulea dolens. *Arch Surg 86:*256, 1963.

133. Haimovici, H. *Ischemic Forms of Venous Thrombosis: Phlegmasia Cerulea Dolens Venous Gangrene.* Springfield, IL, Thomas, 1971.

134. Godin, cited by Dionisi, P. J. *Les Gangrènes des Membres d'Origine Veineuse,* thesis. Marseille Medical School, 1938.

135. Hueter, Fall von Gangrän in Folge von Venenobliteration. *Virchows Arch Path Anat 17:*482, 1859.

136. Gaillard, M. L. Gangrène humide du pied gauche par thrombose de la veine femorale, chez une cancereuse de 27 ans. *Bull Soc Med H Paris, 1:*315, 1894.

137. Reyt. *Sur les Gangrènes d'Origine Veineuse,* thesis in medicine, Paris, 1897.

138. Pons, H. Gangrène de la jambe consecutive à une thrombose de la veine femorale. *Bull Soc Anat 7:*645, 1905.

139. Buerger, L. The circulatory disturbances of the extremities. Philadelphia, Saunders, 1924, pp 158, 479.

140. Trémolières, F., and Véran, P. Syndrome d'oblitération artérielle du membre inférieur droit apparu au cours d'une phlébite superficielle et profonde avec embolies pulmonaires effect de l'acétylcholine. *Bull Méd Paris 43:*1101, 1929.

141. Grégoire, R. La phlébite bleue (phlegmatia caerulea dolens). *Presse Méd 2:*1313, 1929.

142. Tilley, J. M. Gangrene of the extremities in puerperal thrombophlebitis. *Am J Obstet Gynecol 36:*157, 1938.

143. Pringle, J. M. Massive ischaemic gangrene with thrombosis of veins and patent arteries. *Glasgow M J 129:*126, 1938.

144. DeBakey, M. E., and Ochsner, A. Phlegmasia cerulea dolens and gangrene associated with thrombophlebitis. *Surgery 26:*16, 1949.

145. Vasko, J. S., and Brockman, S. K. Massive venous occlusion of the lower extremity. *Surg Forum 45:*233, 1964.

146. Brockman, S. K., and Vasko, J. S. Observations on the pathophysiology and treatment of phlegmasia cerulea dolens with special reference to thrombectomy. *Am J Surg 109:*485, 1965.

147. Brockman, S. J., and Vasko, J. S. Collective review: Phlegmasia cerulea dolens. *Surg Gynecol Obstet 121:*1347, 1965.

148. Brockman, S. K., and Vasko, J. S. The pathologic physiology of phlegmasia cerulea dolens. *Surgery 59:*997, 1966.

149. Läwen, A. Ueber Thrombektomie bei Venenthrombose und Arteriospasmus. *Zbl Chir 61:*1681, 1934.

150. Veal, J. R., Dugan, T. J., Jamison, W. L., and Bauersfeld, R. S. Acute massive venous occlusion of the lower extremities. *Surgery 29:*355, 1951.

151. Burton, A. C. On the physical equilibration of small blood vessels. *Am J Physiol 164:*319, 1951.

152. Haller, J. A., and Mays, T. Experimental studies on iliofemoral venous thrombosis. *Am Surg 29:*567, 1963.

153. Lansing, A. M., and Davis, W. H. Five-year follow-up study of iliofemoral venous thrombectomy. *Ann Surg 168:*620, 1968.

154. Fogarty, T. J., and Krippaehne, W. W. Catheter technique for venous thrombectomy. *Surg Gynecol Obstet 121:*362, 1965.

155. Fogarty, T. J., Dennis, D., and Krippaehne, W. W. Surgical management of iliofemoral venous thrombosis. *Am J Surg 112:*211, 1966.

155a. Hafner, C. D., Cranley, J. J., Krause, R. J., and Strasser, E. S. Venous thrombectomy: Current status. *Ann Surg 161:*411, 1965.

156. Krause, R. J., Cranley, J. J., Strasser, E. S., and Hafner, C. D. Caval ligation in thrombo-embolic disease. *Arch Surg 87:*184, 1963.

157. Cranley, J. Obliterative arterial disease. In *Vascular Surgery.* Hagerstown, MD, Harper & Row, 1972, vol. 1, p 13.

3

Diagnostic Tests for Venous Thrombosis

PHLEBOGRAPHY

Phlebography is the standard by which all other modalities of diagnosis are tested. There is nothing quite so scientifically certain as a directly visualized pathologic condition. Even when the clot is not visible, one can sometimes make the diagnosis with certainty by the presence of dye in an area where the vein is known to be, coupled with the presence of multitudinous dilated collateral veins around this point.

Used experimentally by Franck and Alwens[1] and introduced in humans by Berberich and Hirsch[2] in 1923, phlebography was advocated in the 1930s and 1940s by influential spokesmen like Dos Santos,[3] DeBakey *et al.,*[4] Mahorner,[5] and Felder;[6] yet, it has lagged behind arteriography as a widely used diagnostic modality. In the past, physicians usually were reluctant to employ the technique for a variety of reasons: some technical, some concerned with difficulties of interpretation, others concerned with discomfort and risk to the patient, and, finally, some due to a lack of conviction that a phlebogram was needed at all for establishing the diagnosis of thrombophlebitis.

Technical difficulties no longer discourage the use of phlebography. The quality of films has improved: sheet film with long cassettes enabling visualization of the veins from the foot to the upper abdomen (Fig. 3-1) are standard equipment.

DIAGNOSTIC CRITERIA

Interpretation of the phlebogram still presents certain difficulties. However, when a thrombus is actually visualized, as is usually the case (Figs. 3-2 to 3-7), the diagnosis can be made without equivocation. The criteria we use closely parallel those of Rabinov and Paulin[7] and may be summarized as follows: The primary sign of deep venous thrombosis in a phlebogram is the actual demonstration of a clot. This is a constant filling defect, outlined by contrast material on one or both sides. It may give the impression of a railroad track (railroad track sign) or may appear serpiginous, like "a worm in a tube" (Fig. 3-8). It is our opinion that this represents a relatively acute sign. The clot is probably no older than 2 or 3 weeks. The second x-ray feature of deep venous thrombosis is complete obliteration of the deep system or a significant part of it. This is particularly true if a previous phlebogram has shown the actual, visible clot. The importance of a deep system that does not fill is magnified by the presence of many collateral ves-

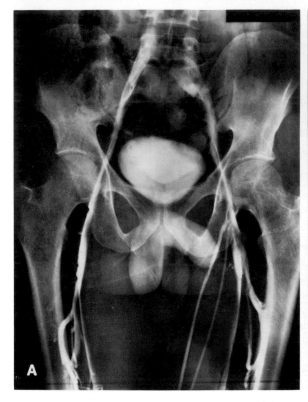

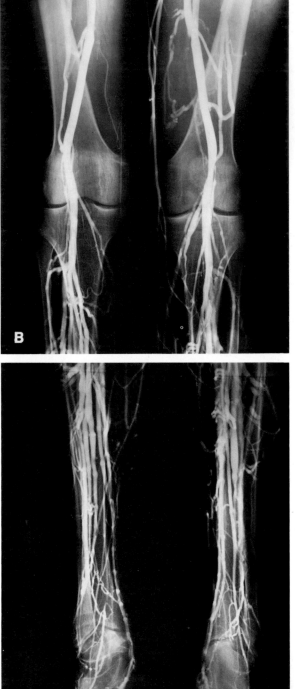

Figure 3-1. Normal phlebograms. **A.** Pelvis. **B.** Thighs.
C. Legs.

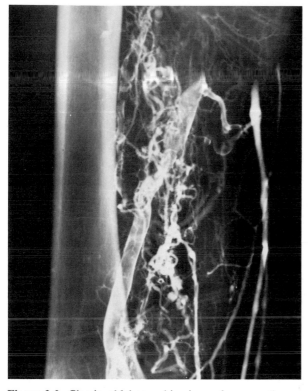

Figure 3-2. Classic phlebographic signs of venous thrombosis; note visible soft clot in mainstream, visualization of extensive collateral veins, and abrupt termination of dye column.

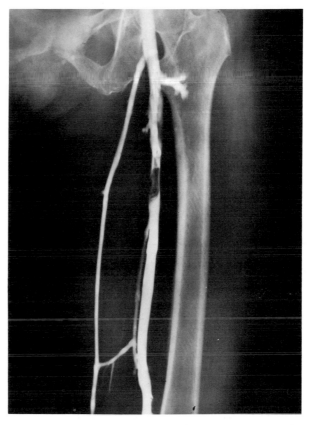

Figure 3-3. Phlebogram demonstrating localized fresh clot in superficial femoral vein.

Figure 3-4. Intraluminal clot is clearly visible.

Figure 3-5. Phlebogram demonstrating abrupt termination of dye column, visualization of the thrombus, and slightly increased collateral circulation, diagnostic features of thrombophlebitis.

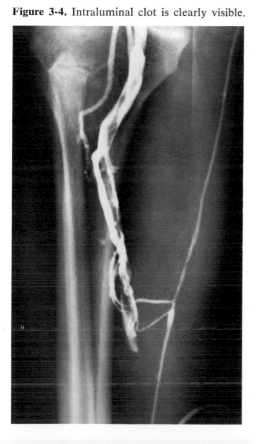

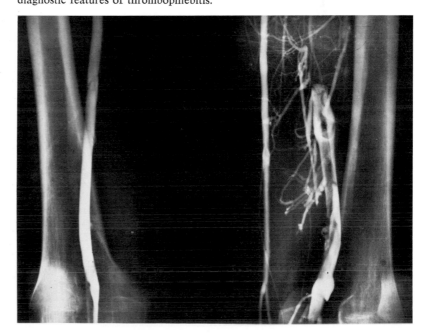

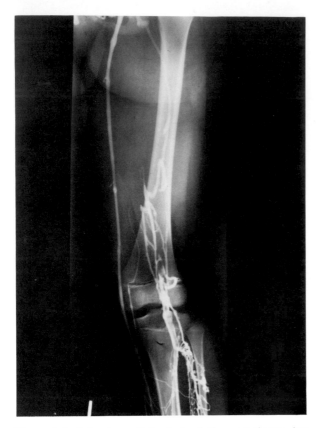

Figure 3-6. Extensive collateral circulation not shown, but visualization of clot combined with abrupt termination of dye column is diagnostic.

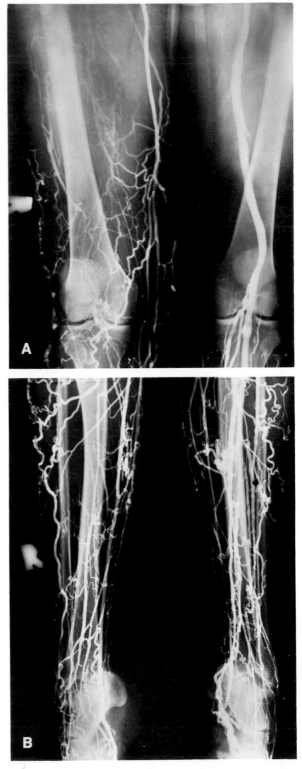

Figure 3-7. A. Phlebogram showing acute deep thrombophlebitis of right thigh. Note increase in collateral circulation of thigh, associated with absence of femoral vein. **B.** Lower right leg.

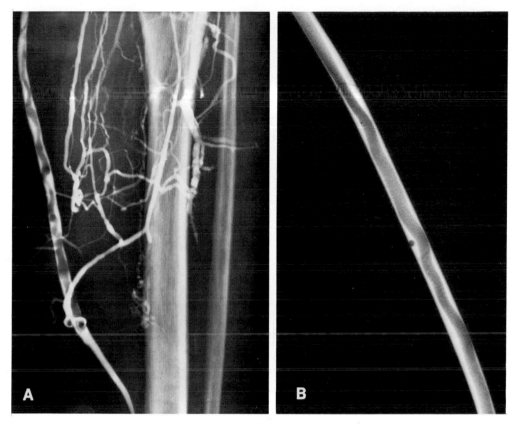

Figure 3-8. A. Superficial thrombophlebitis. "Worm-in-tube" effect clearly visible in saphenous vein. B. Reproduction of "worm-in-tube" radiologic appearance of intravenous clot. Radiolucent catheter was filled with blood, and dye was then injected after the clot had had time to retract. (*Courtesy of Dr. R. B. Mulvey.*)

sels. When nonfilling occurs in the absence of collateral veins, it is best not to consider the diagnosis to be certain.

The abrupt termination of the column of dye is believed to be a less significant finding, and it is one on which we would hesitate to make the diagnosis. It is not unusual for a single vein to be obliterated on one view of the lower extremity and to be well visualized on a later film. This is the most tenuous diagnostic possibility and, fortunately, the most unusual.

Misleading Phlebographic Phenomena

A frequently encountered artifact is that of apparent venous occlusion due to extension of the leg at the knee[7a] (Figure 3-9 A-E). When the phlebogram is repeated with the knee flexed slightly, the vein is shown to be patent.

A second pitfall is that one may make the diagnosis of venous thrombosis because of a sharp gap in the column of dye in the vein; this phenomenon is due to the fact that dye is heavier than blood. Consequently, if the film is taken with the patient in the semierect position, the dye may rest on the valve, and the area beneath the valve may appear to be clotted. By repeating the film with the patient in the supine position, the veins may be shown to be widely patent (Figs. 3-10 to 3-11.)

Figures 3-12 through 3-17 are illustrative phlebograms.

Kjellberg in 1943[8] drew attention to the risk of incomplete mixing and layering when contrast medium is injected into the vascular system. The different specific weights of the contrast medium and blood, their relative viscosity, the rate of injection, the velocity of the bloodstream, and the caliber and position of the vessels are all contributing factors to phlebographic phenomena that may be falsely read as clots. Boyd *et al.*[9] noted an artifact that they refer to as a "streamlined" effect (called by others a "streaming" effect) which takes

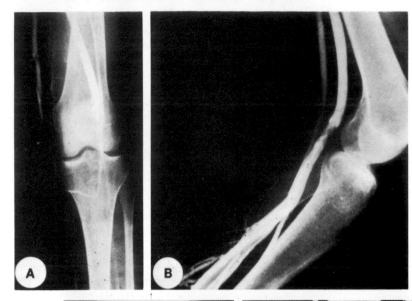

Figure 3-9. A. A 36-year-old female with clinical evidence of superficial thrombophlebitis. On examination with patient supine and leg extended, there is failure to visualize the deep venous system below the level of the femoral condyle, simulating deep venous occlusion. B. A patent femoropopliteal system is readily opacified in lateral examination with leg flexed. C and D. A 19-year-old female with unilateral leg edema. Deep venous thrombosis was considered when anteroposterior supine and attempted lateral recumbent studies, both with the leg extended, showed no filling of deep venous system. E. Third injection in same patient in lateral position and with slight flexion of knee results in good delineation of normal deep venous structures. (*From Arkoff,* et al. Radiology 90:*66, 1968.*)

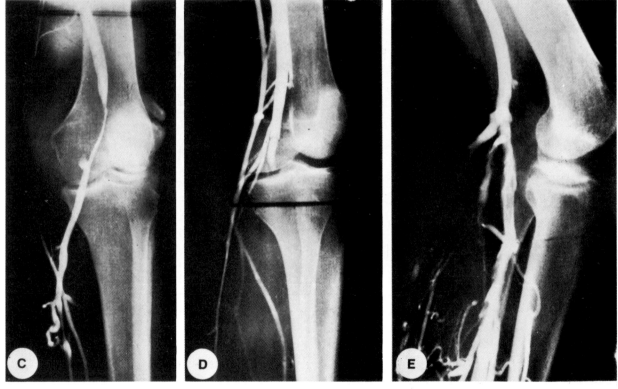

Figure 3-10. Since dye is heavier than blood, if the film is taken with patient in semierect position, dye may rest on valve and the area distal to valve may appear clotted. A. Phlebogram taken with patient in semierect position. B. Phlebogram with patient in supine position, showing veins to be widely patent.

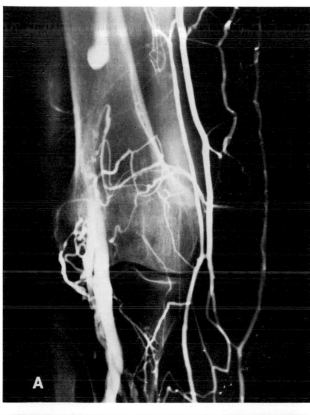

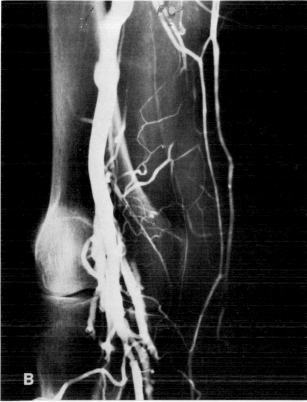

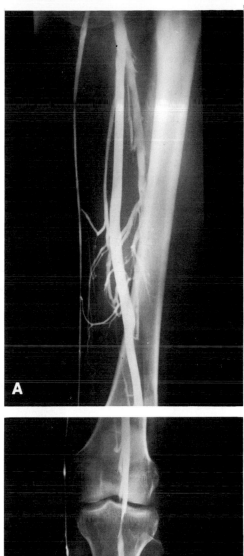

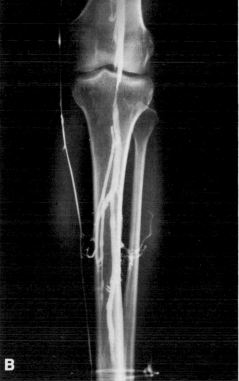

Figure 3-11. A and **B.** Compression of the popliteal vein by muscles of the popliteal fossa when the knee is extended. The leg shows compression, while rest of extremity is normal.

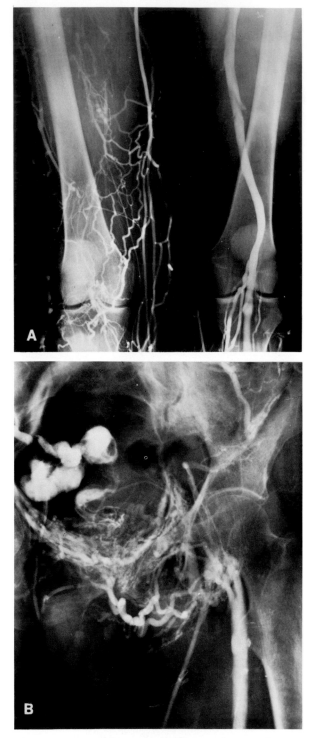

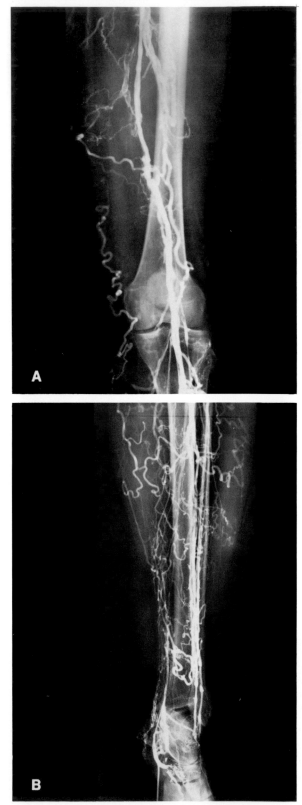

Figure 3-13. Phlebogram of patient with deep thrombophlebitis of the leg and thigh. **A.** Thigh. **B.** Leg.

Figure 3-12. A. Phlebogram showing acute deep thrombophlebitis of right thigh. Note increase in collateral circulation of the thigh, associated with absence of femoral vein. **B.** Occlusion of left iliac vein with extensive pelvic collateral circulation.

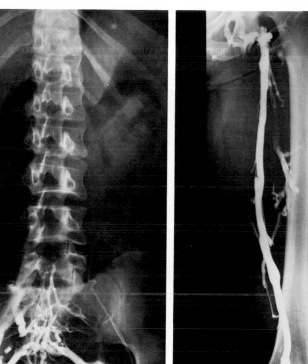

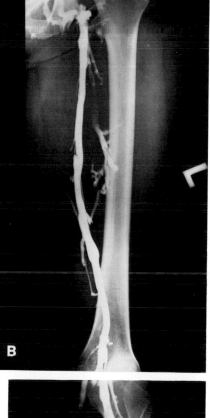

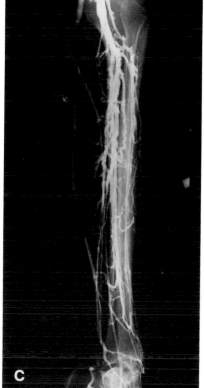

Figure 3-14. A, B, and **C.** Left iliac thrombophlebitis. The veins of the leg (**C**) are normal. The femoral vein is patent but ends abruptly (**B**) at common femoral vein, where the dye passes across the pelvis to the right iliac vein.

place when the contrast medium, entering a main vessel from a tributary, remains entirely on one side of a segment of the vessel; this results in one wall of the vein being clearly contrasted while the opposite wall remains undemonstrated. They caution against misinterpreting this phenomenon as a thrombus. Rabinov and Paulin[7] also discussed the pitfalls in phlebographic interpretation, commenting on the ways in which water-soluble radiopaque media differ from blood. To avoid such diagnostic difficulties, they now carry out phlebographic examination with the patient in the predominantly upright position. The best filling of the veins is accomplished by having the patient stand on one limb while the opposite leg, bearing no weight, is being x rayed in the dependent position. With the muscles relaxed under this technique, and using large amounts of radi-

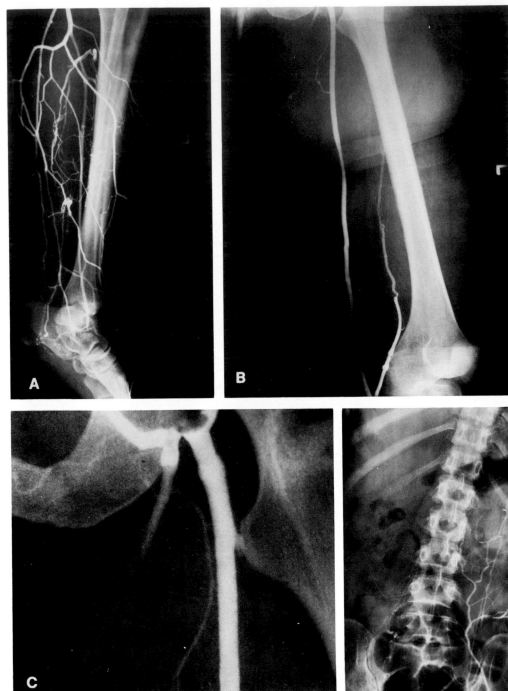

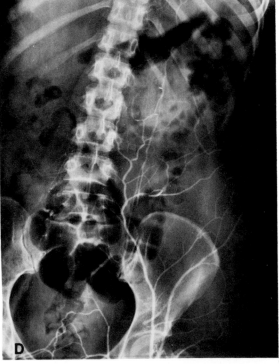

Figure 3-15. A. Leg. Deep veins are obliterated and superficial veins are patent. **B.** Thigh. Saphenous vein patent in thigh. Top of dye column is shut off but is shown by close up (**C**). **C.** Close up. Dye of saphenous vein enters common femoral vein and ends abruptly, then courses over to the right, medially and laterally. **D.** Iliac system is totally obliterated on left side.

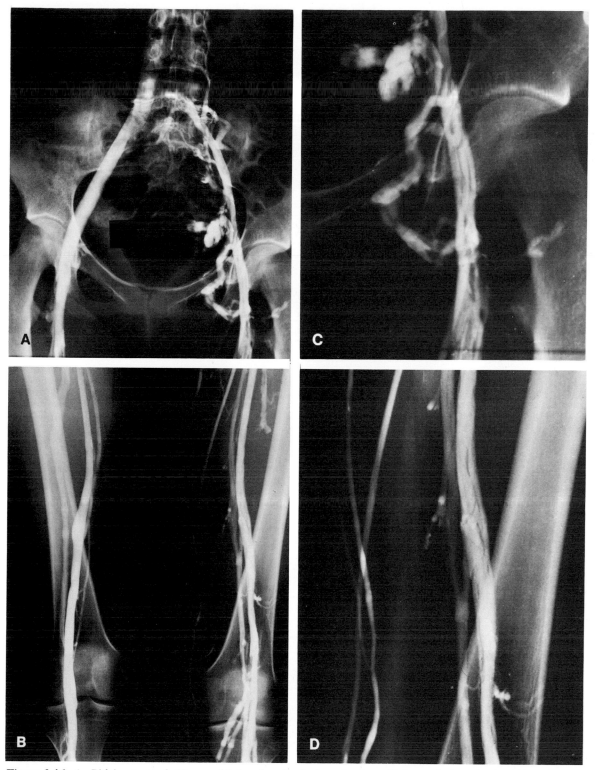

Figure 3-16. A. Phlebogram of 19-year-old female who had postpartum iliofemoral thrombophlebitis of left lower extremity. Area where left common iliac vein passes under iliac artery is obliterated. **B.** The left superficial femoral vein has recanalized. Faint striae in dye column represent "tree-barking," a sign of recanalization of previously thrombosed vein. **C** and **D.** Close up film of left common femoral and superficial femoral veins, showing the typical "tree-barking" x-ray appearance of recanalized vein.

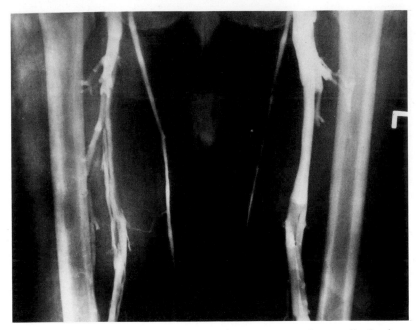

Figure 3-17. Another example of "tree-bark" appearance of recanalized vein.

opaque medium, nearly all of the veins of the lower extremity, including the soleal sinuses, are clearly demonstrated.

Venous Thrombosis Secondary to Phlebography

The value of phlebography can be so great at times as to overshadow all objections. Nevertheless, the difficulties may be listed as follows: Phlebography is invasive. It may be allergenic or thrombogenic. In early years, pulmonary embolus was reported[10] 1 day after a normal phlebogram. Deaths due to Diodrast have also been reported.[11, 12] In our own practice, pulmonary embolism secondary to phlebography has not been encountered; nevertheless, thrombophlebitis has been observed following this procedure. For many years it was our practice to obtain phlebograms on the day before operation for recurrent ulceration of the limb following previous surgical treatment. Our purpose in so doing was to visualize the remaining veins in hope of accomplishing a more thorough extirpation. In an estimated 50 per cent of the patients, veins containing fresh thrombi were found during the operative procedure; these were found not only in the superficial veins but also in the veins deep to the

fascia of the leg. In all instances thrombosis was obviously fresh and soft. There was no doubt that this was secondary to the phlebogram taken the day before, even though following phlebography the veins were routinely flushed with heparinized saline solution (Fig. 3-18).

Case Report 3-1

A young male with huge varicose veins in one leg (Fig. 3-18*A*) was admitted for excisional therapy. Because the disease was unilateral, we thought it desirable to obtain a phlebogram in order to inspect the status of his deep veins (Fig. 3-18*B*). The radiopaque medium was Renografin 70%. The rinse solution following the phlebogram contained 5000 units heparin in 500 cc saline solution, as well as 100 mg Solu-Cortef. The patient's leg was wrapped snugly with rubberized bandages, and the limb was elevated. Despite these precautionary measures, at operation the next morning innumerable clotted veins, filled with soft, fresh clot, were found in the subcutaneous tissue (Fig. 3-18*C*). This clotting was very extensive and involved many of the varices below the knee.

In the hope of reducing the incidence of the chemical type of thrombophlebitis, it is now our practice to add cortisone to the rinse solution along

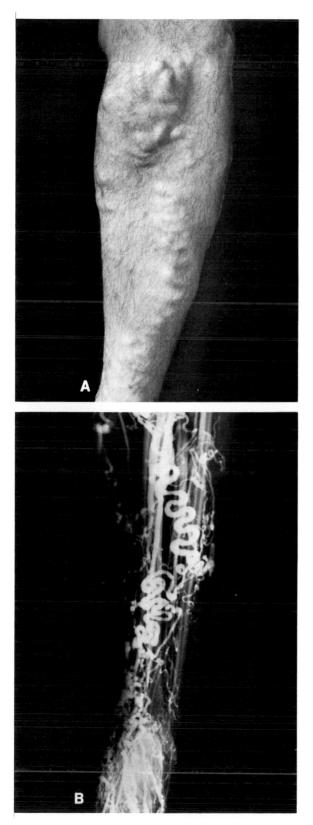

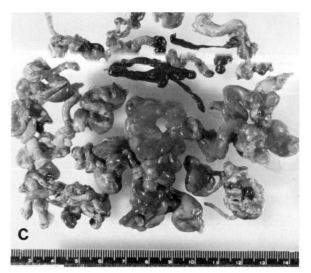

Figure 3-18. Thrombophlebitis caused by phlebography. **A.** Extensive varicosities. **B.** Phlebogram showing absence of clots in varices. **C.** Extensive thrombosis of varices excised next day despite the facts that at the time of phlebography the rinse solution contained 5000 units heparin and 100 mg Solu-Cortef and that the leg was tightly wrapped from toes to groin and the limb elevated overnight.

with heparin. Nevertheless, 2 patients have been encountered with extensive thrombophlebitis of the lower extremity following diagnostic phlebography. We remain skeptical of the claims of others[9, 13-15] that neither superficial nor deep venous thrombosis occurs after phlebographic examination.

Phlebography is at times a painful procedure, particularly if deep venous thrombosis is present in the limb; the pain is probably a pressure effect. Despite the disadvantages of phlebography, however, widespread recognition of the defects inherent in clinical diagnosis did not become apparent until phlebography became a common practice.

Technique

The first studies[1] were carried out on experimental animals in the semierect position. In the 60 years since then, patients have been studied in various positions, viz., horizontal, supine, prone, semierect, and erect, and with or without a tourniquet.[13-27] In the earlier described techniques,[3, 5, 6, 16] the contrast medium was injected into a vein at the foot or ankle, with the patient in a horizontal position (either prone or supine) on the radiographic table.

Mark[17] used a tourniquet at the groin to delay the emptying of the venous system. Mahorner[5] placed a tourniquet at the ankle to direct the dye into the deep veins of the leg. Felder[6] also elevated the head of the table 15 degrees. Bauer[18] introduced a catheter into the distal femoral vein; with the foot of the table lowered, contrast medium was injected through the catheter. Scott and Roach[19] and Rogoff and DeWeese[13] demonstrated that placing the patient in the semierect position (the former without a tourniquet at the ankle, the latter with one) improved visualization of the veins. The horizontal position likewise had its advocates. DeBakey et al.[4] as early as 1943 described the technique with the patient lying flat on the table. The tourniquet was placed below the fossa ovalis and the thigh and leg were rotated internally to separate the shadow of the tibia and the fibula. Eyler[14] and Lesser and Danelius[20] likewise positioned the patient on a horizontal table, the latter team turning the patient prone and injecting the medium into the posterior tibial vein.

Another variation in general technique is concerned with the direction of flow of the contrast medium. In 1938, Dos Santos[3] described ascending phlebography. He made injections into the superficial veins behind the external malleolus, taking films as the radiopaque material ascended in the leg and thigh with an entirely free circulation. Since then, the value of using a tourniquet above the ankle to force the dye into the deep venous system has been demonstrated. Ascending phlebography performed with free circulation has been described by Boyd et al.,[9] Dow,[21] and Cockett and Thomas.[22] Moore[23] varied the technique by occluding the arterial inflow with a sphygmomanometer cuff. In descending phlebography, the contrast material is injected into the femoral vein at the groin with the patient in the erect position. The dye is allowed to descend the vein. Bauer,[18] Luke,[24] and Moore[23] used this method to show the presence or absence of valves in the femoral and popliteal veins.

In 1967, Thomas and Fletcher[25] reported intra-

Figure 3-19. A. Opacification of pelvic veins and inferior vena cava by turning patient to prone position after injecting dye. **B.** Pelvic varicosities demonstrated by turning patient prone. (*From Mulvey, R. B. Radiology 97:51, 1970*).

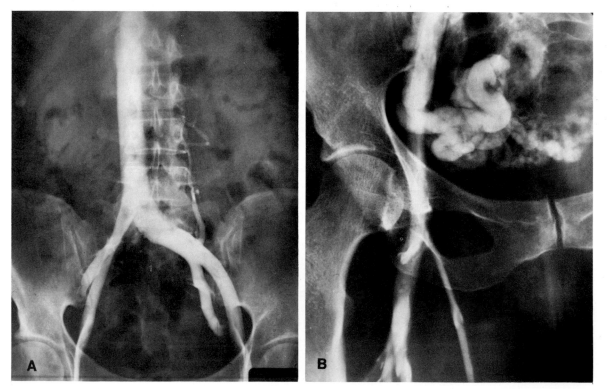

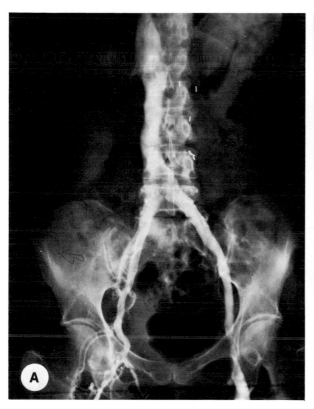

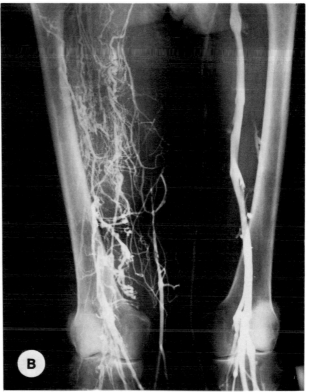

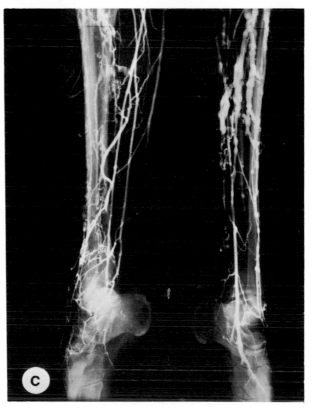

Figure 3-20. Full length visualization of venous tree of lower extremities obtained by method of Mulvey. **A.** Opacification of the iliac veins showing obstruction of right iliac vein and flow of dye through the hypogastric vein to the common iliac where faint clots can be seen. **B.** Complete occlusion of superficial femoral vein and deep femoral vein with extensive collateral circulation. Patient is in prone position. **C.** Deep veins of the leg do not fill. Patient is in supine position.

osseous injection for demonstration of the iliac vein, with the patient in the prone position. In 1970, Mulvey[26] described opacification of the iliac vein by placing the patient in the prone position and obtaining a film after phlebography of the legs (Figs. 3-19 and 3-20). The investigations of Kjellberg[8] and others[27,28] have led some physicians to prefer performing phlebographic examinations with the patient in the upright position to avoid diagnostic pitfalls. We recognize certain advantages in this technique as reported by Rabinov and Paulin;[7] nevertheless, we prefer the horizontal technique.

We have used various methods in which dye is injected with the patient in the semierect or the erect position rather than supine; we have also had the patient elevate himself on his toes 10 times between the first and the second injection.[13, 15, 29] These methods were satisfactory, but at times we were disturbed by the possibility that the dye, being heavier than blood, might "hang up" on a valve and thus mislead us into believing that an area of vein not visualized might represent a thrombus. However, the most compelling reason for our change in technique was the fact that the RIL table, which permits films 51 inches long, must be flat for the sensitive mechanism to work satisfactorily; therefore, most recently we have consistently obtained phlebograms with the patient supine on this table.

TECHNICAL POINTS

A foot vein is used. If a vein cannot be found, one may be made visible by having the patient sit up or by inflating a venous tourniquet and wrapping the foot in warm towels. If one must use the saphenous vein in the foot, a tourniquet is placed tightly around the ankle to force the dye into the deep system. The larger the needle used, the better the filling. This is especially obvious when it is necessary to use a smaller needle in one limb than in the other when bilateral phlebograms are being obtained. Therefore, if at all possible, a 19-gauge thinwall needle is used. A tourniquet is placed tightly around the thigh just above the knee. The

intravenous fluid is then allowed to drip in as rapidly as possible, until it slows down precipitously. Thus the veins of the limb are relatively filled with blood and fluid. Injection of dye is then begun. After 35 cc of dye has been injected, the first film is taken; this is usually the best film of the leg veins. The thigh tourniquet is then removed and the remaining 15 cc of dye is injected as rapidly as possible. The second film is taken; this is usually the best film of the veins of the thigh and pelvis. As soon as this film is taken, the patient (having been instructed earlier) draws a deep breath and bears down as hard as possible; at the same time, the limbs may be elevated if one is particularly interested in the pelvic area. At this time, the third exposure is made. This usually gives the best reflux into the deep femoral veins and, at times, into the internal iliac as well. An alternate technique for demonstrating the veins below the knees is to have the patient sit on the table with his legs dangling, thus relaxing the muscles as much as possible, a method similar to the technique of Rabinov and Paulin.[7] The dye is injected without using a tourniquet. After 50 cc of dye has been injected, the patient lies back, his legs are placed on the table, and the first film is taken. A second exposure is made, followed as soon as possible by a third, with or without elevation of the legs or the Valsalva maneuver.

NONINVASIVE DIAGNOSTIC TEST FOR DEEP VENOUS THROMBOSIS

Because of the invasive nature of phlebography and the attendant discomfort to the patient, clinicians are continually interested in finding alternative objective methods of diagnosing deep venous thrombosis. Among those currently available are the radioactive fibrinogen uptake test, the Doppler ultrasound technique, impedance plethysmography,

and the phleborheographic technique recently developed in our laboratory. Few patients would permit daily or twice-weekly phlebograms, even if the cost were negligible (which it is not). By contrast, phleborheography (see Chapter 4) can be performed daily or even at intervals of several hours if repeated studies are indicated.

RADIOACTIVE FIBRINOGEN UPTAKE TEST

Detection of experimental venous thrombosis by means of ^{131}I-labelled fibrinogen was developed in Britain by Hobbs and Davies[30] in 1960 and by Gomez et al.[31] in 1963 using ^{131}I-labelled plasminogen. The first clinical trials were reported by Palko et al.[32] in 1964; a year later, Atkins and

Hawkins[33] introduced the use of ^{125}I-labelled fibrinogen. The fibrinogen uptake test quickly became an accepted diagnostic measure in some English hospitals, but it is not used widely in the United States. A commercial preparation of radioactive fibrinogen has not yet been approved by the

United States Division of Biologic Standards. In Britain, the fibrinogen uptake test is used extensively for the detection of deep venous thrombosis in prospective clinical trials and to a lesser degree for the diagnosis of the established disease.

From the outset, the proponents[34-37] of this new test frankly admitted the limitations and disadvantages of the method. In their view, these objections are offset by the fact that they now possess a means of detecting early formation of preclinical thrombi that might prove of great value in determining the true incidence of postoperative thrombosis and might also reduce the danger of death from silent venous thrombosis and unheralded pulmonary embolism. (See Chapter 2, Autopsy Studies.)

The main disadvantage of this test lies in its failure to detect the thrombotic process in the pelvic veins (from which emboli are known to originate), the upper thigh, or the lower third of the leg and foot. Because early detection of thrombi depends on the differential count between the two lower extremities and the progressive changes in the affected side, the test fails to differentiate in the upper thigh and pelvis between the count in the more peripheral blood vessels and in the background, due to the radioactive material contained in the urine and the multitudinous visceral veins. Thus, a small clot in a vein cannot be distinguished from the surrounding radioactive tissue.

A further objection is the fact that the test helps detect a clot only in the stage of formation and does not help delineate a clot that has already formed. Because it is linked with fibrinogenesis, it helps detect a wide range of lesions. Browse[36] points out that a false-positive result may occur when any inflammatory fibrinous exudate is present in an extremity. This includes ulcers of the leg, wounds, hematoma, cellulitis, and active arthritis. Furthermore, since it detects any clot in its early formation, it detects superficial thrombophlebitis, the benign form of the disease, thus interfering with the diagnosis of deep venous thrombosis. Gomez et al.[31] stated that a false-positive result may also be recorded over the site of a recent operation. A patient with lymphedema may also have a positive test. This test indeed warns of the presence of a forming clot, detecting preclinical thrombi in minor veins, e.g., the soleal veins, that even phlebography fails to visualize. However, the significance of such small clots, out of the mainstream of venous bloodflow, is questionable.

The greatest value of this test would seem to be as a research tool for establishing the true incidence of postoperative thrombosis.

This is an invasive test. The thyroid gland must be blocked by the oral administration of 100 mg of sodium iodide 24 hours prior to the injection of ^{125}I-fibrinogen (dose to be given daily for one month after test) to prevent excessive uptake of radioactive material in this gland. Strict precautions must be taken to screen the donors of the fibrinogen so hepatitis is not transferred to the patient. In the limited area in which the test is effective, i.e., in the midthigh to midleg segment of the lower extremity, for detecting established thrombosis, Browse[36] found 80 per cent correct correlation with phlebography. Kakkar[37] reported an accuracy of 92 per cent confirmed by phlebography; although he has improved the instrumentation to make it less unwieldy than originally, the fibrinogen uptake test is still less convenient than the use of phleborheography.

THE DOPPLER ULTRASOUND TECHNIQUE

The ultrasonic Doppler method for diagnosing deep venous thrombosis of the lower extremity was developed and popularized by Strandness et al.[38] in Seattle and by Sigel et al.[39] in Philadelphia at nearly the same time. The latter group introduced the concept of squeezing the calf muscle and dorsiflexing the foot to produce augmented sounds over the major veins, caused by the increased velocity of the blood flowing by the probe with these maneuvers.[40]

The Doppler ultrasound method is noninvasive and can be used at the bedside or in the laboratory; in experienced hands it has been very effective in diagnosing various types of peripheral vascular disease on the basis of whether or not bloodflow is present in the vessel under study. The Doppler transducer contains two piezoelectric crystals.[41] One crystal transmits an ultrasonic beam into the tissue, and the other crystal receives back scattered sound reflected from density interfaces. If the reflector of the sound is in motion (e.g., blood cells within vessels), the frequency of the received sound signal will be shifted in proportion to the velocity of the reflector because of the Doppler effect.[41] The sound signal may be heard with earphones or a loudspeaker, or it may be recorded graphically. By monitoring the common femoral vein, the popliteal vein, and the posterior tibial vein and in compressing[42] the calf distal to the point at which one is listening, a distinct, brief, high-pitched signal is produced, corresponding to the acceleration of bloodflow passing beneath the transducer secondary to the compression.

We have been impressed by the fact that the principles involved in impedance plethysmography[43-46] in the diagnosis of thrombophlebitis are similar to those employed by the Doppler technique. Indeed, our own phleborheographic technique (see Chapter 4) for diagnosing deep venous thrombosis is based on the same fundamental principle, with this difference: Sigel et al.[40] have been concentrating on the changes in velocity of bloodflow caused by compression of the calf,

whereas in our technique, a change in volume of the limb produced by compression of the calf in the presence of obstruction of the venous outflow is detected.

The Doppler method is portable, simple, atraumatic, and the least expensive of the techniques. In the hands of those familiar with it, it is quite accurate. Sigel et al.[40] reported that 75.9 per cent of extremities with clots proved by phlebography can be detected by the Doppler method; Strandness et al.[42] were able to detect thrombi in 93 per cent of the extremities. The drawback is that the audiometric technique yields better results when the person carrying out the test is motivated and expert. Considerable experience seems to be necessary to achieve the maximum reliability obtained by Sigel and Strandness. Only due to persistent prodding have our resident surgeons used the instrument. Recently, however, a pocket-size model was introduced. It is so convenient to use that a far wider interest on the part of practicing physicians is anticipated.

IMPEDANCE PLETHYSMOGRAPHY

The word plethysmograph is derived from the Greek plethysmos, "enlargement," plus graphein, "to write"; hence, it refers to an instrument designed to determine and register variations in size of an organ or a limb and thus in the variations in the amount of bloodflow occurring there. By definition, all plethysmographs record volume changes. Therefore, in a strict sense it is incorrect to use the term "impedance plethysmograph,"[47] because impedance is an electrical term that records a combination of ohmic resistance plus reactance and is not a direct measure of volume or pressure.

Impedance plethysmography takes advantage of the fact that the blood is an excellent conductor of electricity, more so than the tissues. If a limb becomes engorged with blood, its total impedance decreases, and when it contains less blood, the total impedance increases. The intrinsic resistance of the tissues is counterbalanced by a resistor placed in the circuit; thus, only the change in impedance is recorded.

Difficulties arise in attempting to calibrate an impedance plethysmograph. The portion being measured, viz., the change in impedance produced by the volume change in the limb, is such a small proportion of the total resistance of the limb that what is being measured, figuratively speaking, is the "inch at the end of the mile," a complicated measurement indeed.

In general, however, the difficulties of impedance plethysmography are inherent; therefore, despite continuing work for over 30 years, the technique has still not obtained wide acceptance. In the opinion of some biomedical engineers,[48-50] this creeping progress results from inadequate understanding of the biologic mechanisms contributing to the measured impedance. A single variable is not being measured; an infinite combination of variables within the tissues can provide electrical characteristics as measured from the body surface. In addition, changes and movements of the electrode contacting the skin or even the distance between electrodes may cause artifacts. It is true that an impedance tracing of a limb has the same appearance as a volumetric recording of the same limb. In conventional geometric reasoning, things *equal to the same thing are equal to each other;* thus, the impedance tracing is considered to be a volume tracing. However, this geometric axiom is not necessarily true in electric circuits; identical waves are not necessarily identical in character or in substance.

Cooley and Lehr[48] suggest the possibility that the excellent results of some researchers[51] in this field might be due to the fact that in spending many years in the investigation of electric impedance fluctuation, they have become expert in its use, and their results reflect their particular artistry rather than the scientific value of the instrumentation.

Impedance plethysmography for the diagnosis of deep venous thrombosis has been given great impetus by the studies of Wheeler and Mullick.[43–46] When the diagnosis of pulmonary embolism was confirmed by pulmonary angiogram and lung scan, impedance plethysmography showed an accuracy rate of 91 per cent. Dmochowski et al.[52] reported an overall accuracy rate of 53.5 per cent in a much smaller series. Steer et al.[53] and Deuvaert et al.[54] have evaluated impedance plethysmography, and

neither group could duplicate the accuracy rate of Wheeler and Mullick. One drawback noted by Steer et al.[53] was that 20 per cent of their patients were unable to lie quietly and supine and to inhale deeply on command without otherwise moving. When we attempted to use the deep breath as a stimulus for volume changes within the limb in phleborheography, we noted that there are three varieties of breathing: primarily with the chest, with the diaphragm, and with a combination of chest and diaphragm. In our experience, these three types of breathing created three types of response in the limb.

Wheeler[55] has since modified his technique so that now the limb is engorged with blood by means of a pneumatic cuff, after which the rate of reduction of engorgement is measured. This is a logical approach, one which we considered using and which Barnes et al.[56] (Strandness' group) have incorporated into their Doppler technique. Gazzaniga et al.[57] also have applied it in their impedance rheographic studies on deep venous thrombosis.

REFERENCES

1. Franck, O., and Alwens, W. Kreislaufstudien am Röntgenschirm. *Münchn Med Wschr 57:*950, 1910.
2. Berberich, J., and Hirsch, S. Die röntgenologische Darstellung der Arterien und Venen im lebenden Menschen. *Klin Wsch 49:*2226, 1923.
3. Dos Santos, J. C. La phlébographie directe: Conception-technique-premiers resultats. *J Internat Chir 3:*625, 1938.
4. DeBakey, M. E., Schroeder, G. F., and Ochsner, A. Significance of phlebography in phlebothrombosis. *JAMA 123:*738, 1943.
5. Mahorner, H. A method of obtaining venograms of the veins of the extremities. *Surg Gynecol Obstet 76:*41, 1943.
6. Felder, D. A. A method of venography. *Radiology 54:*516, 1950.
7. Rabinov, K., and Paulin, S. Roentgen diagnosis of venous thrombosis in the leg. *Arch Surg 104:*134, 1972.
7a. Arkoff, R. S., Gilfillan, R. S., and Burhenne, H. J. A simple method of lower extremity phlebography—Pseudo-obstruction of the popliteal vein. *Radiology 90:*66, 1968.
8. Kjellberg, S. R. Die Mischungs-und Strömungsverhältnisse von wasserlöslichem Kontrastmittel bei Gefäss-und Herzuntersuchung. *Acta Radiol 24:*433, 1943.
9. Boyd, A. M., Catchpole, B. N., Jepson, R. P., and

Rose, S. S. The technic and interpretation of lower limb phlebography. *Ann Surg 138:*726, 1953.
10. Homans, J. Thrombosis as a complication of venography. *JAMA 119:*136, 1942.
11. Goldburgh, H. L., and Baer, S. Death following intravenous administration of diodrast. *JAMA 118:*1051, 1942.
12. Dolan, L. P. Allergic death due to intravenous use of diodrast: Suggestions for possible prevention. *JAMA 114:*138, 1940.
13. Rogoff, S. M., and DeWeese, J. A. Phlebography of the lower extremity. *JAMA 172:*1599, 1960.
14. Eyler, W. R. Lumbar and peripheral arteriography: Technics and radiologic anatomy. *Radiology 69:*165, 1957.
15. DeWeese, J. A., and Rogoff, S. M. Functional ascending phlebography of the lower extremity by serial long film technique. *Am J Roentgen 81:*841, 1959.
16. Doughtery, J., and Homans, J. Venography: A clinical study. *Surg Gynecol Obstet 71:*697, 1940.
17. Mark, J. Venography: I. Its use in the differential diagnosis of the peripheral venous circulation; II. A simplified technic. *Ann Surg 118:*469, 1943.
18. Bauer, G. A venographic study of thrombo-embolic problems. *Acta Chir Scand Suppl 61,* 1940.
19. Scott, H. W., and Roach, J. F. Phlebography of the leg in the erect position. *Ann Surg 134:*104, 1951.

20. Lesser, A., and Danelius, G. Venography: Its value in the diagnosis and management of venous disturbances of the lower extremities. *Ann Surg 119:* 903, 1944.

21. Dow, J. D. Venography of the leg with particular reference to acute deep thrombophlebitis and gravitational ulceration. *J Fac Radiol 2:*180, 1951.

22. Cockett, F. B., and Thomas, M. L. The iliac compression syndrome. *Br J Surg 52:*816, 1965.

23. Moore, H. D. A new method of venography with particular reference to its use in varicose veins. *Br J Surg 145:*78, 1949.

24. Luke, J. C. The deep vein valves: A venographic study in normal and postphlebitic states. *Surgery 29:*381, 1951.

25. Thomas, M. L., and Fletcher, E. W. L. The technique of pelvic phlebography. *Clin Radiol 18:*399, 1967.

26. Mulvey, R. B. Ascending phlebography and iliac vein opacification. *Radiology 97:*51, 1970.

27. Swart, B., and Dingendorf, W. Experimenteller Beitrag zur optimalen Gefässdarstellung. *Fortschr Roentgenstr 97:*637, 1962.

28. Fox, J. A., and Hugh, A. E. Some physical factors in arteriography. *Clin Radiol 15:*183, 1964.

29. Shumacker, H. B., Moore, T. C., and Campbell, J. A. Functional venography of the lower extremities. *Surg Gynecol Obstet 98:*257, 1954.

30. Hobbs, J. T., and Davies, J. W. L. Detection of venous thrombosis with ^{131}I-labelled fibrinogen in the rabbit. *Lancet 2:*134, 1960.

31. Gomez, R. L., Wheeler, H. B., Belko, J. S., and Warren, R. Observations on the uptake of a radioactive fibrinolytic enzyme by intravascular clots. *Ann Surg 158:*905, 1963.

32. Palko, P. D., Nanson, E. M., and Fedoruk, S. O. The early detection of deep venous thrombosis using I 131 tagged human fibrinogen. *Can J Surg 7:*215, 1964.

33. Atkins, P., and Hawkins, L. A. Detection of venous thrombosis in the legs. *Lancet 2:*1217, 1965.

34. Flanc, C., Kakkar, V. V., and Clarke, M. B. The detection of venous thrombosis of the legs using ^{125}I-labelled fibrinogen. *Br J Surg 55:*742, 1968.

35. Negus, D., Pinto, D. J., Le Quesne, L. P., Brown, N., and Chapman, M. ^{125}I-labelled fibrinogen in the diagnosis of deep vein thrombosis and its correlation with phlebography. *Br J Surg 55:*835, 1968.

36. Browse, N. L. The ^{125}I-fibrinogen uptake test. *Arch Surg 104:*160, 1972.

37. Kakkar, V. V. The diagnosis of deep vein thrombosis using the ^{125}I-fibrinogen test. *Arch Surg 104:* 152, 1972.

38. Strandness, D. E., Schultz, R. D., Sumner, D. S., and Rushmer, R. F. Ultrasonic flow detection: A useful technic in the evaluation of peripheral vascular disease. *Am J Surg 113:*311, 1967.

39. Sigel, B., Popky, G. L., Boland, J. P., Wagner, D. K., and Mapp, E. M. Diagnosis of venous disease by ultrasonic flow detection. *Surg Forum 18:*185, 1967.

40. Sigel, B., Felix, W. R., Popky, G. L., and Ipsen, J. Diagnosis of lower limb venous thrombosis by Doppler ultrasound technique. *Arch Surg 104:*174, 1972.

41. Rushmer, R. F., Baker, D. W., and Stegall, H. F. Transcutaneous Doppler flow detection as a nondestructive technique. *J Appl Physiol 21:*554, 1966.

42. Strandness, D. E., and Sumner, D. S. Ultrasonic velocity detector in the diagnosis of thrombophlebitis. *Arch Surg 104:*180, 1972.

43. Mullick, S. C., Wheeler, H. B., and Songster, G. P. Diagnosis of deep venous thrombosis by measurement of electrical impedance. *Am J Surg 119:*417, 1970.

44. Wheeler, H. B., and Mullick, S. C. Detection of venous obstruction in the leg by measurement of electrical impedance. *Ann NY Acad Sci 170:*804, 1970.

45. Wheeler, H. B., Pearson, D., O'Connell, D., and Mullick, S. C. Impedance phlebography: Technique, interpretation, and results. *Arch Surg 104:*164, 1972.

46. Wheeler, H. B., Mullick, S. C., Anderson, J. N., and Pearson, D. Diagnosis of occult deep vein thrombosis by a noninvasive bedside technique. *Surgery 70:*20, 1971.

47. Nyboer, J. Electrical impedance plethysmograph. In Glasser, O. (ed.) *Med. Physics.* Chicago, Year Book, 1950, vol. 1, p. 340; vol. 2, p. 736.

48. Cooley, W. L., and Lehr, J. L. Electrical impedance fluctuation as an indicator of fluid volume changes in a living organism. *Biomed Engineering NY 6:*313, 1972.

49. Cooley, W. L. The calculation of cardiac stroke volume from variations in transthoracic electrical impedance. *Biomed Engineering NY 6:*316, 1972.

50. Impedance measurement: Art or science? Editorial, *Biomed Engineering NY 6:*303, 1972.

51. Nyboer, J. *Electrical Impedance Plethysmography,* ed 2. Springfield, Thomas, 1970.

52. Dmochowski, J. R., Adams, D. F., and Couch, N. P. Impedance measurement in the diagnosis of deep venous thrombosis. *Arch Surg 104:*170, 1972.

53. Steer, M. L., Spotnitz, A. J., Cohen, S. I., Paulin, S., and Salzman, E. W. Limitations of impedance phlebography for diagnosis of venous thrombosis. *Arch Surg 106:*44, 1973.

54. Deuvaert, F. E., Dmochowski, J. R., and Couch, N. P. Positional factors in venous impedance plethysmography. *Arch Surg 106:*53, 1973.

55. Wheeler, H. B. Personal communication, September 1972.

56. Barnes, R. W., Collicott, P. E., Nozersky, D. J., Sumner, D. S., and Strandness, D. E. Noninvasive quantitation of maximum venous outflow in acute thrombophlebitis. *Surgery 72:*971, 1973.

57. Gazzaniga, A. B., Pacela, A. F., Bartlett, R. H., and Geraghty, T. R. Bilateral impedance rheography in the diagnosis of deep venous thrombosis of the legs. *Arch Surg 104:*515, 1972.

4

Phleborheography

"Phleborheography" is defined as the tracing of moving currents within a vein; it was considered to be an appropriate term to designate a plethysmographic technique for the diagnosis of deep venous thrombosis of the lower extremity.[1] This technique is practical and highly accurate and has become a standard clinical test.

CONCEPTUAL DEVELOPMENT OF PHLEBORHEOGRAPHY

Our interest in this particular area was aroused by the work of Wheeler *et al.*[2-5] with the impedance plethysmograph. A visit to Wheeler's laboratory impressed us with the physiologic soundness of the principles involved, and consultation was sought with Simeone and Grass[1] for the purpose of investigating this problem further. In previous collaboration[6] we had considered the impedance technique, but our deliberations led to the choice of mechanical plethysmography. A later review of the possible techniques for measuring changes in volume of limbs and digits again led to the same conclusion.[1] It seemed desirable to attempt to measure venous bloodflow in the healthy limb and in extremities with deep venous thrombosis. It was anticipated that the classic plethysmographic boot would be used for relating volume changes of the limb to the volume changes of the part being measured and to measure changes in limb volume on elevating the extremity or after release of a proximal venous tourniquet. The boot proved to be unwieldy, and elevating and lowering the limb for emptying and filling the veins caused excessive artifacts in the highly amplified recording. The

method which finally evolved proved to be quite different from our original concept, but it has proved highly satisfactory to date.

METHOD

The patient lies quietly in bed with the head of the bed elevated so that the body is at an angle of 10 to 12 degrees from the horizontal (Fig. 4-1). By the patient lying quietly in bed the artifacts are reduced, and by maintaining the limbs below heart level the veins are distended, making their caliber more uniform and the transmission of impulses more effective. Modified blood pressure cuffs are used to encircle the limb, and two are used interchangeably to record volume changes and to act as a pump. Pumping and recording cuffs in use today are half the size originally reported (2×7 in.).[1] The foot cuff is still 4×7 in. An encircling cuff is placed around the upper abdomen to record respiratory waves. One recording cuff is placed around the middle third of the thigh, the second just below the knee. The third is placed just inferior to this, on the bulge of the calf. The fourth is placed just

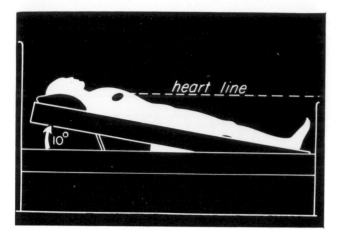

Figure 4-1. Elevation of head of bed.

tory waves in the upper third and in the lower third of the leg, but they still will be absent in the middle of the leg, just at the site of the thrombosis. It seems certain to us that much more remains to be learned about these respiratory waves; however, for the purposes described here, they represent a highly accurate test for the patency of the venous tree. It does require experience to detect the difference between a very small respiratory wave and the absence of respiratory waves. Sometimes this can

Figure 4-2. Normal respiratory waves (**top**) that disappear in the presence of deep venous thrombosis (**bottom**).

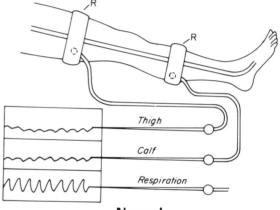

Normal

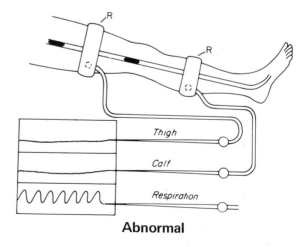

Abnormal

below the third at the junction of the gastrocnemius and soleus muscles, and the fifth is placed on the foot. The two most distal recording cuffs are also used to apply 50 mm Hg of pressure to the calf or 100 mm Hg to the foot. The tracings show respiratory waves, pulse waves (which are ignored), and changes in the volume of the part as produced by application of pressure. By passive compression of muscle and soft tissue, the physiologic effects of walking are produced while the patient's limbs are motionless, thus reducing the artifacts.

Principles Involved

The first principle involved is the reduction of respiratory waves in deep venous thrombosis. The respiratory waves are measured directly by a cuff encircling the upper abdomen. These waves are reflected in the tracings of the thigh and leg (and occasionally the foot) while the patient is lying in bed. In the presence of acute venous thrombosis, the respiratory waves disappear (Fig. 4-2) and then recur in approximately 2 weeks. At this time, however, they are smaller and more rounded, rather than peaked as would be the case in the normal extremity (Fig. 4-3). In a patient with femoroiliac thrombophlebitis, the respiratory waves are completely absent in the thigh but may still be visible in the leg if the veins of the leg are patent. It appears that the respiratory influence passes down the limb through the collateral veins. At times, for example, one can see normal respira-

Figure 4-3. A. Phleborheogram of normal subject (Run B without compression) showing large respiratory waves **B.** Tracing of abnormal phleborheogram showing absence of respiratory waves in a limb with deep venous thrombosis.

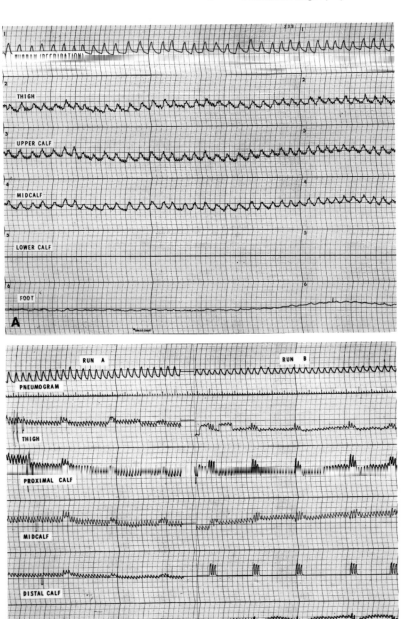

be clarified by asking the patient to breathe more deeply. Large respiratory waves may appear in the foot of a patient with a postphlebitic extremity in which recanalization has taken place.

The second principle is that intermittent compression of the extremity propels blood proximally, just as active muscular contraction does on walking. A recording cuff placed proximal to the site of compression detects the momentary damming up of blood if its exit is blocked by venous thrombosis or extraluminal venous compression; this is evidenced by an abrupt rise in the baseline of the volume recorded. Similar compression of the normal extremity with unimpeded venous outflow does not affect the level of the baseline.

No matter how many times the normal calf, leg,

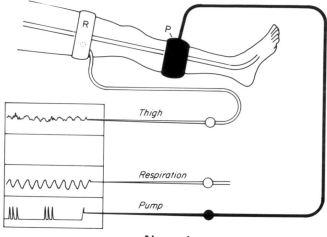

Normal

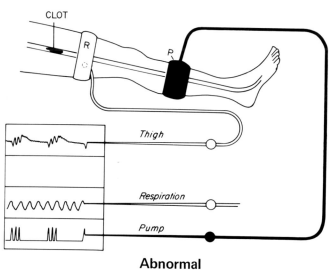

Abnormal

Figure 4-4. Pumping cuff on the midcalf. **Top.** Normal limb. **Bottom.** Limb with clot in femoral vein as evidenced by rising baseline.

or foot is compressed, the baseline remains level (Fig. 4-4 *Top*). The baseline may jiggle due to the transmission of the pressure or slight movement of the extremity, but the baseline does not rise. However, if there is any obstruction to the flow of venous blood above the recording cuff, then compression distally causes a step-wise rise in the base-line (Fig. 4-4 *Bottom*). Thus, if the thigh recording shows a step-wise rise while the calf is compressed, there is obstruction to the deep venous system above the thigh cuff. This obstruction is occasionally due to external compression, but otherwise it indicates intraluminal thrombosis.

Figure 4-5. Pumping cuff on foot. Normal limb (**top**); clot present in femoral and popliteal veins (**bottom**), as evidenced by rising baselines.

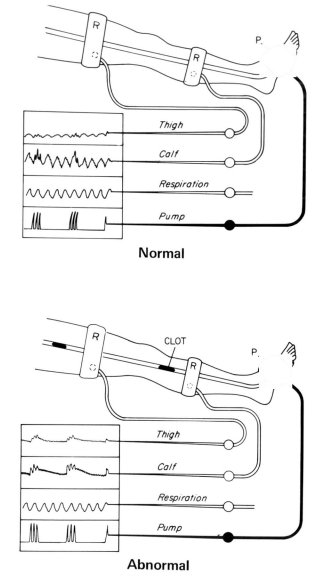

Normal

Abnormal

Similarly, compression of the foot causes a rise in the baseline of the recordings taken in the leg (Fig. 4-5) if there is any obstruction at or above the recording cuffs. When positive, this is the most accurate index of venous obstruction, with no known exceptions. In practice, 50 mm Hg of pressure is applied three times in rapid succession to simulate squeezing the calf with the hand or dorsiflexion and plantar flexion of the foot. If the clotting is limited to the leg, the thigh cuff shows no rise in the baseline but the cuffs on the leg record a rise in the baseline as the foot is compressed.

The third principle is that compression of the calf not only propels blood up the unobstructed extremity but also suctions some blood out of the normal foot. Thus, a recording cuff on the foot shows a fall in the baseline when the calf is compressed (Fig. 4-6). When this was reported, we were not aware of the work of Sakaguchi *et al.*[7-9] who made this same observation. This maneuver is the least sensitive of the three and is most subject to artifact and error. For example, this test may be positive in the limb of a patient with lymphedema, and in many instances it is equivocal. The major reason for not discarding it entirely is that when the limb is normal, venous patency is easily recognizable at a glance from this tracing. Furthermore, the elimination of artifacts that in large part are responsible for its seeming lack of specificity now appears possible, due to the development of an instrument uniquely designed to diagnose deep venous thrombosis. For mass screening, this maneuver can be carried out in a few minutes, and examination of the tracing frequently discloses three criteria of a normal venous tree, thus eliminating the need for further testing. For example, in a tracing of the normal extremity one immediately recognizes the presence of respiratory waves in the thigh, calf, and foot; the absence of a rise in the baseline of the thigh as the calf is compressed; and normal emptying of the foot as the calf is compressed. On the basis of these three findings, one can be certain that the venous drainage of the limb is normal.

TECHNICAL POINTS

The recording cuffs contain a small amount of air at 10 mm Hg in order to effect good coupling with the limb.

When the cuffs are applied (Fig. 4-7), the strap-

ping is placed posteriorly and the bladder or recording portion is placed anteriorly. If the bladder is placed under the limb, the pressure of the limb on the bladder produces large artifacts.

Figure 4-6. A fall in baseline of normal limb when the calf is compressed, thus suctioning some blood from the normal foot (**top**). In the abnormal limb (**bottom**), blood is not suctioned from the foot with compression of the calf since the veins below and above the calf are obstructed by clot.

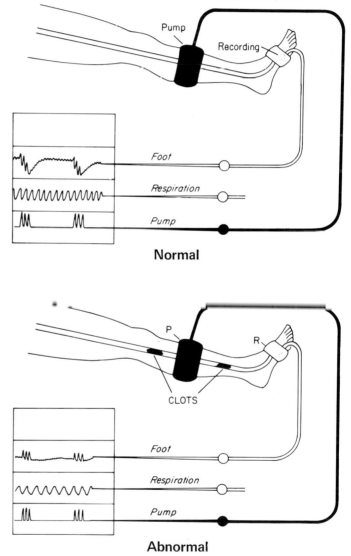

Normal

Abnormal

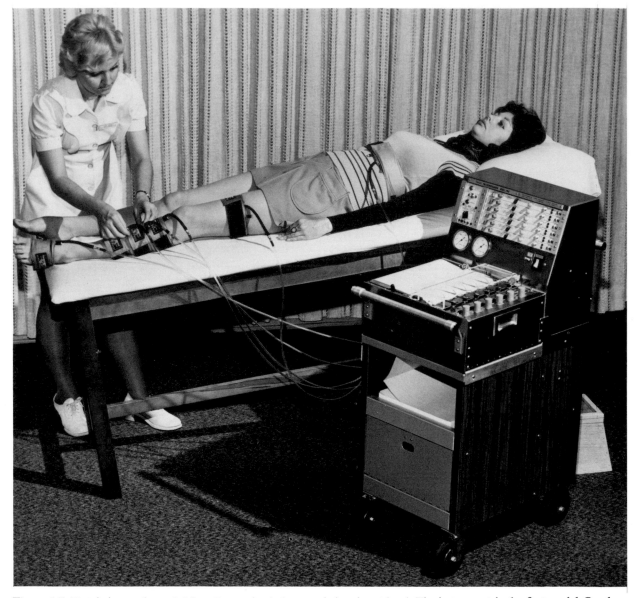

Figure 4-7. Test being performed. Note that patient's legs are below heart level. The instrument is the first model Cranley-Grass phleborheograph.

The pumping cuff must be applied carefully (Figs. 4-8 to 4-13) and must not be made of glossy material, lest it move on the limb as the pressure is applied and produce artifacts.

The patient must lie still. Movement or talking produces artifacts. The technician should continue the tracing until clear responses are obtained. If any questionable responses or artifacts are noted,

the technician merely continues the tracing, making certain that the pens have time to return to the baseline after each maneuver.

ARTIFACTS

The most frequently encountered artifact is one of venous occlusion by extension of the leg at the knee (Figs. 4-14 and 4-15). This artifact has been noted in phlebograms[10,11] and by those using the Doppler[5] and impedance[12] techniques. Accordingly, the technician must recognize the positive tracing and repeat the maneuver with the knee flexed slightly. It would be desirable to study all patients with the knee slightly flexed to avoid this artifact; as yet, however, we have not found a convenient, practical, or comfortable way for the majority of patients to lie with the knee flexed without producing more artifacts. Artifacts produced by deep breathing or breath-holding are easily detected on the pneumogram.

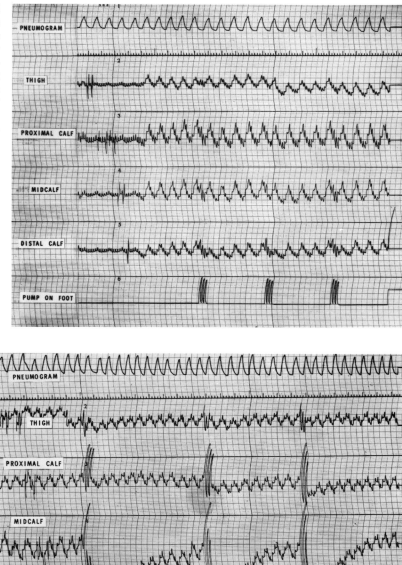

Figure 4-8. Normal tracing, Run A. In the normal extremity large respiratory waves are clearly visible and sharply pointed in the thigh, proximal calf, midcalf, and distal calf. Larger waves are frequently noted in the proximal calf and midcalf than in the thigh; this is believed to be due to more efficient coupling between the cuff and the leg. (This is also true of oscillometric recordings.) When pressure of 100 mm Hg is applied to the foot there is no rise in the baseline of any of the tracings. (Note: The tracings in Figures 4-8 through 4-19 are from the first model of the apparatus specifically designed for this test, now called the phleborheograph. In this apparatus, there is a switch permitting the technician to use "Run A" or "Run B." In Run A the sixth channel is the pump and all other channels are recording. In Run B the fifth cuff is the pump and the sixth channel becomes a recording of the foot.)

Figure 4-9. Normal tracing, Run B. Pressure is being applied to the lower calf. Note emptying of the foot: 0.35 cc of blood is evacuated from the foot under the cuff. (Normal equals 0.3 cc with the size of cuff currently in use.) Similar emptying can be noted in the midcalf. Note absence of rise in baseline of midcalf, proximal calf, or thigh. Also note large respiratory waves visible in thigh, the proximal calf, the midcalf, and even the foot. Large respiratory waves visible in the foot are seen in postphlebitic limbs and in some normal limbs. In the postphlebitic limb, however, the filling time of the foot is shorter, and there is usually some rise in the baseline tracing of the calf or thigh, indicating some degree of obstruction. (See note Figure 4-8.)

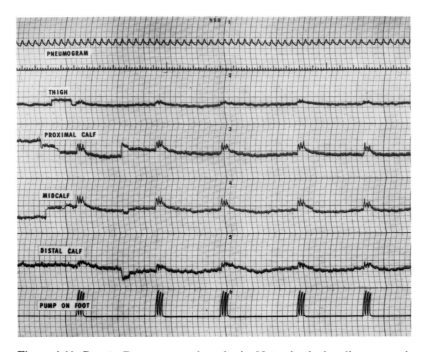

Figure 4-10. Run A. Deep venous thrombosis. Note rise in baseline every time pressure is applied to foot, indicating venous obstruction. Respiratory waves are visible even though greatly diminished in size. They are rounded or blunted rather than peaked. The fact that they are visible at all suggests that the thrombosis is several days old. (See note Figure 4-8.)

Figure 4-11. Run A. Deep venous thrombosis. Note rise in baseline of distal calf, midcalf, and proximal calf. However, there is not a clearly distinct rise in baseline in the thigh tracing, and respiratory waves are visible in the thigh, although they are not of normal size. Respiratory waves are absent in proximal calf and midcalf and scarcely visible in distal calf. This is diagnostic of acute deep venous thrombosis. Its location is centered around the midcalf and knee area. (See note Figure 4-8.)

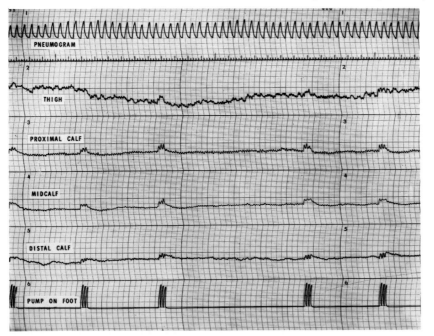

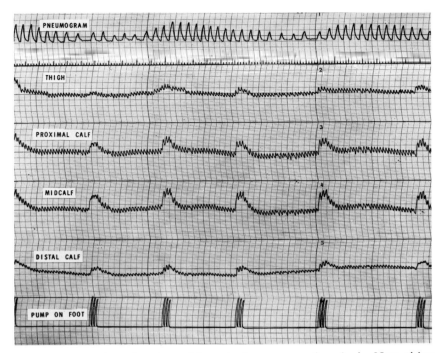

Figure 4-12. Tracing of patient with acute deep venous thrombosis. Note rising baseline clearly seen in all channels and absence of respiratory waves, indicating the acute thrombophlebitic process. (See note Figure 4-8.)

Figure 4-13. Run B. Tracing of patient with acute deep thrombophlebitis. Note absence of normal emptying of foot and rise in baseline in leg and thigh; absence of respiratory waves indicates that the process is acute. (See note Figure 4-8.)

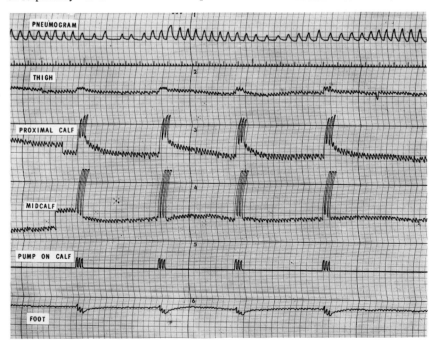

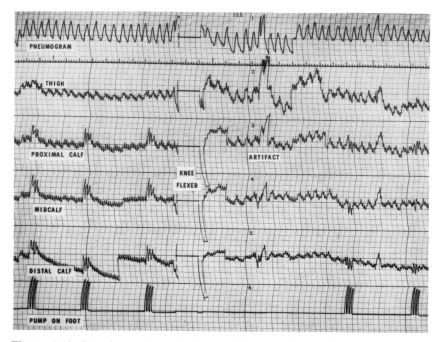

Figure 4-14. Run A. Artifact of the straight knee. Note rise in baseline and diminished respiratory waves on left side of the tracing when knee is straight. However, when knee is flexed (shown on the right side of the tracing), there is no rise in baseline and respiratory waves are clearly visible. (See note Figure 4-8.)

Figure 4-15. Artifact that may be produced by the straight knee, indicating some degree of venous obstruction at the knee which disappears when the knee is flexed. (See note Figure 4-8.)

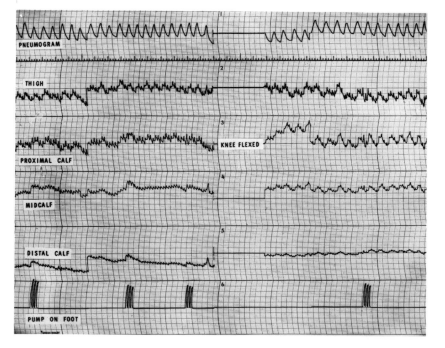

Interpretation

When the entire tracing is inspected and the responses to all three maneuvers are weighed, the diagnosis (Figs. 4-16 to 4-19) can be made in most patients. (See Tables 4-1 and 4-2).

EFFECT OF DEEP BREATHING. At the end of the test, the patient is asked to take several deep breaths. There is frequently a rise in baseline in the presence of deep venous obstruction and a horizontal or declining baseline in a normal subject. Although a confirmatory sign, this maneuver is not necessary.

Limitations

This test cannot be performed in the patient whose lower extremity is in a long-leg cast, nor can it be done satisfactorily in a patient with coarse tremors. At times it is difficult to carry out in elderly patients who are restless. In these instances, mild sedation may be used.

Only thrombi in the mainstream of the venous return are detected by the phleborheograph; clots in the tributaries and small veins are not discovered. Isolated clots in the deep femoral, saphenous, and hypogastric veins, as well as clots in the soleal veins, would not be expected to produce positive tracings (Fig. 4-20).

RESULTS

In February 1974, a multichannel phleborheograph specifically designed for diagnosing deep venous thrombosis became available and replaced the standard Grass polygraph in our laboratory, on which our tests were carried out during the exploratory period from late 1971 to early 1975. From experience with this new instrument, we are confident that the results of phleborheography (Table 4-1), already comparing favorably with other standard diagnostic tests for venous thrombosis, are certain to improve because of the high degree of standardization of the technique that was not possible earlier. Errors traceable to artifacts have been markedly reduced. False-positive tests have been virtually eliminated. Interpretation has become freer of ambiguities. The major remaining problem

Figure 4-16. Run B. Acute deep venous thrombosis. Note that rise in baseline occurs at all levels and is unchanged whether the knee is flexed or straight. Note minimal emptying of the foot (< 0.1 cc of blood). (See note Figure 4-8.)

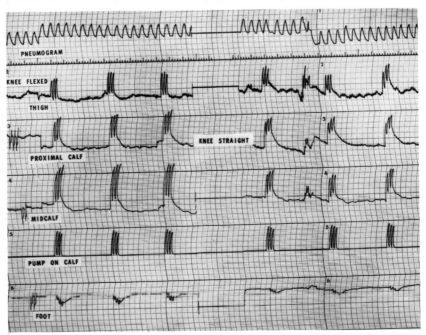

TABLE 4-1. Phlebographic Correlations: 504 Extremities

	POLYGRAPH	PHLEBORHEOGRAPH
False—negative	13/127 (10%)	3/36 (8.0%)
Equivocal	2 (1.6%)	0
Error in interpretation	4 (3.2%)	0
Test error	7 (5.5%)	3 (8.0%)
In below-knee thrombi	8/34 (24%)	
False—positive	13/294 (4.5%)	0/47 (0%)
Equivocal	2 (0.7%)	0
Technical	3 (1.0%)	0
Error in interpretation	3 (1.0%)	0
Test error	5 (1.7%)	0

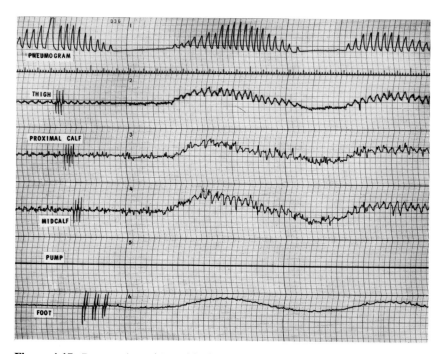

Figure 4-17. Run B. A patient with Cheyne-Stokes respiration. Note that during periods of apnea, the respiratory waves disappear from the thigh, calf, and midcalf. Also note increase in volume of limb as evidenced by rise in baseline associated with deep breathing, which even shows down at the foot level. (See note Figure 4-8.)

is the difficulty of diagnosing small clots, particularly those that are nonocclusive, that occur in one or two of the veins below the knee. In this group, false-negative tests by phlebography have numbered approximately 25 per cent in the past. The phleborheograph fails to detect them easily because due to their small size they do not cause sufficient obstruction to the flow of venous blood (Figs. 4-21 to 4-23). Attempts are in progress to solve this problem by increasing the sensitivity of the technique.

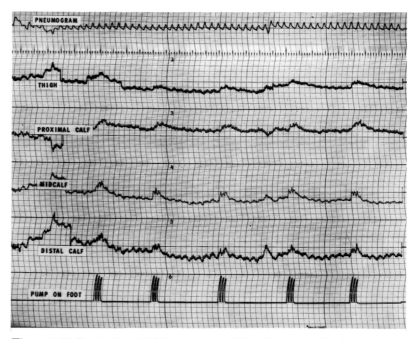

Figure 4-18. Run A. Postphlebitic syndrome. Note that on application of pressure to the foot there is a rise in baseline in distal calf, midcalf, and proximal calf, with the presence of respiratory waves. Thus, there is chronic obstruction. (See note Figure 4-8.)

Figure 4-19. Postphlebitic syndrome. (See note Figure 4-8.)

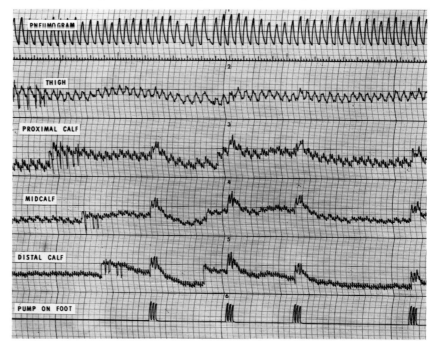

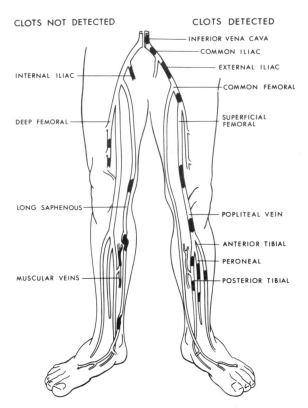

CLOTS NOT DETECTED | CLOTS DETECTED

INFERIOR VENA CAVA
COMMON ILIAC
EXTERNAL ILIAC
INTERNAL ILIAC
COMMON FEMORAL
DEEP FEMORAL
SUPERFICIAL FEMORAL
LONG SAPHENOUS
POPLITEAL VEIN
ANTERIOR TIBIAL
PERONEAL
MUSCULAR VEINS
POSTERIOR TIBIAL

Figure 4-20. Limitations of phleborheography.

Figure 4-21. Clot in a deep vein of the leg missed by phleborheography in a patient whose saphenous system had been stripped out at an earlier date.

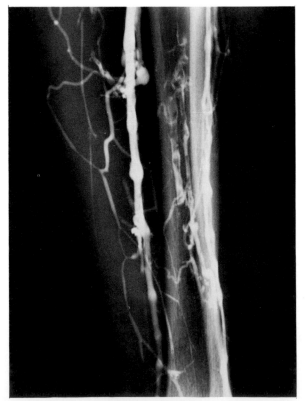

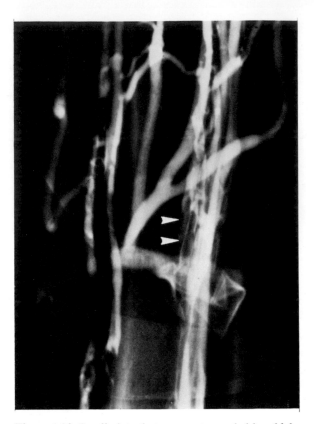

Figure 4-22. Small clots that were not revealed by phleborheography.

Phleborheography-Phlebography Correlations

FALSE-NEGATIVES

While less exact than phlebography in detecting the presence of small clots in the minor veins below the knee, phleborheography has the advantage that it can be repeated daily or more frequently, if called for, therefore providing the physician with an unsurpassed clinical tool for making the diagnosis and following the progress of the patient with deep venous thrombosis of the lower extremity.

Phleborheography was carried out on 127 extremities in which deep venous thrombosis was detected by phlebography (Table 4-1). The phleborheogram was positive in 114, leaving a gross error of 13 (10 per cent). All of the 7 true errors reflected a small thrombus in one vein and its tributaries below the knee. There have been no false-negatives whenever two of the major veins below the knee have been involved, and none with any thrombosis of the popliteal, femoral, or external iliac veins or the vena cava.

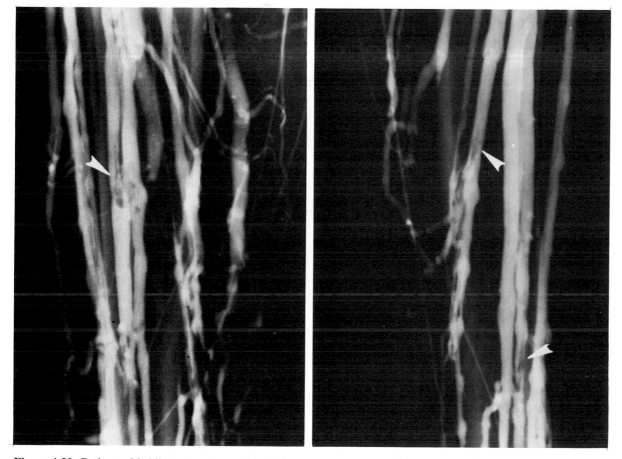

Figure 4-23. Patient with bilateral small clots in the deep venous system that were not detected by phleborheography

FALSE-POSITIVES

There have been 294 extremities that have had a negative phlebogram in which a phleborheogram was also obtained; 281 of the latter were negative, leaving an error of 13 (4.5 per cent). Three of these errors were due to the straight leg compression of the popliteal vein (see Artifacts); all three tests became negative when repeated with the knee flexed. In one other extremity this was believed to be the cause of error, but it was impossible to prove it by repeat testing.

NONTHROMBOTIC OBSTRUCTION. There were 6 positive tests in extremities in which no evidence of venous thrombosis could be found but in which evidence of venous compression was present. In 2 there was compression of the left common iliac vein by the right common iliac artery[13,14] (Fig. 4-24); in 1 there was compression of the right common iliac vein by metastatic tumor (Fig. 4-25). All three of these were demonstrated by phlebography. There was also one patient in this group in the last trimester of pregnancy with hydramnios. Her phleborheogram was intermittently positive when she would lie on her back and reverted to normal when she would lie on her side.[15,16] One false-positive was found in a patient with great swelling of the entire extremity, cardiac decompensation, cirrhosis, and a functioning splenorenal shunt. The patient had a very high venous pressure. The test reverted to normal when the patient's heart became compensated.

One patient was studied prior to removal of an artificially created AV shunt in the femoral artery (see Volume I, Chapter 6). The phleborheogram was positive, which was considered to be reason-

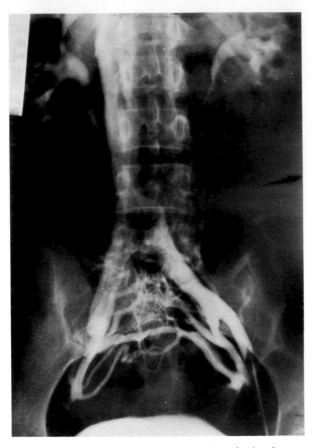

Figure 4-24. Phlebogram showing nonthrombotic obstruction of left common iliac vein by right common iliac artery, producing a false-positive phleborheographic tracing. Note that vein is markedly increased in its transverse diameter or "splayed out" by the artery. This in itself would not indicate obstruction, but the presence of such large pelvic collateral veins indicates obstruction in the main channel.

able due to the high venous pressure. However, at operation we were surprised to find complete fibrosis of the portion of the vein anatomically proximal to the AV fistula.

Clinical Testing

In addition to the above, the test has been positive in 296 (13 per cent) of 2245 extremities that were believed to have deep venous thrombosis (Table 4-2). It was not possible to obtain phlebograms on these extremities, so they are considered in a separate group. As of this time, 1813 normal extremities have been studied; in all of these the phleborheogram was negative.

The test has been used clinically in 137 office

patients not included in the above statistics. Occasionally it has not been possible to interpret the initial tracing; however, these tracings have almost invariably become clear on repeat testing. It is impossible to say whether or not errors have been made in this clinical group; at least, no proven errors have been brought to our attention.

Special Studies with the Phleborheograph

A group of 26 pregnant women in the third trimester have been studied; all tests were negative with the exception of that of a patient with hydramnios (see *Nonthrombotic obstruction*) whose test repeatedly was positive while she was lying on her back and negative when she was lying on her side.

Forty seven patients with ligation of the inferior vena cava were studied at an average of 9 years postoperatively; 77 per cent of thigh tracings were normal, a finding interpreted as indicating that minimal or no obstruction existed to the outflow of blood from the thigh veins through the pelvis or

Figure 4-25. Phlebogram showing compression of right iliac vein by metastatic carcinoma of the prostate, producing a false-positive phleborheogram.

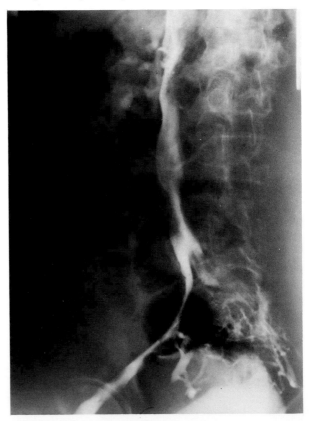

TABLE 4-2. Grass Polygraph Vs. Phleborheograph

	POLYGRAPH	PHLEBORHEOGRAPH
Clinical tests	2245	1354
Positive	296 (13%)	186 (13.8%)
Negative	1929 (86%)	1159 (85.5%)
Equivocal	20 (1%)	9 (0.7%)

abdomen. Of the leg tracings, 65 per cent were abnormal. This finding indicates residual obstruction in the veins at and below the knee level. (For a detailed discussion, see Chapter 6, section on phleborheography following vena cava ligation.)

Avenues of future investigation include phleborheographic quantification of the postphlebitic lower extremity utilizing a slight modification of the present technique, by means of which the postphlebitic limb is readily identifiable by certain criteria, viz., the rise in baseline due to an obstructed vein, the presence of large respiratory waves, and the rapid filling of the foot (indicating absence of venous valves) following emptying secondary to calf compression. Conversely, delayed filling of the foot is observed after compression of the calf in patients with obliterative arterial disease. Rheographic investigative studies are projected for patients seen in our arterial laboratory preoperatively and postoperatively, as well as for those managed conservatively. Also on the agenda is the continued development of techniques for study of thrombotic problems of the upper extremity.

REFERENCES

1. Cranley, J. J., Gay, A. Y., Grass, A. M., and Simeone, F. A. A plethysmographic technique for the diagnosis of deep venous thrombosis of the lower extremities. *Surg Gynecol Obstet 136:*385, 1973.
2. Mullick, S. C., Wheeler, H. B., and Songster, G. P. Diagnosis of deep venous thrombosis by measurement of electrical impedance. *Am J Surg 119:*417, 1970.
3. Wheeler, H. B., and Mullick, S. C. Detection of venous thrombosis in the leg by measurement of electrical impedance. *Ann NY Acad Sci 170:*804, 1970.
4. Wheeler, H. B., Pearson, D., O'Connell, D., and Mullick, S. C. Impedance phlebography: Technique, interpretation, and results. *Arch Surg 104:* 164, 1972.
5. Wheeler, H. B., Mullick, S. C., Anderson, J. N., and Pearson, D. Diagnosis of occult deep vein thrombosis by a noninvasive bedside technique. *Surgery 70:*20, 1971.
6. Simeone, F. A., Cranley, J. J., Grass, A. M., Linton, R. R., and Lynn, R. B. An oscillographic plethysmograph using a new type of transducer. *Science 116:*355, 1952.
7. Sakaguchi, S., Tomita, T., Endo, I., and Ishitobi, K. Functional segmental plethysmography: A new venous function test: Preliminary report. *J Cardiov Surg 9:*87, 1968.
8. Sakaguchi, S., Tomita, T., Endo, I., and Ishitobi, K. Functional segmental plethysmography: Clinical application and results. *Angiology 21:*714, 1970.
9. Sakaguchi, S., Ishitobi, K., and Kameda, T. Functional segmental plethysmography with mercury strain gauge. *Angiology 23:*217, 1972.
10. Arkoff, R. S., Gilfillan, R. S., and Burhenne, H. J. A simple method for lower extremity phlebography: Pseudo-obstruction of the popliteal vein. *Radiology 90:*66, 1968.
11. Britton, R. C. In Schobinger, R. A., and Ruzicka, F. F., Jr. (eds.) *Vascular Roentgenology.* New York, Macmillan, 1964, pp 658–661.
12. Sigel, B., Popky, G. L., Wagner, D. K., Boland, J. P., Mapp, E. McD., and Feigl, P. A Doppler ultrasound method for diagnosing lower extremity venous disease. *Surg Gynecol Obstet 127:*339, 1968.
13. Cockett, F. B., and Thomas, M. L. The iliac compression syndrome. *Br J Surg 52:*816, 1963.
14. Cockett, F. B., Thomas, L. M., and Negus, D. Iliac vein compression: Its relationship to iliofemoral thrombosis and the post-thrombotic syndrome. *Br Med J 2:*14, 1967.
15. McRoberts, W. A. Postural shock in pregnancy. *Am J Obstet Gynecol 62:*627, 1951.
16. Howard, B. K., Goodson, J. H., and Mengert, W. F. Supine hypotensive syndrome in late pregnancy. *Obstet Gynecol 1:*371, 1953.

5

Nonoperative Management of Thrombophlebitis and Venous Thrombosis

THE CONCEPT OF PROPHYLAXIS IN THE MANAGEMENT OF POTENTIAL VENOUS THROMBOSIS AND/OR PULMONARY EMBOLISM

Strictly speaking, the only treatment of venous thrombosis is extraction of the clot by mechanical means (thrombectomy) or its dissolution by thrombolytic agents; however, considering the large number of patients with thrombophlebitis, these techniques are indicated only on rare occasions. The main thrust of our efforts to overcome this potentially lethal condition is in the area of prophylaxis. Attempts are made to prevent the development of thrombophlebitis in patients at risk by either augmenting the rate of venous bloodflow through the lower extremities or altering the coagulability of the blood. Once venous thrombosis is established, treatment is largely symptomatic, except for the prophylaxis of pulmonary embolism. The major method of prophylaxis is the use of anticoagulants to prevent the propagation of the clot to a larger size while waiting for it to become firmly attached to the vein wall. At this stage in the disease, thrombolytic therapy appears to be desirable if safe and effective agents are available.

Only very occasionally is mechanical prophylaxis against pulmonary embolism indicated, i.e., some type of barricade is placed in the venous tree between the thrombus and the lung. When the thrombus is of such size as to seriously impair the venous drainage of the limb, as in massive femoro-iliac thrombophlebitis, extraction of the clot by thrombectomy or dissolution by fibrinolytic agents is indicated.

The following is an outline of the overlapping roles of prophylaxis of venous thrombosis, of pulmonary embolism, and of recurrent venous thrombosis and pulmonary embolism.

I. Prophylaxis of Venous Thrombosis
   A. Augmentation of the rate of venous bloodflow in the lower extremity (compare Virchow's third postulate: stasis of venous blood as an etiologic factor in venous thrombosis)
     1. By physical measures

a. Active means
  (1) Preoperatively the patient is advised to be as active as possible until the day of operation.
  (2) Intraoperatively, galvanic stimulation to produce *forced* active contraction of the muscles.
  (3) Soon after operation while the patient is confined to bed, he is instructed to exercise by means of dorsiflexion and plantar flexion of his feet to activate the soleal pump.
  (4) Postoperatively, ambulation is encouraged, brisk enough to exercise the soleal muscles.
  (5) At all times, sitting in a chair or sitting up in bed with the limbs below heart level is to be avoided.
b. Passive means
  (1) Intraoperatively and throughout the postoperative period extremities to be elevated above heart level.
  (2) Use of rubberized bandages or elastic stockings.
  (3) Intermittent pneumatic compression of the limbs.
B. Alteration of the coagulability of the blood (compare Virchow's second postulate: changes in the coagulability of blood as an etiologic factor in venous thrombosis)

  1. Prevention of platelet adhesiveness by administration of aspirin, dextran, etc.
  2. Augmentation of capillary flow (dextran)
  3. Prophylactic use of anticoagulant agents or defibrinating agents
II. Management of Patient With Established Acute Venous Thrombosis
  A. Physical measures
    1. Elevation of limbs above heart level
    2. Rest
    3. Heat
    4. Active exercises: dorsiflexion and plantar flexion of the feet to exercise the soleal pump
  B. Therapeutic doses of heparin, prothrombin-depressant agents, defibrinating agents, etc.
  C. Thrombectomy (See Chapter 6)
III. Prophylaxis Against Pulmonary Embolism
  A. All measures listed above
  B. Placement of a barricade between the thrombus and the lung (See Chapter 6)
IV. Management of Patient With Pulmonary Embolism (See Chapter 8)
V. Long-Term Prophylaxis Against Recurrent Venous Thrombosis and Pulmonary Embolism
  A. Encouragement to patient to be as active as possible (Caution against prolonged sitting with inactive muscles, e.g., on long bus rides, automobile trips)
  B. Use of elastic stockings to control edema
  C. Anticoagulant therapy

PROPHYLAXIS OF DEEP VENOUS THROMBOSIS

AUGMENTATION OF THE RATE OF VENOUS BLOODFLOW IN THE LOWER EXTREMITY

Elevation of the Limbs

In 1895 Hill[1] observed that in animals the flow of blood increased when the body was tilted with the head downward; he attributed this to the effect of gravity. These observations led to elevating the foot of the bed as prophylaxis against thrombophlebitis in bedridden or postoperative patients for at least part of the day until they have recovered sufficiently to contract their leg muscles voluntarily.[2] Wright

et al.[3] reviewed many of the objective studies carried out to demonstrate the value of elevation of the lower extremities; Wright and Osborn[4] also contributed a well-documented study of the comparison of flow rates as measured by injecting radioactive sodium into the foot and timing its arrival in the groin vessels. Their studies demonstrated that the venous flow rate is approximately halved when a person stands or sits as compared with the rate when he is supine. In contrast, the venous bloodflow rate is doubled when a person is tilted head downward or after vigorous dorsiflexion and plantar flexion of the feet.

Intraoperative Elevation of the Limbs

Two opposing methods of augmenting the return of venous blood from the limbs are based on the findings of Wright and Osborn.[3, 4] Elevation of the extremities has been shown to be a reasonable method and probably should be begun in the operating room, as recommended by McLachlin *et al.*[5] and later by Lewis *et al.*[6] The work of these investigators clearly indicates that the extremities should be elevated while the patient is on the operating table, as well as in the postoperative period. It is possible that the low incidence of thrombophlebitis following excisional therapy for varicose veins is related to the fact that such patients are customarily operated on while the extremities are in the elevated position. Gibbs, however, believes that in order to be effective, elevation would have to be more than 60 degrees[7] or the patient would have to lie on his side or assume the prone position for dependent drainage of the intramuscular veins of the soleus muscles to take place. The basis for this opinion is his anatomic dissection of 253 patients,[8] in which he demonstrated that the soleal veins drain upward into an anatomic bottleneck in the anterior and posterior tibial veins. While we accept the accuracy of Gibbs' observations, despite the fact that the drainage from the sural veins is indirect, rapid drainage of the blood in the posterior tibial, anterior tibial, and peroneal veins still should exert a siphoning effect on the drainage of the soleal veins by the Venturi principle. Moreover, clinical experience seems to bear out the beneficial effects of elevation.

Elevation of the Head of the Bed and Dorsiflexion of the Feet

Frykholm,[9] in the belief that two etiologic factors were primarily involved in deep venous thrombosis in bedridden patients, viz., injury to the calf veins by their walls being pressed together in the collapsed state due to the horizontal position and the decrease in the rate of bloodflow (Fig. 5-1), recommended that the head of the bed be elevated several hours a day and that a footboard be used. Thus, the position of the legs below heart level would maintain the veins in the distended condition and contraction of the gastrocnemius and soleus muscles necessary to keep the patient from sliding down the bed would provide active exercise forcing intermittent emptying of the calf muscles. The patient was kept in this position for one or two hours daily. Linton[10] adapted this practice by keeping the head of the bed elevated on all his postoperative patients, again using a footboard to induce the patient to use his gastrocnemius muscles.

In our experience, many elderly patients are not able to maintain the position advocated by Linton; with the head of the bed raised, instead of bearing down on their feet, they bend their knees and slide down on the bed. Therefore, our preference has been to elevate the lower extremities so that, at least from the midthigh down, the legs lie in a plane above heart level. However, the patient is also instructed to dorsiflex his feet 100 times every hour that he is awake. Such treatment is not outmoded; even today, it is the treatment of choice for the patient who is at home awaiting a hospital bed or when anticoagulant therapy is contraindicated. Elevation helps not only by reducing the postoperative swelling but probably also by accelerating bloodflow through the venous channels, thus lessening the tendency for thrombus to propagate.

Elastic Compression

Elastic support of the lower extremities is a rational procedure, and laboratory evidence bears out its value. Stanton *et al.*[11] demonstrated that the application of 20 to 35 mm Hg of pressure to the lower extremities of the human subject increased the velocity of venous flow, as measured by fluoroscopy, serial roentgenograms, foot-to-tongue circulation times, and limb venous circulation times. In their view, the mechanism of increased velocity of venous flow during local compression is the concomitant decrease in the total cross-sectional area of the venous beds. In a later communication from the same laboratory, Wilkins *et al.*[12] suggested that 10 to 15 mm Hg of pressure applied smoothly to the limb was effective and preferred. Paulsen *et al*[13] reported that the rate of venous flow of the lower extremities may be increased by application of elastic compression bandages to the horizontal limb, by elevation of the limb 8 inches above heart level, or by application of elastic compression to the elevated limbs. Husni *et al.*[14 17] studied venous hemodynamics with phlebography with and without elastic compression; pressure of 15 to 20 mm

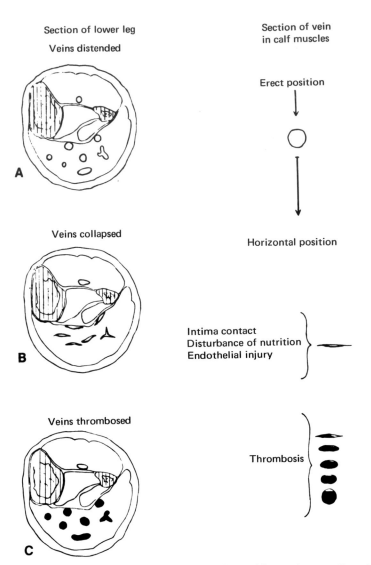

Section of lower leg

Veins distended

Section of vein
in calf muscles

Erect position

Veins collapsed

Horizontal position

Intima contact
Disturbance of nutrition
Endothelial injury

Veins thrombosed

Thrombosis

Figure 5-1. When patient is in the upright position, veins are distended with blood. In the horizontal position, veins are collapsed; the intimal contact may be a cause of thrombosis. (*From Frykholm, R.* Surg Gynecol Obstet 71:*309, 1940. By permission of Surgery Gynecology & Obstetrics.*)

Hg (similar to that of Wilkins) caused significant reduction in the venous pool of the leg with improved venous return. He also pointed out that wrapping the knee joint may easily compress the popliteal vein and seriously interfere with the venous return of the limb. For prophylaxis, the elastic bandage or stocking should be used on the leg only and should not include the knee. When the knee must be bandaged (as after a knee operation) or when an entire extremity is swollen, care should be taken not to apply excessive pressure to the popliteal area. We have seen a number of patients in whom thrombophelebitis of the leg developed secondary to venous engorgement from wrapping of the knee. In every case in which the knee is bandaged, the wrapping should begin at the metatarsal heads and be applied smoothly to well above the knee. Husni's suggestion that a "G" air splint be used after knee surgery is commendable. In the anesthetized patient, the value of elastic compression has not been proved.

Elastic Stockings

Caution likewise must be exercised in prescribing elastic stockings for the hospitalized patient. The amount of pressure needed to control edema in the ambulatory patient (see Chapter 9) cannot be applied to the extremity of the patient who is confined to bed. The compression rapidly becomes painful. A less heavy stocking must be substituted. If prescribed for a patient with advanced obliterative arterial disease as prophylaxis against deep venous thrombosis, the stockings should be worn only during the daytime and be removed at night. We know of 5 patients with severe arteriosclerosis obliterans in whom gangrene of the heel developed as a consequence of wearing heavyweight elastic stockings round-the-clock as prophylaxis of venous thrombosis.

Intraoperative Galvanic Stimulation of the Calf Muscle

In 1964 Doran and associates[18–22] began a series of studies on the effectiveness of galvanic stimulation of the calf muscles of the leg in the augmentation of venous flow from the leg and the prevention of thrombophlebitis. In their first report[18] they concluded that during operation under general anesthesia the velocity of venous return from the lower extremities was increased in at least three-fourths of the patients who were operated on; secondly, they also concluded that of patients whose venous return slowed during operation, approximately one-half developed a degree of venous stasis similar to that found to occur when a patient is confined to bed for 10 to 14 days, as reported by Wright *et al.*[3] in 1951. In the remaining patients who developed venous stasis, the degree of slowing is two or three times as severe as that produced by 14 days in bed and comparable only to that which occurs in paraplegia. The venous stasis which develops in the lower extremities during operation can be effectively counteracted in most patients by electrical stimulation of the calf muscles intra-operatively. In their subsequent reports, Doran *et al.*[19–22] have confirmed their original findings; they

have also found that 15 degrees elevation above the horizontal is roughly as effective as galvanic stimulation. Galvanic stimulation can be carried out only on anesthetized patients; it would not be tolerated by the awake patient because it is painful.

Intermittent Pneumatic Compression

McCarthy *et al.* in 1949 published a preliminary report[23] on a new method of preventing pulmonary embolism and in 1957[24] enlarged on this method of pneumatic compression of the calf as a means of intraoperative and postoperative massage to alter the venous bloodflow in the legs. Calnan *et al.*[25] devised a similar apparatus. In 1972,[26] these investigators suggested that the electric pump inflate each legging alternately at a pressure of 45 mm Hg for 1 minute, followed by 1 minute of relaxation. Roberts *et al.*,[27] while working on external pneumatic compression, determined that peak femoral vein flow could be increased sixfold and the pulsatility be increased thirtyfold. The maximum values occur when the interval between successive compressions is approximately 60 seconds; this appears to be related to the time required for the venous system to refill following release of leg compression. Allenby *et al.*[28] suggested that this beneficial result might be due to fibrinolysis rather than to augmentation of the bloodflow alone.

In the United States a pneumatic system has been devised that compresses the calf intermittently in a manner similar to that of ambulation. The pressure is applied quickly for 12 seconds, then relaxed for 48 seconds. The amount of pressure applied can be varied[29] (Table 5-1). In our studies (Tables 5-2 to 5-4), 50 mm Hg have been used. At Massachusetts General Hospital, Raines and Harris[30] have demonstrated by using this pneumatic system on patients undergoing phlebography that the entire calf is effectively emptied and that the dye which tends to collect in the area just beyond the valves is swept out. The conditions for optimum emptying of the venous tree were found to be a rapid rise (1 second) at pressures between 40 and 50 mm Hg and a 45-second rest period (Figs. 5-2 and 5-3).

Early Ambulation

Wright *et al.*,[3–4] using the laboratory techniques mentioned in the section on elastic compression,

TABLE 5-1. Alternating Pneumatic Pressure

AUTHOR	YEAR	CYCLE (SEC)	PRESSURE (mmHg)
McCarthy et al.[23]	1949	20	100
Calnan et al.[25]	1970	60	40–45
Calnan et al.[26]	1972	60	40–45
Roberts et al.[27]	1972	60	30
Lipson[29]	1972	12–48	±50
Cranley	1974	12–48	50

TABLE 5-2. Alternating Pneumatic Pressure as Prophylaxis Against Venous Thrombosis in 190 Patients Undergoing Total Hip Replacement*

Right hip	100
Left hip	90
Treated group	95
Control group	95

*Treated an average of 5 days.

TABLE 5-3. Results of Alternating Pneumatic Pressure in Prophylaxis of Deep Venous Thrombosis in 95 Patients Undergoing Total Hip Replacement

	NO. PATIENTS
Postoperative deep venous thrombosis	22
Treated group	8 (8.4%) of 95
Control group	14 (14.7%) of 95

TABLE 5-4. Complications of Alternating Pneumatic Pressure in 26 Patients

Minor blister formation	6
Heel pain	9
Generalized leg pain	1

measured the flow rate in 117 surgical patients on different days after operation. In those that were ambulatory during convalescence no slowing of venous flow rate was apparent in either legs or arms. In patients confined to bed, a reduction of flow rate occurred which was most marked at 10 to 12 days after operation. Variations in rate were always greater in the leg than in the arm. Observations on patients from whom pelvic masses were

removed suggested that alleviation of intra-abdominal pressure had a greater influence than postoperative ambulation on venous flow rate. Browse[31, 32] conducted interesting studies in this area. In his first study, he investigated the bloodflow in the calf in 29 healthy male patients; 12 of the 29 were living a normal ward life and the rest were confined to bed. Measurement of calf muscle bloodflow was remarkably constant. Of the 17 remaining patients, there was no day-to-day variation in the rate of flow change when 12 were confined to bed for 12 hours or when 5 of them were confined for a period of 2 to 5 days. He found that the calf bloodflow reaches the resting level before an hour of rest has elapsed. He viewed this finding as the answer to why early ambulation after an operation has no effect on the incidence of deep vein thrombosis. One should remember that the subjects under investigation were healthy, normal males and that only 5 of them were confined to bed for a period of 2 to 5 days. In his second study,[32] he demonstrated that 75 per cent of patients who undergo surgical procedures have a marked diminution of their calf bloodflow for 6 to 8 days postoperatively. In 53 per cent of the patients this drop in bloodflow occurred in the immediate postoperative period, and in 22 per cent it occurred gradually. The average drop in flow was to a level of 47 per cent below the preoperative level and lasted for 8 days. Drops in flow of 70 to 80 per cent were encountered. The remainder of the patients showed either a rise in flow (15 per cent) or a rise followed by a fall (9 per cent). He concluded from both studies that resting calf bloodflow is remarkably constant from day to day in a patient living a normal ward life; it is unaffected by long periods of bed rest; it is unchanged after general anesthesia alone; and changes in bloodflow following an operation performed with the patient under general anesthesia also occur after those performed with the patient under local anethesia. Browse comes to the "unavoidable conclusion that the changes in bloodflow are the result of surgical trauma alone. Bed rest and general anesthesia are blameless."[32]

The effectiveness of early ambulation[33, 34] cannot be judged as long as a clean-cut definition of "early ambulation" is lacking. *Ambulation* means to walk; from the prophylactic standpoint it means contraction of the soleus muscle, known to augment venous bloodflow. This in turn depends on

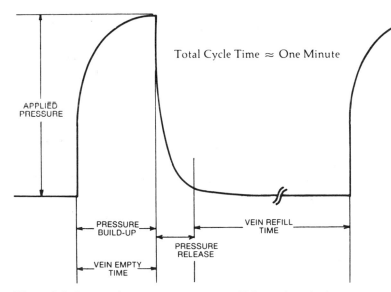

Total Cycle Time ≈ One Minute

APPLIED
PRESSURE

PRESSURE
BUILD-UP

VEIN EMPTY
TIME

PRESSURE
RELEASE

VEIN REFILL
TIME

Figure 5-2. Pneumatic system compresses calf intermittently in a manner similar to ambulation. Pressure is applied quickly for 12 seconds, then relaxed for 48 seconds; cycle is repeated at 1-minute intervals.

Figure 5-3. Investigative pneumatic system used to apply intermittent pressure to the lower extremities.

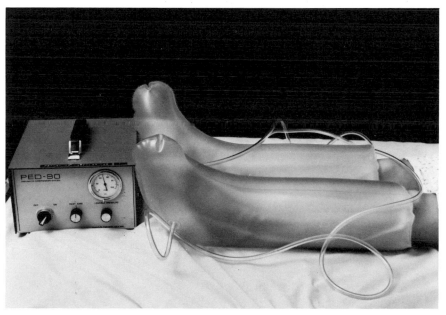

the number of steps taken and whether the patient is walking properly. Using a walker, shuffling, walking with a stiff leg, and taking a few steps to the bathroom supported by a nurse or an orderly are not effective ambulation. Forcing a patient who is in pain to get out of bed the first postoperative day and shuffle around the room a few times can hardly be considered a means of accelerating the drainage of blood from the lower extremities. Similarly, sitting in a chair with the legs dependent is worse than lying in bed. We see no point in stressing early ambulation unless the patient can actually walk down the corridor several times a day in a relatively normal manner.

Therefore, to be effective in the prophylaxis of deep venous thrombosis, both elastic compression and early ambulation must improve the venous return. Sufficient pressure must be applied to reduce the venous pool of the leg, and ambulation must be brisk enough to exercise the soleus muscles in order to increase the bloodflow out of the lower extremities. The degree of compression and the nature of the ambulation both must be taken into account when assessing the value of these measures. It was an unforgettable experience while on a visit to a world-famous medical center to be escorted through the wards and to be told that an elderly gentleman who was seated in a chair, restrained only by shoulder straps, partially conscious and falling forward, with his legs dependent and half-wrapped with loosely applied cotton-type "elastic" bandages was a patient in a controlled study of the effectiveness of compression bandages and early ambulation in the prophylaxis of phlebothrombosis! It would be unthinkable when speaking of a medication such as digitalis or morphine not to be concerned with dosage, yet it is commonplace to ignore the amount of pressure to be applied when "elastic support" is prescribed. If the lower extremities are to be wrapped, rubberized elastic support should be used. The minimum width should be 4 inches for below the knee and 6 inches for above the knee. For really effective support, the bandage must be applied tightly and smoothly, so that the entire leg is covered from the metatarsals to the knee. If the limb is greatly swollen, it is frequently better to double the bandage.

Prevention of Platelet Adhesiveness

ASPIRIN

Aspirin was given in a controlled trial as a prophylactic agent against thrombophlebitis and proved to be equally effective as either dextran or warfarin sodium.[35] In a trial conducted in Britain,[36] however, conflicting data were reported.

DIPYRAMIDOLE

Dipyramidole also affects platelet function; however, in 2 controlled trials,[36, 37] it was proved ineffective in the prevention of deep venous thrombosis and pulmonary embolism.

HYDROXYCHLOROQUINE

This drug is thought to alter platelet activity and has been reported effective in preventing venous thromboembolism.[38]

Augmentation of Capillary Flow

DEXTRAN

Dextran is thought to work prophylactically by a combination of mechanisms, i.e., by suppression of platelet activity and by expansion of the plasma volume through infusion, thereby increasing the cardiac output and venous bloodflow.

CHEMISTRY AND PHARMACOLOGY OF DEXTRAN. Dextrans are glucose polymers of high molecular weight produced by the fermentation of sucrose by *Leuconostoc mesenteroides*. The molecular weight of the polymer may vary from a few thousand to several million.[39] There are two preparations of dextran suitable for clinical use. Dextran 70 (Macrodex) is the earlier preparation that has been commercially available for years. Its average weight is 70,000, with 90 per cent of the molecules falling between 25,000 and 125,000. It is usually made up in a 6 per cent solution of normal saline.[40–42] Dextran 40 (Rheomacrodex) has been introduced more recently for clinical application. Its average molecular weight is 40,000, with 90 per cent of the molecules falling between 10,000 and 80,000. It is usually made up in a 10 per cent solution in normal saline or in 5 per cent dextrose and water.[40] There is an overlap of their molecular spectrums.

Dextran was originally investigated by Swedish surgeons[43–46] as a blood-volume expander and for use as a blood substitute; however, it was soon found to have other effects, including improvement of the microcirculation, antilipemic effects, and antithrombogenic effects.[47–49] Only its antithrombogenic effects will be discussed here. According to Berman,[50] dextran acts differently from classic anticoagulants in that it does not interfere with thrombin clot formation but reduces platelet adhesiveness and aggregation, which are considered to be the initial phase of intravascular thrombosis. The effect of dextran on the platelet *in vivo* is thought to be the result of interference with some factors in plasma which affect platelets, rather than interference with the platelets themselves, since *in vitro* dextran does not affect platelet adhesiveness. Infusing patients with dextran reduces an elevated plasma fibrinogen level; however, the effect of the recommended dose of dextran on the normal amount of plasma fibrinogen is minimal. In addition to specific effects on platelets and fibrinogen, dextrans inhibit intravascular thrombosis by dilution of clotting factors and improvement of bloodflow in general.[51-53] Moncrief and his associates in a series of experiments[54-56] produced a standard clot in the jugular vein of dogs using the method of Williams and Carey;[57] they found that dextran 70 with an average molecular weight of 77,500 was superior to all other molecular weights of dextran in the prevention of thrombus propagation. On the other hand, Atik, in a large, personally followed clinical series, could recognize no difference in the effectiveness of dextran 40 and dextran 70; he believes that since there is an overlap of molecular sizes in the two preparations, any differences between them are a matter of degree rather than of exclusive quality.[40-42]

TOXICITY OF DEXTRAN. Adverse side-effects include bleeding,[58,59] overloading,[41] anaphylactoid reactions,[60-64] nephrotoxicity, and interference with typing and cross matching of blood.

EXCESSIVE BLEEDING. In Atik's opinion,[41] excessive bleeding should be a rare problem if dextran 70 and dextran 40 as presently prepared are administered at the recommended dose, not exceeding 15 cc/kg body weight in 24 hours. Dextran should not be given to patients with preexisting thrombocytopenia, deficient clotting factors, or consumptive coagulopathy. Dextran potentiates the effect of heparin; therefore, these drugs should not be given simultaneously for prolonged periods of time. If such pairing is unavoidable, then the heparin should be reduced to one-half or one-third the recommended dose.

THE OVERLOADING SYNDROME. This complication likewise is avoidable.[41] Infusion of dextran at the recommended dose of 10 to 15 cc/kg body weight in 24 hours, given over a period of 1 to 2 hours in the presence of established hypovolemia and 4 to 8 hours in normovolemic

patients, rarely causes difficulty. Monitoring the central venous pressure is a further safeguard.[41]

HYPERSENSITIVITY REACTIONS. Rash and urticaria may occur. When minor, these are of negligible clinical significance.

There may be anaphylactoid reactions. Sudden collapse, hypotension, arrhythmia, respiratory difficulty, and choking sensations have been reported.[60-64] With one exception (the third patient of Kohen et al.[63]), this type of reaction has occurred in patients who have received only a few cubic centimeters of the initial dose of dextran. The nature of the anaphylactoid reaction, therefore, remains unclear. Sensitivity may have been acquired by ingestion of dextrans in food or through dextrans manufactured in the body by bacteria. Certain of the pneumococcal polysaccharides may incite cross sensitivity with dextran. As a safeguard, Atik recommends that the first infusion of dextran be started by a physician and that the preparation be given very slowly over the first few minutes.[41]

NEPHROTOXICITY OF DEXTRAN 40. Matheson and Diomi[65] have reviewed the case reports of 34 patients with oliguria or anuria associated with the administration of dextran 40. In at least 4 patients, a causative relationship was suspected between dextran and acute renal failure. In their review, Thomas and Silva[66] state that approximately 50 cases of acute renal failure have been reported after administration of dextran 40.[67-72] They themselves report a death from renal shutdown in a patient receiving dextran 40 in the recommended dose of 100 ml/per hour for 24 hours and then 50 ml/hour. This therapy had been used for 72 hours after arterial embolectomy. Following this experience they modified the recommended dose formula and titrated the dose according to the individual tolerance of the patient. However, the dose tolerance proved to be unpredictable. Atik[72] suggests that dextran may be wrongfully implicated in cases of renal failure, the anuria being due to severe dehydration, interruption of blood supply, and reflex vasospasm. He[72] and others[73] have shown that dextran actually improves perfusion of the kidneys and helps prevent acute renal failure. Nevertheless, he cautions that it may be hazardous to administer dextran to a patient with established renal failure because of the possible overloading that might result.

INTERFERENCE BY DEXTRAN 70 WITH TYPING AND CROSS MATCHING OF BLOOD.

Dextran 70 (not dextran 40) has been known to interfere with accurate typing and cross matching of blood for transfusion.[41] The potential hazard can be avoided by drawing blood before starting the infusion. If this is not possible, the blood bank should be notified. In Hunnicutt's[74] experience the Rh negative factor has been masked by the dextran.

Clinical Studies

Atik has conduced a long-term study of dextran and believes that both dextran 70 and 40 are effective antithrombogenic agents.[40–42] He has noted no apparent difference between the two preparations for this purpose; however, one should note that dextran 70 is used in his studies on the prevention of pulmonary embolism. It is also important to note that in using dextran for the prevention of thrombophlebitis and pulmonary embolism, Atik begins the infusion preoperatively and continues it during the surgical procedure, 200 ml of 6 per cent dextran 70 in saline; 300 ml is administered in the next 6 to 8 hours, after which the patient receives an infusion of 500 ml daily for 3 days postoperatively and every other day thereafter until he is ambulatory or discharged. Since there is evidence that thrombophlebitis may begin during the operation, it is possible that Atik's early and continued use of dextran may help explain his superior results. His series included 126 patients with fractures of the pelvis, hip, or shaft of the femur, admitted to the orthopedic service of the University of Louisville. All patients were randomized into two groups. Patients whose charts were odd-numbered were treated as described above. The patients with even numbers served as controls and received daily equivalent amounts of saline solution or lactated Ringer's solution, given in a similar manner. The diagnosis of thrombophlebitis was made on clinical evidence; pulmonary embolism was diagnosed only if findings were confirmed by positive lung scan in conjunction with an otherwise negative chest x ray or if it was found at autopsy. In 9 patients, pulmonary embolism occurred; 8 of these were patients in the control group and 1 in the group treated prophylactically. It is to be noted, however, that pulmonary embolism in the patient in the treated group developed 7 weeks postoperatively and 5 weeks after discontinuation of the dextran.

EFFECTIVENESS AS PROPHYLAXIS IN CONTROLLED SERIES

Other investigators in the United States and in Europe have reported on the effectiveness of dextran in controlled series. Jansen[75] conducted a double-blind study in which dextran 40 and dextran 70 were compared with 5.5 per cent glucose. He infused the dextran intraoperatively but did not use it postoperatively. The patients were followed carefully with daily clinical examination of the lower extremities; ascending phlebography was performed in all patients with even a slight suggestion of venous thrombosis. In all, 901 patients were studied; 301 in the control group, 304 in the group given dextran 70, and 296 in the dextran 40 group. In the control group there were 30 cases (10 per cent) of phlebographically verified postoperative thrombophlebitis, with six pulmonary emboli, five of them major. The incidence in the dextran 70 group was 18 cases (5.9 per cent) of venous thrombosis, with four pulmonary emboli, one of them major. In the dextran 40 group, there were 14 cases (4.4 per cent) of thrombophlebitis with no pulmonary emboli. The dextran 40 group seemed to be superior, but the difference between this group was not statistically significant. In a later study in which the test solution was given the day after operation, the frequency of postoperative embolism was equal in all three groups.

COMPARISON WITH WARFARIN SODIUM PROPHYLAXIS. Lambie et al.[76] compared dextran 70 with warfarin sodium in a controlled prospective trial in a group of 80 women undergoing gynecologic surgery; the women were randomly allocated to the dextran or the warfarin treatment. These at-risk patients were well matched in age, weight, and other predisposing factors. The diagnosis of venous thrombosis was made by means of the fibrinogen uptake test starting on the first postoperative day. In the warfarin group, 30 per cent developed thrombophlebitis, half of them with thrombi in the calf area. In the dextran 70 group, 10 per cent developed thrombophlebitis, in all instances confined to veins below the knee. There was one pulmonary embolism, occurring in a patient on warfarin sodium. Venous thrombosis was apparent on the first postoperative day in 62.5 per cent of the dextranized patients and in 58 per cent of the warfarinized patients. This suggests that if anticoagulation is to be of prophylactic value it must be effectively established at the time of operation. Many clinicians are reluctant to adopt this suggestion, made as long ago as 1959 by Sevitt and Gallagher,[77] out of fear of possible intraoperative bleeding and because of the ingrained belief that thrombophlebitis develops 5 to 7 days postoperatively.

From Denmark, Stadil[78] reported on 821 patients scheduled for general surgical procedures who were randomized into two well-matched groups according to sex, age, and other predisposing factors. One group was infused with dextran 70 intraoperatively and again 24 hours postoperatively; the other group was not given this treatment. Of those who had been dextranized, 3 per cent developed thrombophlebitis, compared with 7 per cent of the other group. Postmortem studies were done on 41 cases, evenly divided between controls and dextranized patients. At autopsy thrombophlebitis was present in 20 per cent of the dextranized group and 57 per cent of the control group. Stadil[78] looks on dextran therapy as a reasonable alternative to anticoagulants.

At the Massachusetts General and New England Baptist Hospitals, a prospective randomized study of thromboembolic disease was carried out on 227 patients on the orthopedic services who underwent total hip replacement.[79] The first group was infused with dextran 40 either intraoperatively or in the recovery room immediately after operation. Therapy was continued for 3 days postoperatively and then on every third day until the patient was ambulatory. The second group received warfarin sodium, usually 15 mg, intramuscularly in the recovery room or the evening after operation. The drug was continued in the therapeutic range of 1½ to two times the control value until the patient was ambulating. The diagnosis of postoperative venous thrombosis was made primarily from clinical criteria augmented by phlebography, radioactive

lung scan, and pulmonary angiography. The rate of venous thrombosis was 2.6 per cent in the warfarinized group and 6.1 per cent in the dextranized group. The rate of pulmonary embolism was 5.3 per cent for those on warfarin sodium and 6.1 per cent for those on dextran. Including 2 patients with both thrombophlebitis and pulmonary embolism, the incidence of thromboembolic disease was 10 per cent for patients on dextran and 7.9 per cent for those on warfarin. The difference is not statistically significant. Bleeding complications were essentially equal in both groups, 9 instances in the warfarinized and 10 in the dextranized patients. There was one death in the series, a patient on dextran who died of Gram-negative septicemia. Micropathologic examination of the kidneys indicated that the acute tubular necrosis was independent of the effect of dextran on the kidneys. To these authors, warfarin and dextran appear comparable in terms of effectiveness and complications.

COMPARISON WITH MECHANICAL PROPHYLAXIS. Renney *et al.*[80] set up a study to evaluate dextran 70 in the prevention of venous thrombosis. This study of 190 matched operative patients is of special interest in that the first (control) group of patients received routine preoperative and postoperative physiotherapy as practiced in most English hospitals and the second group received *intensive* prophylaxis and physiotherapy, including leg elevation and elastic stockings, while in the hospital. In other words, mechanical, external antithrombogenic measures were being tested against the endogenous chemical prophylaxis designed for the third group, who were infused with dextran, 500 ml 4 hours preoperatively and again 36 to 48 hours postoperatively. The rate of venous thrombosis, as diagnosed by the radioactive fibrinogen uptake test, was 35 per cent in the control group, 25 per cent in the intensive physiotherapy group, and 29 per cent in the dextranized group. The differences are not significant. These authors concluded that intensive physiotherapy, designed to prevent venous stasis in the leg, is effective in reducing the incidence of venous thrombosis in patients undergoing major operations but dextran 70 is ineffective. It is to be pointed out that in this study, dextran was given preoperatively but was given only once in the postoperative period, a departure from the standard manner in which this drug is administered.

INEFFECTIVENESS OF DEXTRAN PROPHYLAXIS

Brisman and associates[62, 64] contributed a highly negative report on the prophylactic value of dextran. They carried out a randomized double-blind prospective study at Johns Hopkins Hospital among 179 surgical patients with a high risk of developing pulmonary embolism. Coded solutions, either dextran 70 or dextrose 5 per cent water, were administered as an initial 500 ml intravenous infusion during a 3- to 5-hour period. The first infusion was begun by a physician at least 5 minutes before induction of anesthesia. Infusion therapy was continued until 24 hours after the patient began active ambulation. A diagnosis of thrombophlebitis was made if calf tenderness, swelling, and Homans' sign were present. A diagnosis of pulmonary embolism was based on clinical impression, a "typical" enzyme pattern, and positive lung scan in the presence of a normal chest x ray. In the control group, 6.7 per cent developed pulmonary embolism and 10 per cent developed clinical thrombophlebitis. One case of pulmonary embolism was diagnosed at autopsy. In the dextranized group, 9 per cent had pulmonary emboli and 3.4 per cent thrombophlebitis. One of the emboli was unsuspected and was diagnosed at autopsy. In the control group five deaths occurred and three autopsies performed. In the dextran group, eight deaths occurred, followed by six autopsies. In none of the autopsied cases was pulmonary embolism the immediate cause of death. Dextran apparently did not contribute to any of the deaths. There was no instance of bleeding diathesis.

In the group receiving dextran therapy, the only complication was severe anaphylactoid reaction[62] occurring in 3 patients within 30 seconds of initial infusion. Two of these three were the last two patients to be enrolled in the study. The test was accordingly abandoned. Any possible beneficial prophylactic effect of the dextran was offset by the known severe iatrogenic anaphylactoid reactions, one of which was nearly fatal. In this regard, it is of interest to review Kohen et al.'s[63] experience with anaphylactoid response to dextran therapy. By chance, 2 of their 3 patients who reacted were young physicians under treatment for thrombo-phlebitis of the lower extremities. Numbness and tightness in the chest and difficulty in breathing, followed by a severe anaphylactoid reaction were described by the doctor who was receiving the first infusion of dextran. Within 5 minutes of receiving a second infusion of dextran the other physician-patient became flushed and developed sneezing, rhinorrhea, and swelling of the eyelids. He is the only patient reported in the literature who showed a severe allergic reaction to other than an initial infusion.

Rothermel et al.[59] conducted a prospective randomized study of dextran 40 in patients undergoing total hip replacement. Dextran 40 (500 ml) was given immediately as soon as the patient left the operating room, followed by 500 ml each morning for the first 3 mornings postoperatively and then 500 ml on alternate mornings until the patient became ambulatory. Elastic bandages were wrapped about both legs twice daily and the foot of the bed was elevated 15 degrees. Careful muscle exercises were begun on the evening after surgery and isotonic quadriceps exercises were started on the third postoperative day. The diagnosis of thrombophlebitis was made on clinical examination performed at least twice daily. Pulmonary embolism was suspected on clinical grounds and confirmed by electrocardiographic changes, elevation of serum enzymes, and lung scan. Thrombophlebitis occurred in 4 of the 60 patients treated with dextran 40 and in 6 of the 60 patients in the control group. Three patients on dextran 40 had pulmonary emboli, one of which was fatal. Pulmonary embolism occurred in 4 patients in the control group. Two cases of congestive failure developed in patients on dextran 40. There were two wound seromas and five hematomas in the treated group; in the control group, two hematomas occurred. The authors therefore concluded that dextran 40 given as described does not reduce the incidence of thrombophlebitis and pulmonary embolism in patients following hip surgery. Evarts[81] and Atik and Harkness,[82] however, point out that these results are not entirely contradictory to previous findings, the real difference lying in the fact that dextran 40 was begun after operation, too late to alter thrombus formation that occurs during operation and in the perisurgical period. Also, dextran 40 was given in less than optimum doses.

It is Evarts'[81] belief that dextran 40 remains the antiplatelet agent of choice while physicians await the availability of a "safe agent to administer prophylactically to abolish thromboembolic disease." The British Medical Journal[83] advises that the numbers of patients involved in various studies of dextran and the other anticoagulant agents are too small for any definite conclusions to be drawn as to their value. Continued research is urged into methods to prevent the occurrence of even the small thrombi that are detectable only by phlebography or screening with the fibrinogen uptake test. While subclinical, these may nevertheless cause damage to the vein walls, extend to produce massive venous thrombosis with embolization to the lung, and threaten the loss of limb and, possibly, life itself.[83]

It is difficult to draw conclusions on the effectiveness and safety of dextran as prophylaxis against thrombophlebitis. In most of the studies reported, the protocols are not standardized and differ in one or more possibly significant points. The two series that have impressed us most and which seemed to be comparable are those of Atik[40-42] and Brisman and associates.[62, 64] Yet these two studies come to opposite conclusions in respect to the effectiveness and the safety of the drug. Because we have never been able to assure ourselves of its safety or its effectiveness, we have not used dextran. For prophylaxis we have relied on elevation of the foot of the bed, exercises (dorsiflexion and plantar flexion of the feet), and ambulation; heparin has sometimes been prescribed in high-risk patients.

ANTICOAGULANT THERAPY

Heparin as Prophylaxis

MINIDOSE HEPARIN

Wessler and Yin[84] recently summarized the status of the theory and practice of minidose heparin administration in surgical patients. The theory started with the suggestion of DeTakats[85] who stated that "it takes much less heparin or dicumarol to prevent clotting than to treat it." The concept was enlarged upon by Bauer in 1954[86] and Leggenhager in 1957[87] and has been vigorously propagated by Sharnoff[88, 89] for many years. Wessler and his associates identified a potent, naturally occurring inhibitor to activated factor X (antithrombin III and "heparin cofactor") in rabbit and human plasma.[90-93] They noted that the anticoagulant effect of the inhibitor against activated factor X is profoundly augmented by trace amounts of heparin; $1\mu g$ of the inhibitor prevents the potential generation of 1600 NIH units of thrombin. To neutralize this amount of thrombin, $1000\mu g$ of inhibitor are required. More heparin is necessary to bring about the instantaneous but readily reversible blockade of fibrinogen reaction by the inhibitor than is required to irreversibly neutralize activated factor X. Finally, they point out that activated factor X is a more potent thrombogenic agent than thrombin itself. On this basis, Wessler *et al.*[90-93] proposed a theory that the efficacy of minidose prophylaxis among surgical patients is not "anticoagulation" in the classic sense, because no state of hypocoagulability is induced.

"Circumstantial evidence strongly suggests that during and after the operation the state of hypercoagulability not previously present is initiated but remains "nonthrombotic" as long as the rate of activated factor X neutralization exceeds that of the generation of this activated species. Since this reaction rate is dependent on the inhibitor concentration, the latter becomes rate limiting. Thus, as the inhibitor becomes increasingly utilized, there will come a point in time at which some activated factor X will escape its inhibitor, combine with lipid, calcium ion, and factor V, and rapidly generate vast quantities of thrombin that, once formed, cannot be prevented by low doses of heparin from converting fibrinogen to fibrin. It is, in essence, the presence of small amounts of plasma heparin augmenting severalfold the rate of normal activated factor X neutralization prior to the development of hypercoagulability that can prevent venous thrombosis in patients undergoing operation."[84]

"Six clinical trials, five of them randomized, despite variabilities in design, have each demonstrated that minidose heparin begun prior to surgery and continued through the first 5-7 or more postoperative days significantly reduced the incidence (and in some instances the progression cephalad) of isotopically positive lower limb scans."[84]

The dose in these trials was 5000 units heparin administered subcutaneously beginning 2 hours prior to operation, based on the fact that it was demonstrated in Wessler's laboratory[84] that it takes 30 minutes for heparin of this dose to become demonstrable in the plasma. In Kakkar et al.'s second clinical trial,[94] heparin was resumed 12 hours instead of (as originally given) 24 after the 2-hour preoperative dose; the twice daily dose of 5000 units heparin subcutaneously is now extended from 5 to 7 days. Wessler[84] points out, however, that the data available from the six studies do not constitute proof that minidose heparin prevents postoperative pulmonary emboli and, in turn, death. It is estimated that the actual risk of death from pulmonary embolism is so low in patients over 40 that it would require a patient population in excess of 50,000 for a prospective multicenter randomized trial to establish the value of minidose heparin in the prevention of postoperative pulmonary embolism. Nevertheless, in his opinion it is a reasonable project and one that should be implemented. A final recommendation is that minidoses of heparin be administered to hemostatically competent adults prior to, during, and following operation.[94]

Contrary evidence has been reported by Evarts and Alfidi.[95] They used minidoses of heparin subcutaneously in the prophylaxis of 25 patients consecutively undergoing total hip replacement. Seven (28 per cent) patients developed deep venous thrombosis, and in 6 of these, pulmonary embolism was a complication. Their experience emphasizes the point raised by Salzman,[96] viz., that the dose of heparin perfectly adequate for the "hemostatically competent" adult patient may be ineffective in high-risk patients, such as those undergoing elective hip operations.

HEMORRHAGIC COMPLICATIONS. Wessler[84] is confident that minidose heparin essentially eliminates the drug risk of hemorrhage except for human error in administering an overdose. Hume et al.,[97] on the contrary, recently gave a series of 18 patients heparin, 5000 IU subcutaneously 2 hours preoperatively and every 8 hours postoperatively; of this group, 10 (56 per cent) developed a wound hematoma, which was of major proportion in 39 per cent. This serves as a reminder that hemorrhagic risk is not limited to therapeutic doses of heparin; this drug in doses of any potency whatever may complicate the course of operative patients.

In our practice, we have consistently refrained from using heparin in the perioperative period on even our best surgical candidates; despite its great efficacy, intravenous heparin increases the possibility of hemorrhage in the early postoperative period. As a calculated risk, however, we have excepted from this rule patients who have undergone arterial embolectomy or thrombectomy. In such instances, we have begun heparin therapy 6 to 8 hours postoperatively, 5000 IU intravenously every 6 hours. The dose may be increased or decreased in response to the monitoring method in use.

The Prothrombin-Depressant Agents as Prophylaxis of Thrombophlebitis

WARFARIN SODIUM

Reports of wide experience in the use of oral anticoagulant agents in surgical patients have now accumulated.[98–106] "Operation during anticoagulation therapy is safe and offers few problems provided the prothrombin time is not excessively long."[107] Despite a positive evaluation of their own experience, Clagett and Salzman acknowledge that prophylactic use of warfarin has not gained widespread acceptance among surgeons.[107] Objections include the difficulty sometimes encountered in regulating dosage and the need for careful laboratory control; surgeons also object to the risk of bleeding, no matter how low the incidence is among patients in whom there is no overt contraindication, such as active peptic ulcer, intracranial or visceral injury, hemorrhagic diathesis, gastrointestinal bleeding, severe diastolic hypertension, gross hematuria, and hemoptysis.[107] Warfarin therapy is usually begun several days before operation in order to afford maximum protection, since thrombi frequently develop intraoperatively and perioperatively. A loading dose of warfarin is not necessary; 10 to 15 mg are administered daily, and the dose is adjusted as needed to bring the prothrombin activity within 1½ to two times the control value. Prophylaxis is continued until the patient is ambulatory. Warfarin is the most effective prophylactic agent against thromboembolism; it is especially useful in patients at risk when prophylaxis has been delayed for whatever reason. Warfarin has been shown to be of use in overcoming established, as well as incipient, thrombi.[107]

MEASURES TO REDUCE THE COAGULABILITY OF BLOOD

Prophylactic Use of Defibrinating Agents

When used early, before organization of thrombi has occurred, lysis of fibrin can take place. Defibrinating agents are used in conjunction with anticoagulant drugs.

SUMMARY OF PROPHYLAXIS OF VENOUS THROMBOSIS. In our experience, the most practical method of prophylaxis of venous thrombosis is elevation of the lower extremities above heart level, elastic support as described above, active exercise in the form of dorsal and plantar flexion of the feet while the patient is confined to bed, and early ambulation, brisk enough to activate the soleal pump. These simple prophylactic measures have been studied by Tsapogas et al.[34] in a group of 95 patients undergoing operation; 51 patients were randomly chosen for prophylaxis, and 44 were placed in the control group for whom elevation, elastic stockings, active foot exercises, and early ambulation were not provided. The effectiveness of active and passive physical measures was clearly demonstrated; in the control group, 6 of 44 patients (14 per cent) developed postoperative deep venous thrombosis, while in the test group, only 2 of 51 patients (4 per cent) developed thrombosis. The diagnosis was confirmed by phlebography. Presently it is our practice to rely on phleborheography for early detection of deep venous thrombosis (see Chapter 4). If thrombophlebitis is detected, heparin therapy is instituted, followed by warfarin sodium in therapeutic doses.

MANAGEMENT OF PATIENT WITH ESTABLISHED DEEP VENOUS THROMBOSIS

PHYSICAL MEASURES

Elevation and Bed Rest

Elevation of the limbs above heart level combined with bed rest is a prime therapeutic measure. (See preceding section on prophylaxis.)

Heat

When treated by elevation of the limb and anticoagulant therapy, most patients with deep venous thrombosis of the leg progress so well that only occasionally must one revert to the time-honored technique of applying moist heat in the form of wet packs, to induce vasodilatation. Practically all patients in bed are already vasodilated to a certain degree, due to blankets and to the relaxation and loss of tone in the leg muscles at rest. However, if the swelling is extensive and the limb engorged, particularly in a patient with femoroiliac thrombophlebitis, the application of moist heat is greatly beneficial. By this means, prolonged vasodilatation is produced by relaxation of the arterioles and venules and by a decrease in the tone of the superficial vessels. Thus, the arterial inflow and outflow are augmented. There may be other as yet unclarified beneficial effects of heat; those of us who have treated femoroiliac thrombophlebitis prior to the era of use of heparin and the prothrombin-depressant drugs are mindful of the dramatic overnight improvement that may occur in the affected extremity after the application of warm wet packs.

Active Exercise

Dorsal and plantar flexion of the feet to exercise the soleal pump is recommended, 100 times every waking hour. (See the section on prophylaxis.)

MEASURES TO REDUCE THE COAGULABILITY OF THE BLOOD

Heparin Therapy

Heparin stands unchallenged—for now at least—as the most effective of the anticoagulant drugs, especially during the acute phase of venous thrombosis. However, the venom of the Malayan pit viper, now under clinical trial, may prove to be the treatment of choice in venous thromboembolic disease. (See discussion on Arvin, Reptilase, and Venacil in subsequent section on fibrinolytic agents.)

CHEMISTRY AND PHARMACOLOGY

Heparin is a mucoitin polysulphuric acid originating in the mast cells of Ehrlich.[108–112] It is found in abundance in any organ in which mast cells abound. Accordingly, these cells have also been called *heparinocytes,* which have a predilection for surrounding the finer blood vessels. For this reason, heparin has been called the natural anticoagulant. Although originally extracted from the heart and liver,[113] today the gastrointestinal tract is a rich source of heparin, as are the liver, pancreas, and lungs. Chemically, heparin is a polysaccharide derived from glucosamine and glucuronic acid and contains many sulphate groups. Thus, it is related to mucoitin sulphate of mucus and to chondroitin of cartilage. It derives its anticoagulant action from a strong electronegative charge due to the sulphuric acid group.[114] Electropositive substances, such as toluidine blue and protamine, neutralize the negative charge of heparin and completely destroy its anticoagulant action. The antithrombin effect of heparin is specifically pronounced, making it a strong anticoagulant. Under normal conditions, this is due to combination with a plasma globulin, discovered and named by Howell[113] as the heparin cofactor of plasma. This heparin cofactor, now referred to as α_2 antithrombin, is extremely important. When deficient due to heredity, liver disease, disseminated intravascular coagulation, or pulmonary embolism, it may be an important factor in the response to a given dose of heparin and may explain the so-called resistance to heparin encountered under certain circumstances. Heparin also blocks plasma thromboplastin generation by interfering with the activation of factor IX. Some investigators[115–117] believe that once the coagulation mechanism of the blood is retarded or blocked, the lytic effect of plasma comes into play and may possibly be catalyzed[112] by the presence of heparin.

Because of its extraordinarily strong electric charge, when heparin is present in suitable concentration, it may interfere with almost any reaction in which the proteins are concerned. It is known to combine not only with the positively charged protein molecules but also with the amino groups of the proteins which are on the basic side of the isoelectric point. Consequently, it interferes with numerous types of specific reactions, e.g., the complement-fixation reaction of the Wassermann test, and it exerts a more general influence on cellular permeability, allergic and inflammatory reactions, and tissue growth. In antigen-antibody reactions, it can interfere by taking up histamine or by neutralizing histamine liberators.

In massive pulmonary embolism, it is possible that heparin prevents the accumulation of platelets (and thus their subsequent breakdown) on the thrombus (see Chapter 8).

The incidental discovery of heparin in 1916 and its later development into a clinical tool provides a unique chapter in medical history since it involves a pair of celebrated medical students, Jay McLean and Charles Herbert Best. Having endured great privation in order to enter Johns Hopkins Medical School, McLean asked the renowned Dr. Howell to give him a "problem he could reasonably hope to finish and publish in one academic year entirely by himself."[113] The assignment was to determine the value of the thromboplastic substance of the body, thought by Dr. Howell at that time to be cephalin. While the second-year student was extracting cephalin from the brain, heart, and liver, he found that the liver portion in particular contained a potent anticoagulant,[118] which proved to be heparin. Best, who in 1922 was the codiscoverer of insulin while still in medical school, later determined to study the physiology and chemistry of heparin. Under his leadership, a team, which included such famed investigators as Gordon Murray, Louis Jaques, and T. S. Perrett, was organized at the University of Toronto for the purpose of obtaining and purifying heparin.[111] While they were scoring great success in the clinical use of heparin,[119–127] the Swedish school, led by Jorpes[112] and Bauer,[128] likewise was making clinical progress.

Methods of Heparin Administration

CONTINUOUS INTRAVENOUS ADMINISTRATION

Continuous intravenous administration was the method originally used by Murray[119–127] and appears to be the ideal technique. For a number of reasons, it failed to gain popularity; most importantly, it proved to be difficult to maintain a constant intravenous infusion. Today this is no longer true: many methods of providing a constant intravenous infusion are available,[129] and perhaps this means of administration will achieve widespread application. This method is preferred in the patient who has sustained one or more thromboembolic episodes or who requires a high dose of heparin.

INTERMITTENT INTRAVENOUS INJECTION OF HEPARIN

From the beginning, intermittent intravenous injection was the method chosen by the Swedish school.[112, 128] For several practical reasons, we adopted this technique. By using an indwelling catheter (we currently use a pediatric scalp-vein set) supplied with a diaphragm and container at one end, it is possible to attach the unit to the patient's forearm and administer the heparin intravenously at 4-, 6-, or 8-hour intervals; this permits the patient to move about freely in bed or to be ambulatory while receiving heparin therapy. In almost all of our patients, this has proved to be entirely satisfactory.

INTRAMUSCULAR ADMINISTRATION

In hospitals where the intravenous administration of heparin by nurses was prohibited,[130] heparin was sometimes given intramuscularly. This type of injection is painful, and frequently large hematomas are formed. Formerly recommended when veins were not accessible, the intramuscular route was abandoned in Scandanavia by 1950[131] and is rarely used today in the United States.

SUBCUTANEOUS USE

Some authors[132, 133] have recommended the use of highly concentrated aqueous solutions of heparin in the subcutaneous tissue. However, absorption is less uniform and hematomas are painful. For these reasons, we have avoided this method.

HEPARIN IN DELAYED ABSORPTION MATERIAL

Attempts have been made to render heparin slowly absorbable by the use of media that would dissolve slowly in the human body.[134] Loewe and others[135, 136] have described the action of sodium heparin incorporated in the Pitkin menstruum. A second preparation is depoheparin, consisting of sodium heparin in gelatin, dextrose, water, and a preservative (sodium ethyl mercuri thiosalicylate).[137] Our experience with such preparations has been limited.

THE DOSE OF HEPARIN

Murray[126] used 200 mg or 20,000 units in 1000 cc saline solution or glucose and water. He allowed it to run in at approximately 30 drops/minute. Before the intravenous infusion was begun, the clotting time of the patient was determined. Thereafter, the rate of infusion was controlled by determining when there was a measurable increase in clotting time. When the clotting time reached approximately 15 minutes, the rate of infusion was slowed.

Jorpes' method, according to Bauer,[128, 138] was to initially administer a dose of 150 mg (15,000 USP units) at 8 A.M., 4 P.M., and 8 P.M. On the second and third day the doses were reduced to 100 mg (10,000 USP units) each. Theorizing that it was not necessary to determine clotting times, the Swedish school made no attempt to control clotting during therapy.

A convenient method is to give heparin at 6-hour intervals and to obtain a clotting time once daily, 5½ hours after an injection. As long as the clotting time is still slightly elevated, the dose is continued. If it is not elevated, the dose of heparin is increased or the time shortened to 4-hour intervals. If the clotting time appears to be excessive (see below), one dose is omitted, and administration is restarted at a slightly lower dose. For most patients, 30,000 USP units is the average daily dose. There should be no hesitancy, however, to give a much larger dose if it seems necessary. Our clinical experience confirms that of others. The patient may appear to be resistant to heparin during the first few days of active treatment, and large doses are needed. However, after the clotting process has come under control, the heparin required to obtain the same effect on the clotting time may suddenly drop, e.g., from 10,000 USP units every 4 hours to 5,000 USP units every 6 hours. This gives credence to the possibility that heparin itself is neutralized as it performs its function. In patients with massive pulmonary embolism, even 15,000 units every 4 hours has only a moderate effect on the clotting time.[139, 140]

The use of the intermittent dose in this manner may produce extraordinarily high concentrations of heparin immediately after administration and inadequate levels toward the end of the 4- or 6-hour period. In the postoperative patient or the patient who is difficult to control, the constant infusion of heparin is the preferred method of administration.

CONTROL OF HEPARIN

The control of heparin has been achieved by various clotting tests that have been modified and improved over the past 35 years. Originally, the Lee-White clotting time method was used. Later, the ground-glass clotting time method[141] supplanted it, its advantage being the reduction in the amount of time required for the test to be performed at the bedside, viz., from 15 to 75 minutes to 2 to 7 minutes. The activated clotting time[142, 143] then became available; this saves still more of the laboratory technician's time, since the therapeutic range of this method is between 4½ and 5½ minutes. In each case, the therapeutic range varies between 1½ and three times the baseline control. Other clotting tests, such as the partial thromboplastin time[143] and the thrombin clotting time, are also used to monitor heparin therapy, but we have no experience with them.

Heparin is neutralized by toluidine blue and protamine. Readily available at the present time, protamine permits one to neutralize heparin immediately if it becomes necessary due to complications, and it allows one to use heparin up to the moment of operation. Widespread use of protamine by cardiac surgeons has demonstrated its effectiveness in neutralizing heparin. One to 1.5 mg of protamine neutralizes 100 units of heparin.

CONTRAINDICATIONS

Heparin is contraindicated in any patient who is actively bleeding, unless the bleeding is due to disseminated intravascular coagulation. Also, heparin should not be used in a patient with suspected bleeding. In some patients a small amount of bleeding might be fatal, as in a patient who may have had intracranial hemorrhage. In the immediate postoperative period, heparin may cause massive bleeding and should not be used except with extreme caution. We have decided to use it at times following embolectomy or thrombectomy; however, in such instances it is believed that a constant infusion of heparin rather than an intermittent injection is the safer procedure, since high peaking soon after injection is avoided. In the pregnant woman, heparin has the advantage of not crossing the placental barrier, due to its large molecular size.

COMPLICATIONS OF HEPARIN THERAPY

Heparin has been widely endorsed as the least toxic of all the anticoagulant agents. Implicit in this endorsement, however, is an element of danger. Heparin is a potent drug, and it should be prescribed with discretion. Some physicians tend to minimize the possibility of spontaneous bleeding, reasoning that heparin is administered only to hospitalized patients, who can be observed for hemorrhagic complications. However, a complicating factor concerned not with treatment but with the current method of measuring and labeling this powerful drug is being overlooked.

It is wrongly assumed that heparin is uniformly potent; this is why official USP units should be employed rather than milligram dosages. Cuono[144] pointed out that today, a heparin solution labeled 10,000 USP units no longer represents 100 mg but represents a variable amount ranging from approximately 83 mg to 60 mg or less (varying further from batch to batch). Some batches of heparin actually require as little as 50 mg of the powder to yield a 10,000 USP unit preparation. Consequently, 100 mg of this particular batch would be equivalent to 20,000 USP units. Unless physicians, pharmacists, and nursing personnel bear this inconsistency in mind when orders are being written, filled, or administered, serious complications may occur.

Recognition that there is not one but instead many heparins has been slow in coming. Jaques,[119, 145] who pioneered the refinement of heparin for clinical use, reported[146] a direct test for antithrombosis activity of heparin preparations in animals. This test showed the striking differences in ability to prevent thrombosis that were found in heparin preparations reputed to have the same USP activity. In 1940, he[147] reported that heparin isolated from tissues of different mammalian species exhibits significant variability in biologic activities. When compared with the International Standard of heparin with different coagulation assay systems, such preparations gave different values for relative biologic activities.[148, 149] It is pertinent, therefore, to ask, "What is a unit or a milligram of 'heparin' in terms of actual antithrombosis activity?" Jaques believes the International Standard of heparin has a relatively low antithrombotic activity. To clear away some of the confusion in reports on the effectiveness of heparin on platelets or in various types of thrombosis, he proposes that the exact heparin preparation used in reported clinical and experimental studies be stated.[148, 149] In the international collaborative study on the assay of heparin sponsored by the World Health Organization, Bangham and Woodward[150] demonstrated the serious weakness in the reproducibility and reliability of present methods for determining the unitage of heparin preparations. They recommend, as does Jaques, a chemical measurement which could be routinely applied in assigning the number of units to each heparin preparation.

ADDITIVE EFFECTS OF HEPARIN AND STRESS

The entire problem of hemorrhagic complications with the use of anticoagulants was thrown into high relief by Jaques' reminiscences[145] of his early work with Murray and Best on experimental animals. These pioneers reported that heparin would successfully prevent thrombus formation, but they did not publish another finding of equal clinical importance that might have dispelled "the universal misgivings regarding the possibility of hemorrhage with the administration of anticoagulants."[145] Although hemorrhage was watched for carefully, it was not found in any of several hundred experimental animals, some of which received very large doses of the anticoagulant. Their experience with the prothrombin-depressant agents was similar (see section on these agents). From 1934 to 1949, spontaneous hemorrhage occurred in only five animals. Foreshadowing the interaction of heparin with other concurrently administered drugs, they encountered an anaphylactic reaction in an animal which had been given antidistemper vaccine.

With the clinical introduction of heparin, sporadic reports of hemorrhage appeared, a few of which occurred in patients maintained within ordinarily therapeutic range. It also became known that other patients could tolerate larger doses of heparin without spontaneous bleeding. This led to the surmise that there was some hemorrhagic factor present in the clinical situation that was absent in the animal experiments. In further work, Jaques[145] and his associates subjected heparinized animals to stresses, including frostbite, 10 per cent sodium chloride administered intraperitoneally, electro-

shock, insulin convulsions, epinephrine, histamine, ACTH, salicylates, removal of the adrenal glands, P[32], and reserpine. On Selye's advice, the stress procedures were preadjusted to give approximately a 10 per cent death rate, and *by themselves,* they resulted in the predicted mortality. However, when heparin was injected into adrenalectomized rats, death by hemorrhage occurred in a few hours in 86 per cent of them and in 36 per cent of the sham-operated controls. The mortality from spontaneous hemorrhage was between 30 and 100 per cent in heparinized rats subjected to suitable combinations of the stress procedures. The number of fatal hemorrhages varied with the time of injection of heparin. If injection was initiated 24 hours prior to the stressing procedure, the mortality was 37 per cent. When added in advance of stress and dicoumarin (Dicumarol), the mortality rose to almost 100 per cent. The role of *stress* was illuminated by studies that demonstrated the absence of spontaneous hemorrhage when heparin was added to completely unclottable blood. For bleeding to result, the additive effects of heparin plus stress or infection were required.[145]

Hemostasis involves not only the platelets and the coagulation of blood but also the blood vessel wall. In the intact vessel, vasoconstriction is a very effective hemostatic mechanism. However, when the blood vessel wall is abnormal, blood leaks into the tissues. If fluid alone is lost, a state of increased permeability exists; if red cells also escape, there is decreased capillary resistance. The measurements of Kramar et al.[151–154] of capillary resistance have shown that stress of any type or a lack of corticosteroid hormones results in a marked decrease in capillary resistance. When stress is severe, there is greater damage to blood vessel walls than mere reduced resistance. Spontaneous hemorrhage is brought about only by simultaneous interference with more than one hemostatic mechanism. Disturbance of one of the hemostatic mechanisms, even if severe, does not produce a great potential for hemorrhage. Disturbance of two of the three mechanisms, e.g., coagulation influenced by heparin plus stress interfering with the blood vessel function or interference with platelet function (administration of aspirin to patient), leads to a much greater likelihood of bleeding.

Clinical Reports: Morbidity from Hemorrhagic Complications

A brief review of the literature indicates that hemorrhage has occurred in all decades since the 1940s, and it has occurred even with the most experienced physicians. In an early report, Aggelar[155] stated that the rate of wound or cerebral hemorrhage and gross hematuria varied between 0 and 12 per cent, averaging approximately 1 per cent. In the series of 80 patients reported by Duff et al.,[134] 2.5 per cent of the patients had hemorrhagic complications while under treatment with depoheparin for venous thrombosis secondary to an operative procedure. Crane[139] reported an 8 per cent incidence of hemorrhage in a group of 100 patients who were also being treated with depoheparin for venous thrombosis and pulmonary embolism. In the remaining 291 patients in his series, of those treated with concentrated sodium heparin, 3.3 per cent had episodes of bleeding. Fuller et al.[156] noted bleeding manifestations in 3.6 per cent of patients treated only with intravenous heparin. In 1971, Martyn and Janes,[129] using continuous intravenous administration of heparin, reported a 9 per cent incidence of bleeding episodes in 53 postoperative patients. While the bleeding was severe in all four instances, they accepted the complication as tolerable since the heparin effect can be readily reversed by the use of protamine sulfate. Harrower and associates[133] reported spontaneous hemorrhage from a tooth socket after an extraction. For a clearer view of hemorrhagic complications, Nichol's[157] comment that most hemorrhagic complications are either not noticed or not reported should be added to the above sporadic reports.

SITE OF HEMORRHAGE

The hemorrhage was into the adrenal gland in 1 of Crane's[139, 140] patients and into the pleural space in the other. The adrenal gland was also involved in cases reported by Knight and Valentine[158] and by McDonald et al.[159] In 1949 Cohen[160] found fatal massive cerebral hemorrhage in 13 patients with subacute bacterial endocarditis. Allen[161] reported hemorrhage into the cerebrum. White[161] treated a series of 28 patients with subacute bacterial endocarditis with heparin and sulfonamide drugs at the

Massachusetts General Hospital, but he concluded that "heparin was too dangerous, because too many of his elderly patients developed cerebral hemorrhage during the course of treatment." Allen's cases[161] were a pair of elderly patients treated with heparin for peripheral arteriosclerosis. Like White, he discontinued the therapy after cerebral hemorrhage occurred.

HEMATOMA FORMATION

Hematoma is a frequent complication in both surgical and nonsurgical patients treated with heparin. Harrower et al.[133] reported three instances of major hematomas at the injection site. In their experience, an injection of more than 1.5 cc heparin solution was especially likely to cause local hemorrhage. Morrison and Wurzel[162] reported on retroperitoneal hemorrhage secondary to heparin therapy when the heparin was administered intramuscularly or subcutaneously in the thigh or buttock.

We became aware of the dangers inherent in anticoagulant therapy early in our practice when a patient being treated with heparin for ascending superficial thrombophlebitis developed massive retroperitoneal hemorrhage. We have seen serious hematoma in the knee of a patient under treatment for coronary artery thrombosis and in the thigh of a patient who had undergone ligation of the femoral vein for deep venous thrombosis. Hemorrhage to the right side of the chest and the soft flank tissues occurred in a patient being treated for ileofemoral thrombophlebitis. Vaginal bleeding has been encountered twice, once in a patient being treated for postpartum ileofemoral thrombophlebitis and once in a patient with deep venous thrombosis of the leg. In our experience, the use of heparin in the immediate postoperative period following venous thrombectomy or arterial embolectomy and thrombectomy has produced a high incidence of hemorrhage. We also are guilty of the fault suggested by Nichol,[157] i.e., many of these complications have been handled as a matter of course and have not been fully documented in our records. We have come to believe that the intermittent intravenous dose of heparin should not be used in the early postoperative period. If heparin is deemed necessary, it is safer to use small doses administered by continuous infusion, to avoid the high peaks of the intermittent injection method.

HEMATURIA AND NOSEBLEED

Hematuria and nosebleed are frequent complications and are usually not considered to be of great consequence.

ANAPHYLACTOID REACTIONS

Chernoff[163] reported two instances and Jorpes[112] four instances of anaphylactoid reactions.

URTICARIA

Chernoff[163] reported a case of urticaria. Grolnich and Loewe[164] described fever and urticaria in a patient receiving penicillin concomitantly with heparin therapy.

Mortality Secondary to Heparin Therapy

Duff *et al.*[134] in 1951 stated that death due to complications of heparin therapy is "very infrequent" and cited a fatality at their hospital in a post-embolectomy patient with extensive intraperitoneal and extraperitoneal hemorrhage associated with regional and systemic heparinization. In Crane's series[139] there were two fatal hemorrhages occurring postoperatively in patients, one into the adrenal glands and the other into the pleural space. Wylie *et al.*[165] refer to a fatal instance of massive wound hemorrhage following arterial embolectomy and report on a patient who, 6 hours after an arterial embolectomy and while receiving therapy of 30 mg heparin/100 cc, developed the clinical picture of shock and died within 18 hours. In 1949 Lilly[166] suggested that fatal hemorrhagic complications secondary to Dicumarol poisoning were going unreported and, possibly, unrecognized; this same observation might be made concerning such deaths in patients on heparin therapy. Fortunately, we have not had a fatality secondary to heparin therapy in our own service; however, in conversation with other physicians we have become aware of several fatal hemorrhagic complications of heparin therapy, alone or in combination with the prothrombin-depressant agents.

SELF-ADMINISTRATION OF ANTICOAGU-LANT AGENTS. Reports[167] have sporadically appeared in the journals of bizarre hemorrhagic disorders that are eventually proven to result from surreptitious self-dosing with anticoagulant agents.

Without exception, the deceivers are members of the medical profession, usually nurses. We have encountered 2 patients, both nurses, with unexplained bleeding who eventually were discovered to be self administering an anticoagulant drug, one heparin and one Dicumarol.

The Prothrombin-Depressant Agents

At this time, heparin still stands alone as the most effective of the anticoagulant drugs. Nevertheless, the prothrombin-depressant agents have earned a place in the management of deep venous thrombosis, as well as in its prophylaxis[98–107] (see preceding section on prophylaxis). They provide a convenient method of continuing anticoagulant therapy on a long-term basis.

CONTRAINDICATIONS TO PROTHROMBIN-DEPRESSANT AGENTS

The contraindications are generally the same as for heparin. Since the patient on oral anticoagulant therapy is out of the physician's sight for long periods of time, great care must be taken in prescribing and administering such agents in the patient with a history of peptic ulcer or ulcerative colitis. The use of prothrombin-depressant agents in pregnancy is controversial. Most authorities agree not to use it in late pregnancy or if premature birth is threatened because of the prothrombinopenic effect on the baby. Its use in early pregnancy and midpregnancy is in dispute. We have avoided prescribing these agents throughout pregnancy.

A laboratory capable of providing accurate determinations of prothrombin levels must be available. Furthermore, since there are significant variations in the prothrombin ratio from laboratory to laboratory, the patient should regularly visit the same facilities. Also, it is important to recognize that the patient's prothrombin ratio must be related to the control of that day; one should not rely on "per cent" prothrombin, which is at best misleading and potentially dangerous. The patient himself must possess the intelligence and desire to cooperate with his physician and to accept the need for obtaining a prothrombin level every 2 weeks. Patients must be warned that uncontrolled anticoagulant therapy is more dangerous than the possibility of developing recurrent thrombophlebitis and that it is preferable, if a risk must be taken, to chance recurrent thrombophlebitis rather than uncontrolled anticoagulant therapy.

Dicumarol

The discovery of Dicumarol is second only to that of heparin in human as well as scientific appeal. This pharmacologic and therapeutic breakthrough resulted from the desperate plight of a Wisconsin farmer in 1933, who braved a blizzard to seek help at the Agricultural Experiment Station.[168, 169] By some misdirection, he arrived instead at the biochemistry laboratory of Karl Link, where he dumped off a heifer which had died of hemorrhage, a can of unclottable blood, and a bundle of spoiled sweet clover, the only hay available to feed his cattle. The problem of hemorrhagic disease of cattle had been under discussion in the early 1920s, and research had reached the stage where it was known that the disease was due to improperly cured sweet clover and that it produced a prothrombin defect in the plasma.[170] Link and associates determined to isolate the substance in spoiled sweet clover causing this hemorrhagic state and were using as their method of assay the Quick one-stage plasma prothrombin test.[171] In 1939, crystals of what turned out to be Dicumarol were isolated; the substance was synthesized by Stahmann, Huebner, and Link[172] in April 1940. The hemorrhagic property was at last traced to bacterial oxydation of natural coumarin in sweet clover into 4-hydroxycoumarin, which on coupling with formaldehyde produced 3,3^{1}methylene-bis(4-hydroxycoumarin) or Dicumarol.[172]

USE IN HUMANS

On February 27, 1941, Bingham *et al.* read the first report of the use of Dicumarol in the human at the University of Wisconsin; their results appeared in print in October 1941.[173] The first published account of clinical trials appeared in June 1941 in the bulletin of the Mayo Clinic.[174, 175]

Coumarin and Indanedione Drugs

Since the isolation of Dicumarol,[172] various compounds have been synthesized that exert a similar effect. The two main categories are the coumarin derivatives and the indanedione group. These differ in their rate of absorption, the time required for maximal efficiency, and the duration of action. Warfarin sodium (Coumadin) is probably the most popular anticoagulant agent for several reasons. It is highly effective, has a relatively quick onset of action, has few side effects, and is suitably merchandized. The tablets are easily divisible, are color coded, and have the dose printed on each one. All these details are useful in preventing errors. Prior to selecting Coumadin as the prothrombin-depressant agent of our choice, phenprocoumon (Liquamar) was used as it was being introduced. It was found to be entirely satisfactory; however, it was abandoned in favor of Coumadin because of the packaging described above and because Coumadin was more widely known by the physicians in our community who referred patients for initiation of treatment.

Warfarin sodium may be given orally, intravenously, or intramuscularly and is relatively fast-acting. The initial oral dose is 30 to 50 mg; subsequent doses are regulated according to the prothrombin times. The average daily maintenance dose ranges from 2.5 to 10 mg. Occasionally, a patient is encountered who requires 15, or perhaps 20, mg daily. Admittedly, this is the exception; when such a refractory patient is under treatment, he is followed with extreme watchfulness because of the possibility of a sudden change in his response to therapy. With such refractory patients who are being treated on an ambulatory basis, it is preferable to accept a therapeutic level that is slightly less than ideal, rather than to increase the dose further.

Since the initial depression of the prothrombin level is largely due to the effect of the drug on factor VII and since 4 to 7 days are required for all the other affected factors (II, VII, IX, and X) to be depleted from the plasma, some physicians prefer to give smaller doses of the anticoagulant initially, i.e., 15 mg the first day, 10 mg the second and third days and so on, and accept the fact that the full effect is not obtained for approximately a week. In this way, it is sometimes easier to obtain smoother control.

Of the indanedione derivatives, which have an action similar to that of the coumarin compounds, our experience has been limited to phenindione (Hedulin). Because of its rapid mechanism of action, the physician can have the patient's prothrombin level within the therapeutic range within 24 hours and reverse it to normal limits within 48 hours after discontinuance of the drug. Its disadvantages, in our experience, include the need for a twice daily dose to maintain a steady state and the increased incidence of reaction to this drug as compared with warfarin sodium.

ANTIDOTES

VITAMIN K_1. Physicians at times still confuse vitamin K (menadione bisulfite) with vitamin K_1 (phytonadione). This is a serious mistake, as vitamin K_1 is far more effective in combatting excessive prothrombin deficiency; one problem with use of vitamin K_1 is its possible overeffectiveness in reversing the hemorrhagic tendency. In the normal course of events, if the patient's prothrombin ratio is more than three times the control level, watchful waiting is best, permitting the prothrombin depression to return to normal without interference. If vitamin K_1 is used, a small dose, between 2.5 and 5 mg, is preferable and may be repeated if necessary. Vitamin K_1 in doses of 25 to 50 mg administered intravenously not only restores the prothrombin level to normal in a person with a normal liver but also makes control of the prothrombin level difficult for several days or even a week thereafter. In this event, it is our policy to reinitiate heparin administration, because on at least two occasions it has been learned that a patient has suffered a fatal massive pulmonary embolus following the administration of a large dose of vitamin K_1 because the prothrombin ratio was deemed low (approximately 10 per cent). If a patient on anticoagulant therapy is hemorrhaging, vitamin K_1 in divided doses of 5 or 10 mg may be given while the patient is watched for cessation of bleeding. Individual response to this drug varies.[176] Fresh blood is also effective as a temporary measure while the physician is waiting for the prothrombin level to rise. Lyophilized plasma, reconstituted with 0.1 per cent citric acid solution, also promptly reduces the prothrombin ratio to therapeutic range.

INTERFERENCE WITH ANTICOAGULANT THERAPY WITH PROTHROMBIN-DEPRESSANT AGENTS

The dose of prothrombin-depressant agents is affected by such things as body weight and rate of absorption, degradation, and excretion of the drug, as well as by increased intake of vitamin K_1, whether it be by pill or by certain foods rich in this vitamin, e.g., vegetables, tomatoes, and grains.[177]

An effect is exerted on the prothrombin-depressant agents by anything that interferes with the absorption of vitamin K_1, such as increased gastrointestinal motility, liver function, and the broad-spectrum antibiotics.[177] The salicylates, particularly aspirin, have been incriminated as having an effect similar to that of prothrombin-depressants.[178, 179] Weiner and Dayton[180] reported that the barbiturates inhibit coumarin metabolism, Kazmier and Spittell[181] describe the interactions of barbiturates with coumarin. Koch-Weser[182] has commented on necrosis secondary to the additive effects of quinine and quinidine combined with coumarin; in 1973, von Hamm and associates[183] reviewed the literature and added a case of their own. They concluded that coumarin-related breast necrosis is probably an immunologic phenomenon. Other drugs that potentiate the coumarin effect include Atromid-S,D-thyroxine, and Northandrolone.[181] Cholestyramine has been shown to bind warfarin in the gastrointestinal tract and to delay absorption in rats.[184]

Table 5-5 enumerates the interacting factors that make frequent procurement of prothrombin levels a necessity. Occasionally, a patient is encountered who has his prothrombin ratio checked monthly or less often. It is believed that such lengthy intervals present an unacceptable risk and the patient is sternly admonished. The effect of the majority of the tabulated interactions with anticoagulant drugs can be minimized if the patient has his prothrombin ratio measured at least every 2 weeks. Wright[185] has summarized matters succinctly: the risk implicit in anticoagulation therapy is not excessive if proper precautions are observed.

Complications of Anticoagulant Therapy with Prothrombin-Depressant Agents

DERMATITIS

Extensive dermatitis secondary to warfarin sodium therapy has been reported by Adams and Pass.[186]

URTICARIA

Urticaria has been documented by Sheps and Gifford.[187]

NECROSIS

The most notable complication is necrosis secondary to coumarin therapy. It has been reported

TABLE 5-5. Adverse Interactions of Drugs*

INTERACTING DRUGS	ADVERSE EFFECT	PROBABLE MECHANISM
Anticoagulants, with:		
Allopurinol (Zyloprim)	Increased anticoagulant effect	Inhibition of microsomal enzyme activity
Anabolic-androgenic steroids	Increased anticoagulant effect	Not established
Antibiotics, oral (mainly chloramphenicol, chlortetracycline, neomycin)	Increased anticoagulant effect	Impairment of prothrombin formation
Barbiturates	Diminished anticoagulant effect	Induction of microsomal enzyme activity
Chloral hydrate (Noctec; and others)	Increased anticoagulant effect	Displacement from binding sites
Chloramphenicol (Chloromycetin; and others)	Increased anticoagulant effect with bishydroxycoumarin	Inhibition of microsomal enzyme activity
Clofibrate (Atromid-S)	Increased anticoagulant effect	Displacement from binding sites
Contraceptives, oral	Diminished anticoagulant effect	Increase in activity of some clotting factors
Glutethimide (Doriden)	Diminished anticoagulant effect	Induction of microsomal enzyme activity
Griseofulvin (Fulvicin-U/F; and others)	Diminished anticoagulant effect with warfarin	Induction of microsomal enzyme activity
Phenylbutazone (Butazolidin; Azolid) & oxyphenbutazone (Tandearil; Oxalid)	Increased anticoagulant effect	Displacement from binding sites
Quinidine & quinine	Increased anticoagulant effect	Additive
Salicylates	Increased anticoagulant effect	Reduction of plasma prothrombin
Sulfonamides, long-acting	Increased anticoagulant effect	Displacement from binding sites
Thyroid hormones	Increased anticoagulant effect	Not established

* The Medical Letter on Drugs and Therapeutics. Published by The Medical Letter, Inc. 56 Harrison Street, New Rochelle, N.Y. 10801. Vol. 15 [No. 19] 383; 78, 1973.

frequently in the European literature but less often in the American.[183] Koch-Weser[182] collected more than 150 cases in 50 reports that described localized necrosis of the skin and subcutaneous tissues of patients on coumarin-compound therapy, including gangrene of the skin and breast.

In our practice, 1 patient with a rash secondary to Coumadin therapy and 3 patients with a scarlatiniform eruption secondary to Hedulin therapy have been encountered. No patient has been observed with severe urticaria, loss of hair,[188] or subcutaneous necrosis.

Hemorrhagic Complications of Prothrombin-Depressant Agents

In short-term therapy (up to 6 weeks), the incidence of bleeding is reported to be from 5 to 10 per cent[189] and is ordinarily minor and of no clinical consequence. Wound hemorrhage accounts for a high percentage of hemorrhagic complications. Major bleeding episodes occur in approximately 1 per cent of medical patients and 2 to 3 per cent of surgical patients on short-term therapy. The hemorrhagic risk is reduced in patients on long-term therapy, because the patients with bleeding tendencies are eliminated early.[189]

THE STRESS FACTOR

Jaques[145] isolated the hemorrhagic factor in clinical trials that had been absent in animal experiments. In a series of well-planned studies, rabbits and rats were subjected to stressful situations, both with and without dicumarolization (see section on heparin-therapy). A low mortality was observed with Dicumarol alone; however, after addition of stress such as 10 per cent sodium chloride administered intraperitoneally, there was a 50 per cent mortality from spontaneous hemorrhage. Some other factor, such as stress or infection, must be present for spontaneous hemorrhage to occur with the use of anticoagulants. Dicumarol is the one exception to this rule; this drug has a number of toxic effects aside from its anticoagulant action. DeBakey[190] in 1943 cautioned against its indiscriminate use. Duff and Shull[191] published 23 reports of deaths from Dicumarol poisoning, collected from the literature. Lilly and Lee[166] commented in 1949 that enthusiastic reports[175, 192] on Dicumarol might actually cause more deaths than they prevent when anticoagulant therapy "permeates to the outposts of medical practice." In a more tempered comment, Rainie,[193] who reviewed the literature and reported a fatality from Dicumarol therapy, blamed not Dicumarol but the method of its use. He emphasized that a reliable laboratory and a competent physician are essential for the correct use of these drugs. Nevertheless, Flaxman[194] reviewed more than 100 cases of fatal drug poisoning over a 5-year period and listed Dicumarol as the most common cause of death resulting from drugs given orally; Klingensmith[195] in 1967 expressed the belief that Dicumarol might still retain this unenviable position.

SITE OF HEMORRHAGE

INTESTINAL TRACT. All large series report hemorrhage of the intestinal tract, many with a fatal outcome.[195] The term "anticoagulant ileus" was coined by Hafner *et al.*[196] in 1962 to describe an acute abdominal condition which may occur during extended anticoagulant therapy. This diagnosis was not readily apparent. On x-ray studies, however, paralytic ileus was revealed. It is a non-surgical condition, and an awareness of its existence and its true nature in this era of extensive prophylactic anticoagulation therapy is imperative in order to obviate needless operative intervention. Treatment includes use of vitamin K₁. Recovery in Hafner *et al.'s* reported cases was uneventful; however, 1 patient in this series developed an embolus to the aortic bifurcation 2 weeks later, after the discontinuation of anticoagulant therapy; the embolus was treated successfully by embolectomy. This patient suffered from rheumatic and arteriosclerotic heart disease, with auricular fibrillation. If the medical condition of the patient warrants it, it is recommended that, despite the anticoagulant ileus, the patient be restored to proper anticoagulant levels as soon as is safely feasible.

URINARY TRACT. Hematuria is the most common of the hemorrhagic complications referred to in all the large series. Acute urinary retention secondary to perivesical hematoma after prostatic massage in a patient on anticoagulant therapy has been reported by Klingensmith.[195]

ADRENAL HEMORRHAGE. If not recognized and treated, adrenal hemorrhage has a fatal outcome. Amador[197] in his review of more than 4300 autopsies on adults at the Peter Bent Brigham Hospital found 30 patients with adrenal hemorrhage, 10 of whom had been receiving anticoagulants; the fact that none of the hemorrhages had been diagnosed clinically gives one food for thought. He found the pathologic changes to be hematoma with resulting necrosis of the outer cortex. Adrenal hemorrhage should be suspected in patients receiving anticoagulant therapy who develop abdominal or flank pain with nausea and vomiting or with fever and lethargy. McDonald *et al.*[159] reported on 35 patients with adrenal hemorrhage secondary to anticoagulant therapy and added 6 cases of their own. A significant finding is the age factor, 75 per cent of the patients being 60 years old or older.

HEMORRHAGE TO THE BRAIN. Barron and Ferguson[198] reported on intracranial hemorrhage with 63 fatalities. Cerebrovascular accident, often with a fatal outcome, has been described.[199] Subdural hematoma is a not uncommon complication[200] in patients receiving anticoagulant therapy for coronary disease. The prognosis is generally poor; the operative mortality in treated patients has been reported[201] as 50 per cent and in non-surgically treated patients as 100 per cent. Dooley and Perlmutter[202] evacuated intracranial hemorrhage proved by arteriography and craniotomy in 3 patients, who then survived. Cerebral aneurysm that ruptured during anticoagulation therapy has been successfully diagnosed and ablated.[203]

HEMORRHAGE TO SPINAL CORD. Cloward and Yuhl[204] recommend surgical exploration and laminectomy for a patient who is receiving anticoagulant therapy and complains of local pain, numbness, and weakness. Early diagnosis and surgical intervention is the only protection against paralysis.[205]

Pollard et al.[206] reported vascular and thromboembolic episodes in patients receiving anticoagulant therapy as prophylaxis for some form of occlusive vascular or thromboembolic disease. Of special interest is the fact that 9 of these 21 patients had also experienced bleeding complications during the period of their treatment with anticoagulants. Six of the 21 patients died as a result of the vascular or thromboembolic episode—four from myocardial infarction and one of cerebral infarction; the sixth death was attributed to acute coronary insufficiency.

Dextran as Therapy for Established Venous Thrombosis

EXPERIMENTAL STUDIES

Moncrief and associates,[54-56] using the method of Williams and Carey[57] to produce a standard venous thrombosis in dogs, were able to demonstrate that clinical dextran (molecular weight, 75,000) offered a high degree of protection against complications of the experimentally produced thrombosis. This protection approximated that provided by heparin; the protection in animals treated with clinical dextran was distinctly better than in the control animals and those in which low molecular weight dextran (40,000) was used. Just-Viera and Yeager[207] came to the same conclusion using a different method of producing thrombosis, i.e., incorporating a polyethylene tube into the vena cava or external jugular vein. In these reports, low molecular weight dextran did not produce the protective effect of clinical dextran.

Using sheep as the experimental animal and using the electric current method of Hunt et al.[208] to induce venous thrombosis, Johnson and associates[209] found that both infusion of low molecular weight dextran and of clinical dextran significantly reduced thrombus propagation and attachment to the vessel wall when infusion was begun 6 hours after femoral venous thrombosis was induced. Although inferior to heparin, these agents contribute significantly to continuous intravenous heparin therapy. In these experiments, clinical dextran was superior to low molecular weight dextran.

CLINICAL STUDIES

Atik has studied the dextrans extensively since 1961, and he is convinced that dextran 70 is useful in preventing deep venous thrombosis and pulmonary embolism; on the other hand, he is less convinced of its value in treating established thrombophlebitis.[40-42] Sawyer et al.[55, 56] report dramatic relief of symptoms, as did Cox and associates,[48, 49] within 24 hours in most patients; time for total resolution was also shortened from approximately 2 weeks to 4 days. Kohen et al.[63] reported three instances of anaphylactoid reaction in patients being treated for acute thrombophlebitis of the lower extremities.

In a prospective double-blind study of clinical dextran in thrombophlebitis, Bernard et al.[210] divided 14 patients with phlebographically proven acute deep venous thrombosis into two groups, one of which received dextran in 0.85 per cent sodium chloride while the other received 0.85 per cent sodium chloride alone. All patients were treated with bed rest and elevation of the lower extremities. All patients were relieved of pain within 18 to 24 hours, most improving greatly almost immediately after elevation. One patient attributed instant relief to the infusion, which was 0.85 per cent sodium chloride. By phlebography performed 3 months to 1 year after the bout, chronic venous disease was evident in 1 patient treated with saline solution and in 2 patients treated with dextran. These investigators suggest that saline and dextran effect similar improvement; therefore, hemodilution and extracellular fluid expansion may play a more important role in treating thrombophlebitis than has been heretofore realized.

The Fibrinolytic Agents

Unlike heparin and Dicumarol, both of which are twentieth-century American discoveries, the fibrinolytic agents have a heterogeneous lineage well-rooted in Western medicine.[211-213] Morgagni in 1769[211, 212, 214] reported an observation, first made in 1725, that human blood may remain liquid following sudden death. Long before this, this finding must have caught the attention of those concerned, legitimately or otherwise, with the inspection of fresh corpses. The therapeutic implications may have led John Hunter to carry out coagulation studies on liquid cadaver blood.

In many modes of destroying life the blood is deprived of its power of coagulation, as happens in sudden death produced by many kinds of fits, by anger, electricity or lightning; or by a blow to the stomach, etc. In these cases we find the blood, after death, not only in as fluid a state as in the living vessels, but it does not even coagulate when taken out of them.[215]

In regard to the liquidity of cadaver blood, one school of thought implicates disseminated intravascular coagulation,[216] although this may be open to question. Virchow[217] confirmed that capillary cadaver blood is always fluid and that venous blood in the limbs, although more often fluid at autopsy than not, is only exceptionally still coagulable. In 1887 Green,[213, 218] noting that clots prepared from human blood obtained by cupping occasionally dissolved within 24 hours, correctly formulated the basic thesis: once fibrin has "dissolved," it can not be clotted by thrombin. The French physiologist Dastre[213, 219] in 1893 proposed that this phenomenon be termed "fibrinolysis." In 1906 Morawitz[220] demonstrated reduction in plasma fibrinogen in cases of sudden death and noted active serum fibrinolytic activity in patients. The next year Opie and Barker,[221] using salt precipitation techniques, separated the albumin and globulin fractions. They found fibrinolytic activity in the globulin fraction. Yudin[222] was the first to put this accumulating knowledge to practical use by transfusing patients with cadaver blood.

FIBRINOLYSIS

The modern concept of fibrinolysis rests largely on the investigative work of Sherry and collaborators. Fibrinolysis is the mechanism almost certainly involved in the dissolution of all fibrinous exudates in the body; it is the mechanism probably involved in maintaining the fluidity of the capillary and microvascular system, which in the opinion of some investigators does not clot unless the fibrinolytic mechanism has been inactivated.[223, 224] In man, fibrinolysis is mediated through the activity of proteolytic enzyme systems surrounding the plasminogen-plasmin system.[225–231] Plasminogen, with a molecular weight of 88,000, is an inactive precursor of the active fibrinolytic enzyme plasmin; it is widely distributed in all body secretions and fluids. Its concentration in plasma is approximately 0.1 to 0.2 mg/ml. Tending to coprecipitate with fibrin whenever fibrin is laid down, significant quantities of plasminogen are incorporated into such deposits.[232] Plasminogen activators (kinases) are proteolytic enzymes highly specific for the activation of plasminogen, which can be found in trace amounts in all body fluids and in most body tissues.[232] Plasminogen activators are especially concentrated in the venous endothelium, particularly in the smaller veins and venules.[232] With increased fibrinolytic activity of the blood, its kinase level in plasma rises sharply. In urine, the activator is called urokinase.

PLASMIN. Plasmin is a proteolytic enzyme with many features similar to but not identical to trypsin. It has the ability to hydrolyze susceptible arginine and lysine bonds in proteins, and it splits arginine and lysine esters with great avidity.[232–234] Plasmin digests fibrinogen at a rate similar to its action on fibrin and also hydrolyzes a number of plasma proteins, including coagulation factors V and VIII. In addition, plasmin digests a great variety of protein substrates; α-casein, which is more soluble and sensitive than casein, is the substrate of choice for laboratory assay.[232]

INHIBITORS. When plasmin is formed in the plasma, it is rapidly inactivated by antiplasmins. Indeed, it is said[235] that there is sufficient antiplasmin activity in the plasma to inactivate 10 times all the available plasmin. This activity is believed due to an α-globulin component (molecular weight, 47,000) probably identical with α-antitrypsin.[232, 236, 237] Platelets also contain antiplasmin activity.[238, 239] The most plausible hypothesis for the normal fibrinolytic mechanism has been provided by Sherry.[232]

In vivo, plasminogen exists as a "two-phase" system, as a soluble phase form in the body fluids (plasma plasminogen), and as a gel phase form in thrombi and fibrinous deposits. The effect of activators in the two phases, and the consequences of plasminogen activation in the two sites, are dissimilar:

minor or slow activation of plasma plasminogen, because of the presence of inhibitors, will not result in detectable signs of plasma proteolysis since the enzyme is effectively inhibited on its formation; however, rapid activation of plasma plasminogen produces excessive plasma proteolytic activity, resulting in the rapid degradation of fibrinogen, the most abundant available substrate. On the other hand, activation of gel phase or clot plasminogen resulting from diffusion or incorporation of the activator into the clot, produces fibrinolysis, for here the enzyme is activated in close spatial relationship with fibrin. The latter is the only substrate available, and the reaction appears, initially, at least, to be independent of inhibitors in the body fluids.

These considerations provide considerable specificity for fibrinolysis, for under physiological circumstances fibrinolytic phenomena appear to be regulated by the concentration of plasminogen activator. Following an appropriate stimulus, activator is transiently released into the circulation and directly raises the clot-dissolving activity of the plasma by its ability to activate gel phase plasminogen, but without invoking the consequences of increased plasma proteolysis. The mechanism is particularly effective when significant quantities of activator are present at the time fibrin formation occurs; under these circumstances the activator is incorporated into the clot while the latter is forming, and the subsequent widespread activation of clot plasminogen leads to very rapid fibrinolysis.

Streptokinase

Fibrinolytic activity of hemolytic streptococci was first reported in 1933.[240] Tillott's group[241–243] incubated plasma clots with β-hemolytic streptococci or their extracts, bringing about rapid fibrinolysis. Milstone[244] observed that instant lysis occurred only in the presence of small amounts of the globulin fraction of the blood protein. In the 1940s, streptococcal fibrinolysis was under intensive investigation.[245–247] It was conclusively demonstrated that the lytic factor of Milstone was a precursor or proenzyme of a proteolytic agent activated by the bacterial filtrate. The activator was termed "streptokinase," the precursor, "plasminogen," and the proteolytic enzyme, "plasmin." The inhibitor present in the albumin fraction was termed "antiplasmin." It has subsequently been shown[248] that bacterial filtrates of staphylococcal origin have similar activating properties.

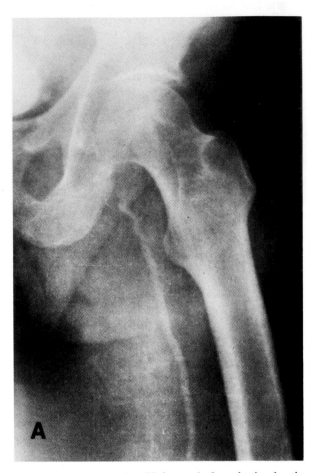

Figure 5-4. A. Massive iliofemoral thrombosis showing occlusion of major venous channels prior to thrombolytic therapy. B. Mid leg. C. Lower leg. (*From Tsapogas*, et al. Surgery 74:973, 1973.)

Streptokinase was originally developed for thrombolytic use in the United States; however, its use for this purpose was abandoned in 1960[249–251] because of its antigenicity and pyrogenic action. In Europe, however, study has continued, and streptokinase is available commercially. Currently, investigation of streptokinase has been resumed,[252] and a preparation has become commercially available in the United States.

The advantage of streptokinase is the fact that it can be produced easily in any quantity desired. Its disadvantages are formidable. It is antigenic to man; antibodies to it are developed after actual streptococcal infection, and thus various degrees of therapeutic resistance are encountered.[253] This variability in response necessitates estimation of the

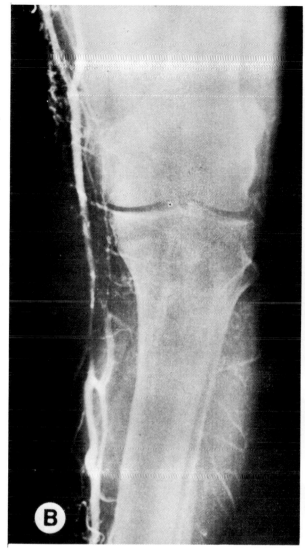

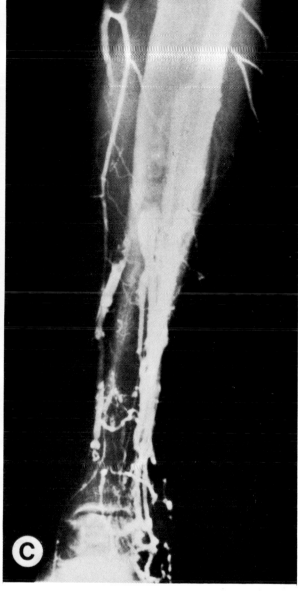

loading dose. Pyrogenic reactions still occur in 15 to 25 per cent of patients, but they are less severe than in the past.

The drawbacks to streptokinase therapy are not dissimilar to those of the prothrombin-depressant agents or heparin. The dose requires individualization and careful monitoring of the therapeutic activity. If the patient has had a previous streptococcal infection, the circulating antistreptokinase must be neutralized before a level of free streptokinase can be maintained in the bloodstream.

UROKINASE

Urokinase is a normal component of human urine. It is not antigenic; therefore, there is no problem with dosage. However, procurement poses a problem: it has been estimated that between 200 and 300 gallons of human urine yield enough urokinase to treat 1 patient.[249] Progress is now being made toward producing urokinase in the laboratory from embryo kidneys.

Clinical Trials of Fibrinolytic Agents

STREPTOKINASE

As far as clinical practice is concerned, thrombolytic therapy seems to be entering a second stage

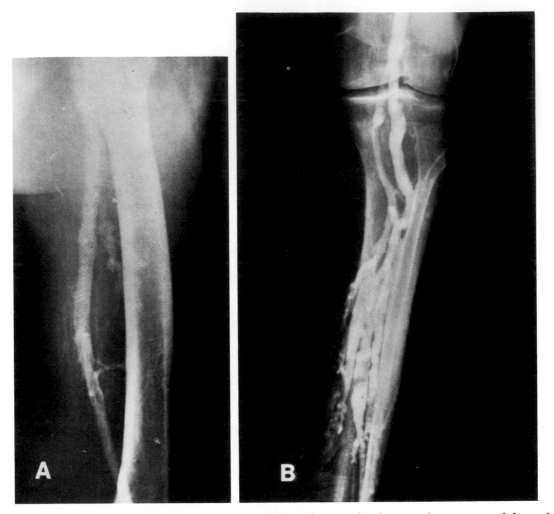

Figure 5-5. A. Phlebogram 48 hours after streptokinase therapy, showing complete patency of femoral vein. **B.** Phlebogram 48 hours after streptokinase therapy, showing complete patency of deep veins of the leg. (*From Tsapogas,* et al. Surgery 74:*973, 1973.*)

in the 1970s.[254] Advances have been made.[255] Streptokinase has been highly purified, and the former pyrogenicity has been removed. It still is antigenic; however, its antigenicity can be circumvented by using a fixed dose large enough so that, on the basis of past experience, it can be predicted that 80 to 90 per cent of the patients will achieve an active thrombolytic state despite the presence of antibodies in some of the patient population.[255]

Diaz and LeVeen,[256] reporting on enzymatic lysis of venous and arterial occlusions, caution that favorable response from fibrinolytic agents can be expected only from patients who are treated early, when clots are fresh. Furthermore, in their experi-

ence, venous thrombosis offers a fine possibility for therapy since the primary defect is in the clotting of blood rather than the disturbances in the vessel wall which can be responsible for occlusion in arterial cases. The great advantage of streptokinase over other forms of therapy is that it leaves the venous valves unscarred and competent.[256] When used early, before organization of thrombi has occurred, the medical equivalent of thrombectomy can take place. Lysis therapy shortens the duration of the illness. One complication is the febrile response to the bacteria in the thrombi, which are released during lysis.[256]

Diaz and LeVeen[256] report on 12 patients with

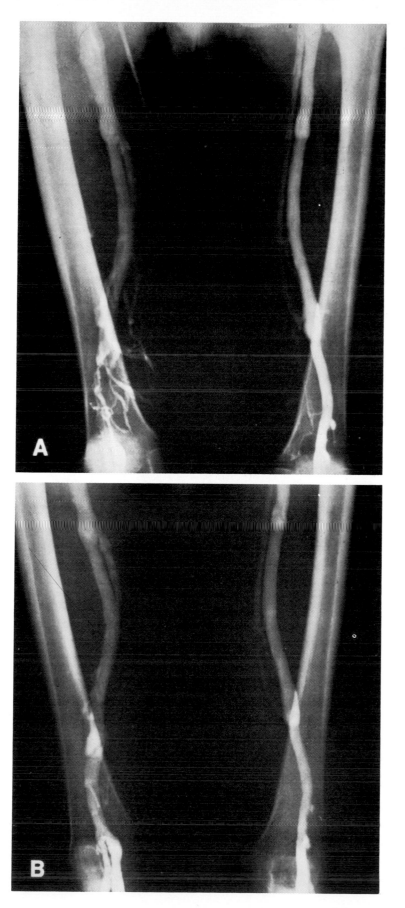

Figure 5-6. A. Thrombus that appeared to be resistant to infusion with streptokinase and was still present above the knee after completion of therapy. **B.** However, phlebogram taken on third day after infusion shows complete dissolution of the clot. (*From Tsapogas,* et al. Surgery 74:*973, 1973.*)

spontaneous venous thrombosis treated with streptokinase at the Brooklyn Veterans Administration Hospital. Three of their patients also had pulmonary emboli. Of the 12, 8 patients showed immediate clinical improvement. Phlebograms showed partial or complete restoration of patency. In 4, the phlebogram demonstrated incomplete resolution of the thrombus. In 3 of the 4, however, there was clinical improvement. The remaining patient, who was not improved by thrombolytic therapy, had a prolonged history of thrombosis with organization of clot and thus was not an ideal candidate.

Timmes et al.[257] have been using streptokinase clinically since mid 1969. They have treated 11 cases of acute arterial or venous occlusion. (Both private patients and physicians have been reluctant to agree to lysis therapy, which is still regarded as experimental.) They describe a patient with subclavian vein occlusion which was resolved and restored to normal with preservation of valves proved by phlebograms taken at 2 and 7 days after therapy. Treatment consisted of streptokinase for 48 hours.

Mavor et al.[258] treated with streptokinase 10 patients with thrombosis which recurred after iliofemoral venous thrombectomy. Phlebographic evidence of significant lysis was obtained in 9 of the 10 patients, including 2 in whom the thrombi were 12 and 30 days old, respectively. Reestablishment of the main channel was obtained in 3 of the 5 patients with occlusive thrombi. Bleeding from the wound occurred in 2 patients and wound hematoma in 5 patients. In their experience, the major theoretic contraindication to the use of streptokinase, i.e., allergic complications, have proved easy to control.

Tsapogas and associates[259] carried out a very carefully controlled study comparing streptokinase and heparin therapy for deep venous thrombosis of the lower extremity. The diagnosis was proven by phlebography in all 34 patients in the series. During the initial period of therapy, daily phlebograms were made. All patients showed clinical improvement, but it occurred earlier in the group receiving streptokinase. Ten of the 19 patients in the streptokinase group showed partial (more than 75 per cent) or complete lysis of the thrombus as demonstrated by phlebography, while only 1 of the 15 patients in the heparin group showed any clot lysis. In a patient with massive ileofemoral venous thrombosis of the phlegmasia cerulea variety in whom treatment was begun approximately 12 hours after onset of symptoms, complete patency of the formerly occluded vein was demonstrated by phlebography (Figs. 5-4 to 5-6). It is important to note that 9 of the 10 patients who showed partial or complete lysis after treatment with streptokinase had symptoms of 2 days duration or less.

Thrombolysin

Boyles and Meyer[260] have treated 23 patients with thrombophlebitis and/or pulmonary emboli with intravenous infusions of a combination of streptokinase and human plasminogen (Thrombolysin). This therapy is begun as soon as the diagnosis is suspected, and it is continued for 24 to 48 hours or longer, depending on the clinical response. After Thrombolysin infusions, anticoagulant treatment is continued with intravenous heparin and/or warfarin sodium for the remaining period of hospitalization. At least 1 million units of Thrombolysin are needed in most patients for effective lytic action. These investigators found it difficult to evaluate the objective value of this drug.

Arvin, Reptilase, and Venacil

Snake venom (Arvin, Reptilase, and Venacil) cleave fibrinogen molecules differently than thrombin.[261] Thrombin splits peptides from each of the alpha and beta chains to form a fibrin monomer. Venom splits peptides from only the alpha chain, and the resulting "monomer" cannot polymerize into fibrin strands. The monomers continue to circulate in soluble form and are cleared by the reticuloendothelial system.[262]

In purifying snake venom, the desired active principle is separated from the hemorrhagic and neurotoxic factors of the venom. After injection of Arvin, platelet count and bleeding time remain normal. More stable than thrombin, Arvin is unaffected by heparin and is not neutralized by fibrin. Degradation products of fibrin or fibrinogen possessing anticoagulant properties have been demonstrated in the blood.[263, 264]

CLINICAL TRIALS

In clinical trials,[264, 265] Arvin is best given intravenously, either by continuous infusion or by repeated injection to maintain the effect. Pitney *et al.*[266] advise a dose of 1 to 2 units/kg, slowly given intravenously over a 6-hour period; doses are repeated every 12 hours. This continuously suppresses the plasma fibrinogen levels. Sensitivity reactions have occasionally been noted. Because Arvin is antigenic, patients may become refractory to a second course of treatment.[266] Sharp *et al.*[264] have found Arvin relatively safe in patients with deep venous thrombosis, pulmonary embolism, and other conditions. It appears to be weakly antigenic. Kakkar *et al.*[267] treated 30 patients with deep venous thrombosis; one group received heparin, another received streptokinase, and the third received Arvin. Complications arose in each group during treatment, but the least occurred with Arvin. Symptoms of venous thrombosis were found to have resolved in most patients before the end of treatment. There seems to have been little difference between heparin and Arvin, although in their experience, Arvin was easier to control and had fewer side-effects.[268] Arvin's advantages are lack of spontaneous bleeding, rapid onset of action, low toxicity, and prompt reversal of its effect by antivenom or fibrinogen.[268] In the United States, snake venom (Venacil) is being investigated under carefully controlled therapeutic trials. To date, approximately 75 patients[269] have been treated with this agent. No complications have been observed. It appears to be as efficacious as heparin. Contrary to expectations, there is an abundant natural source of this material from herpetologic installations. It is possible that this drug will prove to be a therapeutic agent of significant value.

LONG-TERM PROPHYLAXIS AGAINST RECURRENT VENOUS THROMBOSIS AND PULMONARY EMBOLISM

ACTIVITY

The patient is encouraged to be as active as possible and is cautioned against prolonged sitting with inactive muscles, as when travelling.

ELASTIC COMPRESSION

The patient is made aware of the importance of wearing elastic stockings of sufficient weight to control edema and to prevent the postphlebitic syndrome of daily swelling, induration, pigmentation, and ulceration of the lower extremity.

ELEVATION OF THE FOOT OF THE BED

If swelling persists, the patient is instructed to elevate the foot of his bed 6 inches off the floor. This can be done by means of wooden blocks or old magazines and newspapers.

Long-Term Anticoagulant Therapy

A study was undertaken at the Mayo Clinic by Pollard *et al.*[206] involving 139 patients on long-term anticoagulant therapy (Dicumarol). In 47 (34 per cent) of the patients, 61 hemorrhagic complications occurred, including some types of bleeding (epistaxis, ecchymosis, and postmenopausal bleeding) that might have occurred without anticoagulation therapy. Fifteen episodes of bleeding were considered to be major, and three deaths resulted. The lesson to be learned is that these hemorrhagic incidents occurred at the hands of experienced physicians who had available to them the services of a reliable laboratory, yet in only 57 per cent of the 139 patients was the prothrombin activity maintained within the therapeutic range for more than 80 per cent of the time. In extenuation, these patients were treated between 1949 and 1959; yet, after 1957 this figure was raised only to 66 per cent. The majority of the hemorrhagic complications occurred while the prothrombin activity was in the desired therapeutic range. Pollard *et al.*[206] came to the conclusion that the limitations in the practical management of patients on long-term therapy plus the inconvenience, expense, and risks involved compel the physician to scrutinize the indications carefully in each instance. Certainly, there can be no such thing as "routine" use of anticoagulant agents.

Nevertheless, the more recent series[99-106] have been well controlled, and they demonstrate beyond a doubt that anticoagulant therapy by means of the prothrombin-depressant agents is an effective means of reducing the incidence of thrombophlebitis and pulmonary embolism in the postoperative period. Of our several hundreds of patients treated with long-term anticoagulant therapy, one stands out above all others.

Case Report 5-1

First seen in 1952 at the age of 45, this male Caucasian suffered five episodes of intravenous or intra-arterial thrombosis within a year or less, including a stroke, a coronary artery thrombosis, thrombosis of the popliteal artery, and three bouts of superficial thrombophlebitis of the lower extremities. He was placed on anticoagulant therapy and followed until his death, which occurred 17 years later of cardiac failure. Throughout this time, no further episodes of intravenous or intra-arterial thrombosis took place, except progression of his coronary artery disease. Granted that his freedom from further thromboembolic disease while on anticoagulant therapy may have been purely coincidental, this case history is nevertheless impressive.

REFERENCES

1. Hill, L. The influence of the force of gravity on the circulation of the blood. *J Physiol 18:*15, 1895.
2. Ochsner, A. Venous thrombosis. *JAMA 132:*827, 1946.
3. Wright, H. P., Osborn, S. B., and Edmonds, D. E. Effect of postoperative bed rest and early ambulation on the rate of venous blood-flow. *Lancet 1:*22, 1951.
4. Wright, H. P., and Osborn, S. B. Effect of posture on venous velocity measured with ^{24}NaCl. *Br Heart J 14:*325, 1952.
5. McLachlin, A. D., McLachlin, J. A., and Rawling, E. G. Venous stasis in the lower extremities. *Ann Surg 152:*678, 1960.
6. Lewis, C. E., Mueller, C., and Edwards, W. S. Venous stasis on the operating table. *Am J Surg 124:*780, 1972.
7. Gibbs, N. M. Personal communication, 1973.
8. Gibbs, N. M. Venous thrombosis of the lower limbs with particular reference to bed rest. *Br J Surg 45:*209, 1957.
9. Frykholm, R. The pathogenesis and mechanical prophylaxis of venous thrombosis. *Surg Gynecol Obstet 71:*307, 1940.
10. Linton, R. R. Personal communication.
11. Stanton, J. R., Freis, E. D., and Wilkins, R. W. The acceleration of linear flow in the deep veins of the lower extremity of man by local compression. *J Clin Invest 28:*553, 1949.
12. Wilkins, R. W., Mixter, G., Stanton, J. R., and Litter, J. Elastic stockings in the prevention of pulmonary embolism: A preliminary report. *N Engl J Med 246:*360, 1952.
13. Paulsen, P. F., Creech, O., and DeBakey, M. E. Blood vessels and circulation: Observations on the venous circulation time in the lower extremities: Effect of elevation and compression bandages. In Proc 40th Clin Cong Am Coll Surg 1954. *Surg Forum.* Philadelphia, Saunders, 1955, p. 137.
14. Husni, E. A. Elastic support of the lower limb, use and abuse. *Hosp Med 7:*36, 1971.
15. Husni, E. A., Ximenes, J. O., and Hamilton, F. G. Pressure bandaging of the lower extremity. *JAMA 206:*2715, 1968.
16. Husni, E. A., Ximenes, J. O., and Goyette, E. M. Elastic support of the lower limbs in hospital patients: A critical study. *JAMA 214:*1456, 1970.
17. Husni, E. A., and Goyette, E. M. Elastic compression of the lower limbs: Merits and hazard. *Am Heart J 82:*132, 1971.
18. Doran, F. S. A., Drury, M., and Sivyer, A. A simple way to combat the venous stasis which occurs in the lower limbs during surgical operations. *Br J Surg 51:*486, 1964.
19. Doran, F. S. A., and White, H. M. A demonstration that the risk of postoperative deep venous thrombosis is reduced by stimulating the calf muscles electrically during the operation. *Br J Surg 54:*686, 1967.
20. Doran, F. S. A., White, M., and Drury, M. A clinical trial designed to test the relative value of two simple methods of reducing the risk of venous stasis in the lower limbs during surgical operations, the danger of thrombosis, and a subsequent pulmonary embolus with a survey of the problem. *Br J Surg 57:*20, 1970.
21. Doran, F. S. A. Prevention of deep vein thrombosis. *Br J Hosp Med 6:*773, 1971.
22. Powley, J. M., and Doran, F. S. A. Galvanic stimulation to prevent deep-vein thrombosis. *Lancet 1:*406, 1973.
23. McCarthy, H. H., McGuire, L. D., Johnson, A. C., and Gatewood, J. W. A new method of preventing the fatal embolus: Preliminary report. *Surgery 25:*891, 1949.
24. McCarthy, H. H., Organ, C. H., and Giles, W. Thromboembolism and pulmonary embolism: A method of prevention. *Arch Surg 75:*493, 1957.

25. Calnan, J. S., Pflug, J. J., and Mills, C. J. Pneumatic intermittent-compression legging simulating calf-muscle pump. *Lancet 2:*502, 1970.

26. Mills, M. H., Pflug, J. J., Jayasinghe, K., Boardman, L., and Calnan, J. S. Prevention of deep vein thrombosis by intermittent pneumatic compression of calf. *Br Med J 1:*131, 1972.

27. Roberts, V. C., Sabri, S., Beeley, A. H., and·Cotton, L. T. The effect of intermittently applied pressure on the haemodynamics of the lower limb in man. *Br J Surg 59:*223, 1972.

28. Allenby, F., Pflug, J. J., Boardman, L. and Calnan, J. S. Effects of external pneumatic intermittent compression on fibrinolysis in man. *Lancet 2:*1412, 1973.

29. Lipson, C. S. Unpublished data reported to the manufacturer, Clinical Technology Inc., Cambridge, MA 02140, 1972.

30. Raines, J. K. and Harris, W. H. Unpublished data reported to the manufacturer, Clinical Technology Inc., Cambridge, MA 02140, 1972.

31. Browse, N. L. Effect of surgery on resting calf blood flow. *Br Med J 1:*1714, 1962.

32. Browse, N. L. Effect of bed rest on resting calf blood flow in healthy adult males. *Br Med J 1:*1721, 1962.

33. Tsapogas, M. J., Miller, R., Peabody, R. A., and Eckert, C. L. Detection of postoperative venous thrombosis and effectiveness of prophylactic measures. *Arch Surg 101:*149, 1970.

34. Tsapogas, M. J., Goussous, H., Peabody, R. A., Karmody, A. M., and Eckert, C. Postoperative venous thrombosis and the effectiveness of prophylactic measures. *Arch Surg 103:*561, 1971.

35. Salzman, E. W., Harris, W. H., and DeSanctis, R. W. Reduction in venous thromboembolism by agents affecting platelet function. *N Engl J Med 284:*1287, 1971.

36. Report of the steering committee of a trial sponsored by the Medical Research Council. Effect of aspirin on postoperative venous thrombosis. *Lancet 2:*441, 1972.

37. Browse, N. L., and Hall, J. H. Effect of dipyridamole on the incidence of clinically detectable deep-vein thrombosis. *Lancet 2:*718, 1969.

38. Carter, A. E., Eban, R., Perrett, R. D. Prevention of postoperative deep venous thrombosis and pulmonary embolism. *Br Med J 1:*312, 1971.

39. Ingelman, G. The chemistry of dextran and properties of low molecular weight dextran in shock: Pharmacology and pertinent rheology. National Academy of Sciences-National Research Council, 1963, pp 2–5.

40. Atik, M. Dextran 40 and dextran 70: a review. *Arch Surg 94:*664, 1967.

41. Atik, M. The uses of dextran in surgery: A current evaluation. *Surgery 65:*548, 1969

42. Atik, M., Harkess, J. W., and Wichman, H. Prevention of fatal pulmonary embolism. *Surg Gynecol Obstet 130:*403, 1970.

43. Thorsen, G., and Hint, H. Aggregation, sedimentation and intravascular sludging of erythrocytes. *Acta Chir Scan Suppl 154,* 1950.

44. Qulin, L. E. Studies in anemia of injury. *Acta Chir Scan Suppl 210,* 1956.

45. Gelin, L. E., Sölvell, L., and Zederfeldt, B. The plasma volume expanding effect of low viscous dextran and macrodex. *Acta Chir Scan 122:*303, 1961.

46. Thorsen, G. The use of dextrans as infusion fluids. *Surg Gynecol Obstet 109:*43, 1959.

47. Borgstrom, S., Gelin, L. E., and Zederfeldt, B. The formation of vein thrombosis following tissue injury. *Acta Chir Scan Suppl 247,* 1959.

48. Flotte, C. T., and Cox, E. F. Dextran in the treatment of thrombophlebitis. *Tr South SA 74,* 1963.

49. Cox, E. F., Flotte, C. T., and Buxton, R. W. Dextran in the treatment of thrombophlebitis. *Surgery 57:*225, 1965.

50. Berman, H. J. Platelet agglutinability as a factor in hemostasis. *Bibl Anat 4:*736, 1964.

51. Gelin, L. E. Hemato-rheological properties of low molecular weight dextran and other dextrans: Conference on evaluation of low molecular weight dextran in shock: Pharmacology and pertinent rheology. National Academy of Sciences-National Research Council, 1963, pp 6–21.

52. Wells, R. E. Rheology of blood in the microcirculation. *N Engl J Med 27:*832, 1964.

53. Yao, S. T., and Shoemaker, W. C. Plasma and whole blood viscosity changes in shock and after dextran infusion. *Ann Surg 164:*973, 1966.

54. Moncrief, J. A., Darin, J. C., Canizaro, P. C., and Sawyer, R. B. Use of dextran to prevent arterial and venous thrombosis. *Ann Surg 158:*553, 1963.

55. Sawyer, R. B., Moncrief, J. A., and Canizaro, P. C. Dextran therapy in thrombophlebitis. *JAMA 191:*136, 1965.

56. Sawyer, R. B., and Moncrief, J. A. Dextran specificity in thrombus inhibition. *Arch Surg 90:*562, 1965.

57. Williams, R. B., and Carey, L. C. Studies in the production of standard venous thrombosis. *Ann Surg 149:*3, 1959.

58. Nilsson, I. M., and Eiken, O. Further studies on the effect of dextran of various molecular weight on the coagulation mechanism. *Thromb et Diath Haemorrhag 11:*33, 1964.

59. Rothermel, J. E., Wessinger, J. B., and Stinchfield, F. E. Dextran 40 and thromboemoblism in total hip replacement surgery. *Arch Surg 106:*135, 1973.

60. Getzen, J., and Speiggle, W. Anaphylactic reaction to dextran. *Arch Inter Med 112:*168, 1963.

61. Michelson, E. Anaphylactoid reaction to dextran. *N Engl J Med 273:*552, 1968.

62. Brisman, R., Parks, L. C., and Haller, J. A. Anaphylactoid reactions associated with the clinical use of dextran 70. *JAMA 204:*824, 1968.

63. Kohen, M., Mattikow, M., Middleton, E., and Butsch, D. W. A study of three untoward reactions to dextran. *J Allerg 46:*309, 1970.

64. Brisman, R., Parks, L. C., and Haller, J. A. Dextran prophylaxis in surgery. *Ann Surg 174:*137, 1971.

65. Matheson, N. A., and Diomi, P. Renal failure after the administration of dextarn 40. *Surg Gynecol Obstet 131:*661, 1970.

66. Thomas, J. M., and Silva, J. R. Dextran 40 in the treatment of peripheral vascular diseases. *Arch Surg 106:*138, 1973.

67. Chinitz, J. L., Kim, K. E., Onesti, G., and Swartz, C. Pathophysiology and prevention of dextran-40-induced anuria. *J Lab Clin Med 77:*76, 1971.

68. Langsjoen, P. H. Observations on the excretion of low-molecular-weight dextran. *Angiology 16:*148, 1965.

69. Diomi, P., Ericsson, J. L. E., Matheson, N. A. Effects of dextran 40 on urine flow and composition during renal hypoperfusion in dogs with osmotic nephrosis. *Ann Surg 172:*813, 1970.

70. Bergentz, S. E., Falkheden, T., Oslon, S. Diuresis and urinary viscosity in dehydrated patients: Influence of dextran 40,000 with and without mannitol. *Ann Surg 161:*582, 1965.

71. Morgan, T. O., Little, J. M., and Evans, W. A. Renal failure associated with low-molecular-weight dextran infusion. *Br Med J 2:* 737, 1966.

72. Atik, M. Acute renal failure, a preventable complication. *J Trauma 6:*701, 1966.

73. Bryant, M. F., Brewer, S. S., and Bloom, W. C. Use of dextran in preventing thrombosis of small arteries. *Clin Res 10:*49, 1962.

74. Hunnicutt, A. J. In discussion of Atik, M. Dextran 40 and dextran 70: A review. *Arch Surg 94:*664, 1967.

75. Jansen, H. Prevention of venous thrombosis. *Lancet 1:*838, 1970.

76. Lambie, J. M., Barber, D. C., Dhall, D. P., and Matheson, N. A. Dextran 70 in prophylaxis of postoperative venous thrombosis: A controlled trial. *B Med J 2:*144, 1970.

77. Sevitt, S., and Gallagher, N. G. Prevention of venous thrombosis and pulmonary embolism in injured patients. *Lancet 2:*981, 1959.

78. Stadil, F. Prevention of venous thrombosis. *Lancet 2:*50, 1970.

79. Harris, W. H., Salzman, E. W., DeSanctis, R. W., and Coutts, R. D. Prevention of venous thromboembolism following total hip replacement. *JAMA 220:*1319, 1972.

80. Renney, J. T. G., Kakkar, V. V., and Nicolaides, A. N. The prevention of postoperative deep vein thrombosis, comparing dextran-70 and intensive physiotherapy. *Br J Surg 57:*388, 1970.

81. Evarts, C. M. Prevention of thromboembolism: An editorial. *Arch Surg 106:*134, 1973.

82. Atik, M., and Harkess, J. W. Dextran and thromboembolism. *Arch Surg 107:*492, 1973.

83. Prophylaxis of venous thrombosis, editorial. *Br Med J 1:*305, 1971.

84. Wessler, S., and Yin, E. T. Theory and practice of minidose heparin in surgical patients: Status report. *Circulation 47:*671, 1973.

85. DeTakats, G. Anticoagulants in surgery. *JAMA 124:*527, 1950.

86. Bauer, G. Proceedings of the first international conference on thrombosis and embolism. Basel, Schwabe, 1954, p 721.

87. Leggenhager, K. Genese und Prophylaxis der postoperativen Fernthrombose. *Helv Chir Acta 24:*316, 1957.

88. Sharnoff, J. C. Results in prophylaxis of postoperative thromboembolism. *Surg Gynecol Obstet 123:*303, 1966.

89. Sharnoff, J. C., and Kim, E. S. Evaluation of pulmonary megakaryocytes. *Arch Path 66:*176, 1958.

90. Yin, E. T., and Wessler, S. Evidence for a naturally occurring plasma inhibitor of activated factor X: Its isolation and partial purification. *Thromb Diath Hemorrh 21:*398, 1969.

91. Yin, E. T., and Wessler, S. Heparin-accelerated inhibition of activated factor X by its natural inhibitor. *Biochem Biophys Acta 201:*387, 1970.

92. Yin, E. T., Wessler, S., and Stoll, P. Rabbit plasma inhibitor of the activated species of blood coagulation factor X: Purification and some properties. *J Biol Chem 246:*3694, 1971.

93. Yin, E. T., Wessler, S., and Stoll, P. Biological properties of naturally occurring plasma inhibitor to activated factor X. *J Biol Chem 246:*3703, 1971.

94. Kakkar, V. V., Corrigan, T., Spindler, J., Fossard, D. P., Flute, P. T., Crellin, R. O., Wessler, S., and Yin, E. T. Efficacy of low-doses of heparin in prevention of deep-vein thrombosis after major surgery: A double-blind, randomized trial. *Lancet 2:*101, 1972.

95. Evarts, C. M., and Alfidi, R. J. Thromboembolism after total hip reconstruction: Failure of low dose heparin in prevention. *JAMA 225:*515, 1973.

96. Salzman, E. W. Remarks, Symposium on Pulmonary Embolism. American College of Surgeons Meeting, Chicago, October 1973.

97. Hume, M., Kuriakose, T. X., Zuch, L., and Turner, R. H. [125]I fibrinogen and the prevention of venous thrombosis. *Arch Surg 107:*803, 1973.

98. Chalmers, D. G., Marks, J., Bottomley, J. E., and Lloyd, O. Postoperative prophylactic coagulation: Five-year study in an obstetric and gynaecological unit. *Lancet 2:*220, 1960.

99. Eskeland, G. Prevention of venous thrombosis and pulmonary embolism in injured patients. *Lancet 1:*1035, 1962.

100. Tubiana, R., and Duparc, J. Prevention of thromboembolic complications in orthopaedic and accident surgery. *J Bone Joint Surg 43B:*7, 1961.

101. Milch, E. Berman, L., and Egan, R. W. Bisydroxycoumarin (Dicumarol) prophylaxis. *Arch Surg 83:*444, 1961.

102. Fagan, D. G. Prevention of thromboembolic phenomena following operations on neck of femur. *Lancet 1:*846, 1964.

103. Belding, H. H. Use of anticoagulants in prevention of venous thromboembolic disease in postoperative patients. *Arch Surg 90:*566, 1965.

104. Salzman, E. W., Harris, W. H., DeSanctis, R. W. Anticoagulation for prevention of thromboembolism following fractures of the hip. *N Engl J Med* [unclear]

105. Harris, W. H., Salzman, E. W., and DeSanctis, R. W. The prevention of thromboembolic disease by prophylactic anticoagulation: A controlled study in elective hip surgery. *J Bone Joint Surg 49A:*81, 1967.

106. Skinner, D. B., and Salzman, E. W. Anticoagulant prophylaxis in surgical patients. *Surg Gynecol Obstet 125:*741, 1967.

107. Clagett, G. P., and Salzman, E. W. Prevention of venous thromboembolism in surgical patients. *N Engl J Med 290:*93, 1974.

108. Jorpes, J. E. The chemistry of heparin. *Biochem J 29:*1817, 1935.

109. Jorpes, J. E., Holmgren, H., and Wilander, O. Ueber das Vorkommen von Heparin in den Gefässwänden und in den Augen. *Zsch Mikr-Anat Forsch 42:*279, 1937.

110. Holmgren, H., and Wilander, O. Beitrag zur Kenntnis der Chemie und Funktion der Ehrlichschen Mastzellen. *Zsch Mikr-Anat Forsch 42:*242, 1937.

111. Best, C. H. Preparation of heparin and its use in the first clinical cases. *Circulation 19:*79, 1959.

112. Jorpes, J. E. Heparin, its chemistry, pharmacology and clinical use. *Am J Med 33:*692, 1962.

113. McLean, J. The discovery of heparin. *Circulation 19:*75, 1959.

114. Wright, S. *Samson Wright's Applied Physiology,* ed 11. Revised by Keele, C. A., and Neil, E., with the collaboration of Jepson, J. B. London, Oxford [unclear]

115. Halse, T. *Fibrinolyse.* Freib/Breisg & Aulendorf Württ. E. Cantor, 1948.

116. Von Kaulla, K. N., McDonald, S. T., and Taylor, G. H. The effect of heparin on fibrinolysis. *J Lab Clin Med 48:*952, 1956.

117. Hajjar, G. C., and Moser, K. M. Heparin-fibrinolytic synergism in vivo. *Clin Res 10:*26, 1962.

118. McLean, J. The thromboplastic action of cephalin. *Am J Physiol 41:*250, 1916.

119. Murray, D. W. G., Jaques, L. B., Perret, T. S., and Best, C. H. Heparin and vascular occlusion. *Canad Med Assoc J 35:*621, 1936.

120. Murray, D. W. G., and Best, C. H. Heparin and thrombosis: The present situation. *JAMA 110:*118, 1938.

121. Murray, G. D. W., and Best, C. H. The use of heparin in thrombosis. *Ann Surg 108:*163, 1938.

122. Murray, G., and MacKenzie, R. The effect of heparin on portal thrombosis: Its use in mesenteric thrombosis and following splenectomy. *Canad Med Assoc J 40:*38, 1939.

123. Murray, G. Heparin in surgical treatment of blood vessels. *Arch Surg 40:*307, 1940.

124. Murray, G. D. W. Heparin in thrombosis and embolism. *Br J Surg 27:*567, 1940.

125. Murray, G. Heparin in thrombosis and blood vessel surgery. *Surg Gynecol Obstet 72:*340, 1941.

126. Murray, G., Anticoagulant therapy with heparin. *Am J Med 3:*468, 1947

127. Murray, G. Anticoagulants in venous thrombosis and the prevention of pulmonary embolism. *Surg Gynecol Obstet 84:*665, 1947.

128. Bauer, G. Heparin therapy in acute deep venous thrombosis. *JAMA 131:*196, 1946.

129. Martyn, D. T., and Janes, J. M. Continuous intravenous administration of heparin. *Mayo Clin Proc 46:*347, 1971.

130. Coon, W. W., and Willis, P. S. Deep venous thrombosis and pulmonary embolism. *Am J Cardiol 4:*611, 1959.

131. Bauer, G., Kallner, S., Jorpes, J. E., and Boström, H. Intramuscular administration of heparin. *Acta Med Scan 136:*188, 1950.

132. Engelberg, H. Prolonged anticoagulant therapy with subcutaneously administered aqueous heparin. *Surgery 36:*762, 1954.

133. Harrower, H. W., Hurwitz, A., and Yesner, R. The treatment of thromboembolism with aqueous heparin. *Surg Gynecol Obstet 106:*293, 1958.

134. Duff, I. F., Linman, J. W., and Birch, R. The administration of heparin. *Surg Gynecol Obstet 93:*343, 1951.

135. Loewe, L., Rosenblatt, P., and Hirsch, E. Venous thromboembolic disease. *JAMA 130:*386, 1946.

136. Loewe, L. Anticoagulation therapy with heparin/Pitkin menstruum in thromboembolic disease. *Am J Med 3:*447, 1947.

137. Martin, M., Artz, C., and McCleery, R. S. Use of anticoagulants with special emphasis on heparin in retarding media. *Health Center J 1:*119, 1948.

138. Bauer, G. Thirteen years' experience of heparin therapy. In *Thrombosis and Embolism: First International Conference.* Basel, Schwabe, 1954, p 721.

139. Crane, C. Deep venous thrombosis and pulmonary embolism. *N Engl J Med 257:*147, 1957.

140. Crane, C. The diagnosis and treatment of pulmonary embolism. *Surg Clin North Am 46:*551, 1966.

141. Hoffman, G. C., and Snyder, A. The ground-glass clotting time: A sensitive screening test for blood coagulation defects. *Cleve Clin Quart 33:*107, 1966.

142. Struver, G. P., and Bittner, D. L. The partial thromboplastin (cephalin) time in anticoagulant therapy. *Am J Clin Path 38:*473, 1962.

143. Spector, I., and Corn, M. Control of heparin therapy with activated partial thromboplastin times. *JAMA 201:*157, 1967.

144. Cuono, J. D. Heparin dosage and labeling: Editorial. *Surg Gynecol Obstet 125:*598, 1967.

145. Jaques, L. B. Spontaneous hemorrhage with anticoagulants. *Circulation 25:*130, 1962.

146. Jaques, L. B., Kavanagh, L. W., Lavallée, A. A comparison of biological activities and chemical analysis for various heparin preparations. *Arzneimittel-Forsch 17:*774, 1967.

147. Jaques, L. B. The heparins of various mammalian species and their relative anticoagulant potency. *Science 92:*488, 1940.
148. Jaques, L. B. Standardisation of heparin for clinical use. *Lancet 2:*1315, 1972.
149. Jaques, L. B. Heparin from different sources. *Lancet 2:*1262, 1972.
150. Bangham, D. R., and Woodward, P. M. A colloborative study of heparins from different sources. *Bull WHO 42:*139, 1970.
151. Kramar, J. Stress and capillary resistance (capillary fragility. *Am J Physiol 175:*69, 1953.
152. Kramar, J., Meyers, V. W., and Simay-Kramar, M. Contribution to the physiology of capillary resistance in the human. *J Lab Clin Med 47:*423, 1956.
153. Kramar, J., Meyers, V. W., Simay-Kramar, M., and Wilhelmj, C. M. Immediate capillary stress response. *Am J Physiol 184:*640, 1956.
154. Kramar, J. Endocrine regulation of the capillary resistance. *Science 119:*790, 1954.
155. Aggelar, P. M. Heparin and dicumarol-anticoagulants. Their prophylactic and therapeutic uses. *Cal West Med 64:*71, 1946.
156. Fuller, C. H., Robertson, C. W., and Smithwick, R. H. Management of thromboembolic disease. *N Engl J Med 263:*983, 1960.
157. Nichol, E. S. The risk of hemorrhage in anticoagulant therapy. *Ann West Med Surg 4:*71, 1950.
158. Knight, L. L., and Valentine, E. H. Spontaneous bilateral adrenal hemorrhage: Report of a case occurring during heparin therapy. *JAMA 182:*72, 1962.
159. McDonald, F. D., Myers, A. R., and Pardo, R. Adrenal hemorrhage during anticoagulant therapy. *JAMA 198:*1052, 1966.
160. Cohen, S. M. Massive cerebral hemorrhage following heparin therapy in subacute bacterial endocarditis: Report of 2 cases with review of the literature. *J Mt Sinai Hosp NY 16:*214, 1949.
161. Allen, A. W., In discussion of Lilly, G. D., and Lee, R. M. Complications of anticoagulant therapy. *Surgery 26:*957, 1949.
162. Morrison, F. S., and Wurzel, H. A. Retroperitoneal hemorrhage during heparin therapy. *Am J Cardiol 13:* 329, 1964.
163. Chernoff, A. I. Anaphylactic reaction following injection of heparin. *N Engl J Med 242:*315, 1950.
164. Grolnich, M., and Loewe, L. Report of sensitivity to heparin in a patient. *J Allerg 18:*277, 1947.
165. Wylie, E. J., Gardner, R. E., Johansen, R., and McCorkle, H. J. An experimental study of regional heparinization. *Surgery 28:*29, 1950.
166. Lilly, G. D., and Lee, R. M. Complications of anticoagulant therapy. *Surgery 26:*957, 1949.
167. Martin, C. M., Engstrom, P. F., and Barrett, O. Surreptitious self-administration of heparin. *JAMA 212:*475, 1970.
168. Link, K. P. The anticoagulant from spoiled sweet clover hay. *Harvey Lecture 34:*162, 1943–1944.
169. Link, K. P. The discovery of Dicumarol and its sequels. *Circulation 19:*97, 1959.
170. Roderick, L. T. A problem in the coagulation of blood: "Sweet clover" disease of cattle. *Am J Physiol 96:*413, 1931.
171. Quick, A. J., Stanley-Brown, M., and Bancroft, F. W. A study of the coagulation defect in hemophilia and in jaundice. *Am J Med Soc 190:*501, 1935.
172. Stahmann, M. A., Huebner, C. F., and Link, K. P. Studies on the hemorrhagic sweet clover disease: V. Identification and synthesis of the hemorrhagic agent. *J Biol Chem 138:*513, 1941.
173. Bingham, J. B., Meyer, O. O., and Pohle, F. J. Studies on the hemorrhagic agent 3,3¹ methylene bis(4-hydroxycoumarin): I. Its effect on the prothrombin and coagulation time of the blood of dogs and humans. *Am J Med Soc 202:*563 (Oct) 1941.
174. Butt, H. R., Allen, E. V., and Bollman, J. L. A preparation from spoiled sweet clover [3,3¹ methylene-bis (4-hydroxycoumarin)] which prolongs coagulation and prothrombin time of the blood: Preliminary report of experimental and clinical studies. *Proc Staff Meet Mayo Clin 16:*388 (June 18) 1941.
175. Wright, I. S., Marple, C. D., and Beck, D. F. Report of the Committee for the evaluation of anticoagulants in the treatment of coronary thrombosis with myocardial infarction (A progress report on the statistical analysis of the first 800 cases studied by this committee). *Am Heart J 36:*801, 1948.
176. Zieve, P. D., and Solomon, H. M. Variation in the response of human beings to Vitamin K_1. *J Lab Clin Med 73:*103, 1969.
177. Hume, M., Sevitt, S., and Thomas, D. P. *Venous Thrombosis and Pulmonary Embolism.* Cambridge, Harvard University Press, 1970, p 401.
178. Link, K. P., Overman, R. S., Sullivan, W. R., Huebner, C. F., and Scheel, L. D. Studies on the hemorrhagic sweet clover disease: XI. Hypoprothrombinemia in the rat induced by salicylic acid. *J Biol Chem 147:*463, 1943.
179. Weiss, H. J., Aledort, L. M., Kochwa, S. The effect of salicylates on the hemostatic properties of platelets in man. *J Clin Invest 47:*2169, 1968.
180. Weiner, M., and Dayton, P. G. Effect of barbiturate on coumadin activity. *Circulation 20:*783, 1959.
181. Kazmier, F. J., and Spittell, J. A. Coumarin drug interactions. *Mayo Clin Proc 45:*249, 1970.
182. Koch-Weser, J. Editorial notes: Coumarin necrosis. *Ann Intern Med 68:*1365, 1968.
183. von Hamm, E., Seidensticker, J. F., and Hatfield, G. E. Coumarin-related breast necrosis: A case report and review of the literature. *Ohio State Med J 70:*38, 1974.
184. Gallo, D. G., Bailey, K. R., and Sheffner, A. L. The interaction between cholestyramine and drugs. *Proc Soc Exp Biol Med 120:*60, 1965.

185. Wright, I. S. *The Pathogenesis and Treatment of Thrombosis: With a Clinical and Laboratory Guide to Anticoagulant Therapy* New York Grune & Stratton, 1952.
186. Adams, C. W., and Pass, B. J. Extensive dermatitis due to warfarin sodium (Coumadin). *Circulation 22:*947, 1960.
187. Sheps, S. G., and Gifford, R. W. Urticaria after administration of warfarin sodium. *Am J. Cardiol 3:*118, 1959.
188. Rook, A. Some chemical influences on hair growth and pigmentation. *Br J Derm 77:*115, 1965.
189. Hume, M., Sevitt, S., and Thomas, D. P. *Venous thrombosis and pulmonary embolism.* Cambridge, Harvard University Press, 1970, p 405.
190. DeBakey, M. E. Dicumarin and prophylactic anticoagulants in intravascular thrombosis: An editorial. *Surgery 13:*456, 1943.
191. Duff, I. F., and Shull, W. H. Fatal hemorrhage in Dicumarol poisoning: With report of necropsy. *JAMA 139:*762, 1949.
192. Allen, E. V., Hines, E. A., Kvale, W. F., and Barker, N. W. The use of dicumarol as an anticoagulant: Experience in 2,307 cases. *Ann Intern Med 27:*371, 1942.
193. Rainie, R. C. Complications of anticoagulant therapy: Review of the literature and report of a case. *N Engl J Med 250:*810, 1954.
194. Flaxman, H. Drug fatalities. *JAMA 147:*377, 1951.
195. Klingensmith, W. Surgical implications of hemorrhage during anticoagulant therapy: Collective review. *Surg Gynecol Obstet 125:*1333, 1967.
196. Hafner, C. D., Cranley, J. J., Krause, R. J., and Strasser, E. S. Anticoagulant ileus. *JAMA 182:*947, 1962.
197. Amador, E. Adrenal hemorrhage during anticoagulant therapy: A clinical and pathological study of ten cases. *Ann Intern Med 63:*559, 1965.
198. Barron, K. D., and Fergusson, F. Intracranial hemorrhage as a complication of anticoagulant therapy. *Neurology 9:*447, 1959.
199. Wells, C. E., and Urrea, D. Cerebrovascular accidents in patients receiving anticoagulant drugs. *Arch Neurol 3:*553, 1960.
200. Weiner, L. M., and Nathanson, M. Relationship of subdural hematomas to anticoagulant therapy. *Arch Neurol 6:*282, 1962.
201. Strang, R. R., and Tovi, D. Subdural haematomas complicating anticoagulant therapy. *Br Med J 1:*845, 1962.
202. Dooley, D. M., and Perlmutter, I. Spontaneous intracranial hematomas in patients receiving anticoagulation therapy. *JAMA 187:*396, 1964.
203. Finney, L. A., and Gholston, D. Cerebral aneurysm rupture during anticoagulant therapy. *JAMA 200:*1127, 1967.
204. Cloward, R. B., and Yuhl, E. T. Spontaneous intraspinal hemorrhage and paraplegia complicating dicumarol therapy. *Neurology 5:*600, 1955.
205. Strain, R. E. Spinal epidural hematoma in patients on anticoagulant therapy. *Ann Surg 159:*507, 1964.
206. Pollard, J. W., Hamilton, M. J., Christensen, N. A., and Achor, R. W. P. Problems associated with long-term anticoagulant therapy: Observations in 139 cases. *Circulation 25:*311, 1962.
207. Just-Viera, J. O., and Yeager, G. H. Protection from thrombosis in large veins. *Surg Gynecol Obstet 118:*354, 1964.
208. Hunt, P. S., Reeve, T. S., and Hollings, R. M. A "standard" experimental thrombus: Observations on its production, pathology, and response to heparin and thrombectomy. *Surgery 59:*812, 1966.
209. Johnson, D. C., and Reeve, T. S. The effect and clinical significance of low molecular weight and clinical dextran on an experimental venous thrombus in sheep. *Ann Surg 168:*123, 1968.
210. Bernard, H. R., Powers, S. R., Leather, R. P., and Clark, W. R. A prospective double-blind study of clinical dextran in thrombophlebitis. *Surgery 65:*191, 1969.
211. Mole, R. H. Fibrinolysin and the fluidity of the blood *post mortem. J Path Bact 60:*413, 1948.
212. Cooper, J. F. Collective review: The surgical aspects of fibrinolysis. *Int Abst Surg 108:*417, 1959.
213. Cohen, S. A., and Warren, R. Fibrinolysis. *N Engl J Med 264:*79, 1961.
214. Morgagni, J. B. *The Seats and Causes of Diseases.* London, 1769, vol. 3, book 4, letter 53, p 185.
215. Hunter, J. *A Treatise on the Blood, Inflammation, and Gunshot Wounds.* London, 1794, p 26.
216. Weiss, A. E. Personal communication, January 1974.
217. Virchow, R. *Die Cellularpathologie,* ed 4. Berlin, 1871, p 194.
218. Green, J. R. Note on action of sodium chloride in dissolving fibrin. *J Physiol 8:*372, 1887.
219. Dastre, A. Fibrinolyse dans le sang. *Arch de Physiol Norm et Path 5:*661, 1893.
220. Morawitz, P. Ueber einige postmortale Blutveränderungen. *Beitr Chem Phys Path 8:*1, 1906.
221. Opie, E. L., and Barker, B. I. Leucoprotease and antileukoprotease in mammals and birds. *J Exp Med 9:*207, 1907.
222. Yudin, S. S. Transfusion of cadaver blood. *JAMA 106:*997, 1936.
223. Sherry, S., Fletcher, A. P., and Alkjaersig, N. Fibrinolysis and fibrinolytic activity in man. *Physiol Rev 38:*343, 1959.
224. Lewis, J. H., and Doyle, A. P. Effects of epsilon aminocaproic acid on coagulation and fibrinolytic mechanisms. *JAMA 188:*176, 1964.
225. Astrup, T. Fibrinolysis in the organism. *Blood 11:*781, 1956.
226. Johnson, A. J., and Newman, J. The fibrinolytic system in health and disease. *Hemt Sem 1:*401, 1964.

227. Fletcher, A. P., Alkjaersig, N., Sherry, S., Genton, E., Hirsh, J., and Bachmann, F. The development of urokinase as thrombolytic agent. *J Lab Clin Med 65:*713, 1965.

228. Sherry, S. Fibrinolysis in health and disease. *Res Phys 9:*79, 1968.

229. Von Kaulla, K. N. Chemistry of thrombolysis: Human fibrinolytic enzymes. In *American Lecture Series.* Springfield, IL, Thomas, 1963.

230. Sherry, S. Present concepts of the fibrinolytic system. *Scand J Haemat 7:*70, 1965.

231. Selye, H. *Thrombohemorrhagic Phenomena.* Springfield, IL, Thomas, 1966.

232. Sherry, S. Fibrinolysis. *Ann Rev Med 19:*247, 1968.

233. Robbins, K. C., Summaria, L., Elwyn, D., and Barlow, G. H. Further studies on the purification and characterization of human plasminogen and plasmin. *J Biol Chem 240:*541, 1965.

234. Sherry, S., Alkjaersig, N., and Fletcher, A. P. Activity of plasmin and streptokinase-activator on substituted arginine and lysine esters. *Thromb Diath Haemmorrh 16:*18, 1966.

235. Shamash, Y., and Rimon, A. The plasmin inhibitors of plasma: I. A method for their estimation. *Thromb Diath Haemorrh 12:*119, 1964.

236. Rimon, A., Shamash, Y., and Shapiro, B. The plasmin inhibitors of human plasma: IV. Its action on plasmin, trypsin, chymotrypsin, and thrombin. *J Biol Chem 241:*5102, 1966.

237. Shamash, Y., and Rimon, A. The plasmin inhibitors of human plasma: III. Purification and partial characterization. *Biochem Biophys Acta 121:*35, 1966.

238. Alkjaersig, N. In Johnson, S. A., Monto, R. W., Rebuck, J. W., and Horn, R. C. (eds.) *Henry Ford Symposium: Blood Platelets.* Boston, Little, Brown, 1961, pp 329–336.

239. Holemans, R., and Gross, R. Influence of blood platelets on fibrinolysis. *Thromb Diath Haemorrh 6:*196, 1961.

240. Tillett, W. S., and Garner, R. L. Fibrinolytic activity of hemolytic streptococci. *J Exp Med 58:*485, 1933.

241. Tillett, W. S., Johnson, A. J., and McCarty, W. R. The intravenous infusion of streptococcal fibrinolytic principle (streptokinase) into patients. *J Clin Invest 34:*169, 1955.

242. Tillett, W. S., and Sherry, S. The effect in patients of streptococcal fibrinolysin (streptokinase) and streptococcal desoxyribonuclease on fibrinous, purulent, and sanguinous pleural effusions. *J. Clin Invest 28:*173, 1949.

243. Tillett, W. S., Sherry, S., Christensen, L. R., Johnson, A. J., and Hazelhurst, G. Streptococcal enzymatic debridement. *Ann Surg 131:*12, 1958.

244. Milstone, H. A factor in normal blood which participates in streptococcal fibrinolysis. *J Immun Balt 42:*109, 1941.

245. Kaplan, M. H. The nature and role of the lytic factor in hemolytic streptococcal fibrinolysin. *Proc Soc Exp Biol NY 57:*40, 1944.

246. Christensen, L. R. Streptococcal fibrinolysis: A proteolytic reaction due to a serum enzyme activated by streptococcal fibrinolysin. *J Gen Physiol 28:*263, 1945.

247. Christensen, L. R., and MacLeod, C. M. A proteolytic enzyme of serum: Characterization, activation, and reaction with inhibitors. *J Gen Physiol 28:*559, 1945.

248. Lewis, J. H., and Ferguson, J. H. Studies on a proteolytic enzyme system of blood: I. Inhibition of fibrinolysin. *J Clin Invest 29:*486, 1950.

249. Sherry, S. Urokinase. *Ann Intern Med 69:*415, 1968.

250. Johnson, A. J., and McCarty, W. R. Lysis of artificially induced intravascular clots in man by intravascular infusion of streptokinase. *J Clin Invest 38:*1627, 1959.

251. Fletcher, A. P., Alkjaersig, N., and Sherry, S. The maintenance of a sustained thrombolytic state in man: I. Induction and effects. *J Clin Invest 38:*1096, 1959.

252. Fletcher, A. P., Sherry, S., Alkjaersig, N., Smyrniotis, F. E., and Jick, S. The maintenance of a sustained thrombolytic state in man: II. Clinical observations on patients with myocardial infarction and other thromboembolic disorders. *J Clin Invest 38:*1111, 1959.

253. Sherry, S. Streptokinase therapy for thromboembolic occlusive vascular disease, editorial. *Ann Inter Med 74:*437, 1971.

254. Stengle, J. M. Present status of thrombolysis in the United States. In Mammen, E. F., Anderson, G. F., and Barnhart, M. I. (eds.) *Thrombolytic Therapy.* Stuttgart, Schattauer, 1971, p 159.

255. Hirsh, J., O'Sullivan, E. F., and Martin, M. Evaluation of a standard dosage schedule with streptokinase. *Blood 35:*341, 1970.

256. Diaz, C., and LeVeen, H. H. Enzymatic clot lysis in the treatment of venous and arterial occlusive disease. In Mammen, E. F., Anderson, G. F., and Barnhart, M. I. (eds.) Stuttgart, Schattauer, 1971, p 179.

257. Timmes, J. J., Demos, N. J., Chong, S. I., and Müller-Ehrenberg, K. Thrombolysis in acute arterial and venous occlusions. In Mammen, E. F., Anderson, G. F., and Barnhart, M. I. (eds.) *Thrombolytic Therapy.* Stuttgart, Schattauer, 1971, p 193.

258. Mavor, G. E., Bennett, B., Galloway, J. M. D., and Karmody, A. M. Streptokinase in ileofemoral venous thrombosis. *Br J Surg 56:*564, 1969.

259. Tsapogas, M. J., Peabody, R. A., Wu, K. T., Karmody, A. M., Devaraj, K. T., and Eckert, C. Controlled study of thrombolytic therapy in deep vein thrombosis. *Surgery 74:*973, 1973.

260. Boyles, P. W., and Meyer, W. H. Blood changes following thrombolysin therapy. In Mammen, E. F., Anderson, G. F., and Barnhart, M. I. (eds.) Stuttgart, Schattauer, 1971, p 301.
261. Ashford, A., Ross, J. W., and Southgate, P. Pharmacology and toxicology of a defibrinating substance from Malayan pit viper venom. *Lancet 1:* 486, 1968.
262. Weiss, A. E. Personal communication, January 1974.
263. Bell, W. R., Pitney, W. R., Oakley, C. M., and Goodwin, J. F. Therapeutic defibrination in the treatment of thrombotic disease. *Lancet 1:*490, 1968.
264. Sharp, A. A., Warren, B. A., and Paxton, A. M. Anticoagulant therapy with a purified fraction of Malayan pit viper venom. *Lancet 1:*493, 1968.

265. Bell, W. R. Current status of therapy with Arvin. In Mammen, E. F., Anderson, G. F., and Barnhart M. I. (eds.) *Thrombolytic Therapy,* Stuttgart, Schattauer, 1971, p 371.
266. Pitney, W. R., Bray, C., Holt, P. J. L., and Bolton, G. Acquired resistance to treatment with Arvin. *Lancet 1:*79, 1969.
267. Kakkar, V. V., Flanc, C., Howe, C. T., O'Shea, M., and Flute, P. T. Treatment of deep vein thrombosis: A trial of heparin, streptokinase, and Arvin. *Br Med J 1:*806, 1969.
268. Fairbairn, J. F., Juergens, J. L., and Spittell, J. A., Jr., eds. Allen, E. V., Barker, N. W., Hines, E. A. *Peripheral Vascular Diseases,* ed 4. Philadelphia, Saunders, 1972, pp 108–109.
269. Donahoe, J. F. Personal communication, December 1973.

6
Operative Management of Acute Venous Thrombosis and Thrombophlebitis

Raymond J. Krause and

John J. Cranley

Surgical management of venous thrombosis may be prophylactic or therapeutic. Prophylactic procedures include any form of interruption, partial or complete, of a portion of the deep venous system in order to prevent the passage of a detached embolus from the site of origin to the lung. Therapeutic measures include excision of phlebitic veins, thrombectomy, and pulmonary artery embolectomy.

PROPHYLACTIC PROCEDURES

INTERRUPTION OF THE FEMORAL VEIN

Interruption of the femoral vein in the groin was first described by Homans in 1934.[1] It rapidly became a popular method of preventing pulmonary embolus, and Linton reported 15 years later[2] that more than 1000 persons had been treated with this method at Massachusetts General Hospital without a single instance of serious interference with the circulation of the extremity and with an operative mortality of zero. Two deaths occurred following bilateral femoral vein interruption in this series; in 1 patient the superficial vein had been interrupted, and in the other the common femoral vein was interrupted. Neither patient died of a sudden massive pulmonary embolus but instead succumbed to the cumulative effects of relatively small emboli arising from clots in the iliac veins superimposed on thrombi in the veins prior to femoral vein interruption.

Effectiveness of Femoral Vein Interruption

Division and ligation of the superficial femoral vein (the most popular operation) effectively prevents a thrombus formed in the popliteal or superficial femoral vein from embolizing to the lung; in this basic sense, there are no failures. When pulmonary emboli occur following this operation, they come from some other source, e.g., the ipsilateral deep femoral or iliac veins, the contralateral deep venous tree, the vena cava, or the site of ligation itself (in the instance when a thrombus forms just above the ligature and then embolizes). Such failures may be better labeled as secondary to imprecise diagnosis or faulty technique.

It would serve no useful purpose to review the statistics available on femoral vein ligation, since in no true sense can these be regarded as statistically valid. It might be of value, however, to examine the reasons they should be regarded with skepticism.

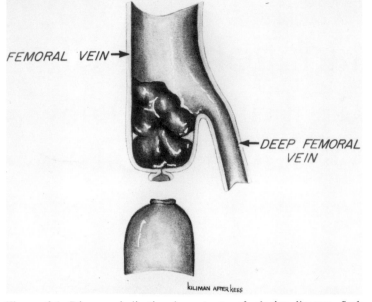

FEMORAL VEIN →

→ DEEP FEMORAL VEIN

KILIMAN AFTER KEES

Figure 6-1. Diagram indicating importance of placing ligature flush with deep femoral vein or large tributary; otherwise, clot may form in the cul-de-sac.

DIAGNOSTIC ERRORS

During the 1940s and 1950s when femoral vein interruption was at the height of its popularity, the diagnosis of deep venous thrombosis was made almost entirely on clinical grounds. As has been seen (Chapters 3 and 4), this introduced a diagnostic error of 30 to 50 per cent. If one-third or one-half of the patients undergoing a procedure such as femoral vein interruption for thrombophlebitis actually had no thrombi in the deep venous system of the distal extremity, the beneficial effects of the operation, as far as the prevention of pulmonary embolism is concerned, would be erroneously magnified. Likewise, the incidence of postphlebitic sequelae in such clot-free extremities would be falsely reduced by the same factor; most vascular surgeons would concur that the degree of postoperative swelling is related more closely to the presence and extent of deep venous thrombosis than to the ligation and division of the vein *per se*. In corroboration of this, O'Keefe *et al.*[3] found minimal, almost undetectable sequelae in patients in whom the superficial femoral vein had been divided and

Figure 6-2. A and **B.** Phlebogram of patient taken 9 years after division and ligation of superficial femoral vein. (*From Hafner,* et al. Ann Surg 161:*414, 1965.*)

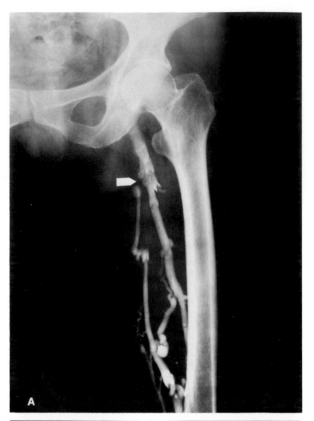

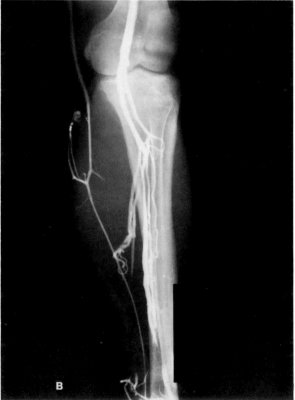

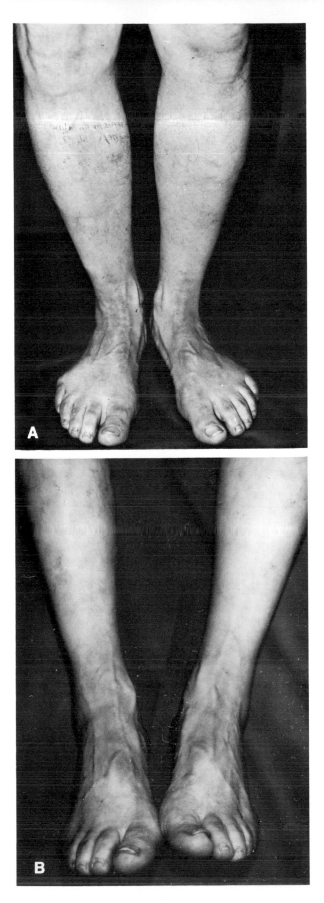

Figure 6-3. A. Photo taken 7 years following division and ligation of superficial femoral veins bilaterally and ligation of left long saphenous vein for superficial thrombophlebitis that extended to the saphenofemoral junction and pulmonary embolism. Patient wore elastic stockings. **B.** Photo taken April 1974, approximately 20 years postoperatively.

Figure 6-4. Photo taken May 1974, 14 years following division and ligation of right common femoral vein near inguinal ligament, thrombectomy of saphenous vein, and partial thrombectomy of common femoral and external iliac veins for superficial and deep thrombophlebitis of right lower extremity. Right limb is only slightly larger than left, on which no surgical treatment of deep veins was performed.

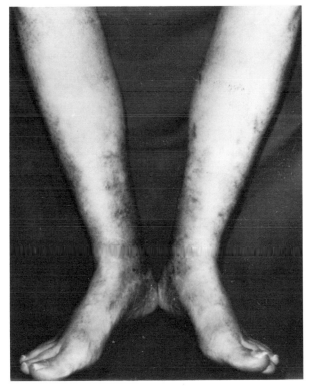

ligated prophylactically. The same source of error is present in reports of successful or unsuccessful treatment of thrombophlebitis by conservative measures if such data come from an era when objective methods of diagnosing venous thrombosis were not readily available. Statistically valid data can be obtained only on patients who are treated for clots in the venous system proved by radiologic evidence or other objective tests.

OTHER PITFALLS

We have seen some patients with pain, swelling, and tenderness of the calf secondary to thrombus in the iliac system whose leg and thigh veins were proved completely patent by phlebography. In this instance, the diagnosis is correct, but the location of the clot is not apparent on clinical examination. Obviously, such a patient is afforded no protection against pulmonary embolism by ligation of the superficial femoral vein.

Not all surgeons who practiced femoral vein interruption ligated the vein at the same location. The most popular choice was to divide and ligate the superficial femoral vein at its termination. Some surgeons placed the ligature on the common femoral vein below one of the large medial collateral tributaries; others ligated it below the saphenous vein; still others actually ligated and divided the vein above the saphenofemoral junction, which would seem to be deliberately inviting disaster as far as postoperative swelling is concerned.

Failure to ligate the vein flush with a large tributary vein will leave a cul-de-sac in which fresh thrombus can form a nidus for a new, large, soft clot (Fig. 6-1).

BILATERAL FEMORAL VEIN LIGATION

The policy of always performing bilateral femoral vein ligation is no longer necessary. If one limb is proved normal by objective diagnostic tests, anticoagulant therapy can be expected to prevent the formation of a thrombus in this unaffected extremity.

Because of the above factors, femoral vein interruption has for the most part been abandoned; however, it is possible that it may regain its role as a clinically useful procedure as more precise diagnoses are made (Figs. 6-2 and 6-3).

Case Report 6-1

This patient was first seen in September 1955 for superficial thrombophlebitis of the right leg. He stated that his mother had varicose veins and that there was a familial history of venous disease, viz., his mother, his aunt, and one of his three sisters had had thrombophlebitis. His own difficulties began in 1944 when he developed "pneumonia," followed by bilateral swelling of the lower extremities. He recalled that he had been off of his feet for 7 months at that time. His legs remained significantly swollen for

approximately 2 years, after which the swelling subsided. He had had varicose veins in his right lower extremity for approximately 8 years; once during this period he had had an attack of superficial thrombophlebitis. The phlebitic veins had been excised by another surgeon.

On physical examination in 1955, the superficial thrombophlebitis was subsiding, and it was recommended that he wear a heavyweight elastic stocking. He was then returned to his family physician. He was seen again in July 1960 while hospitalized for an attack of recurrent chest pain believed by his physicians and ourselves to be due to recurrent small pulmonary emboli. At that time, medical studies were unrevealing, except for chronic duodenal ulcer and diverticula of the colon. His chief complaint was pain and swelling of the right groin, associated with superficial thrombophlebitis extending into the femoral triangle. An operation was performed on the day of consultation. The saphenous vein was thrombosed; when it was opened, the clots were soft and appeared to be recent. The saphenous vein was traced to the saphenofemoral junction; the femoral vein was also thrombosed. The saphenous vein was opened just proximal to its termination, and an effort was made to remove the clots, with only partial success. The common femoral vein was then opened, and it too was filled with clots that appeared to be recently formed and without organization; however, fibrous septums also were present, suggesting earlier thrombophlebitis. The clots extended up to the external iliac vein, and since it was impossible to remove them, the common femoral vein was divided near the inguinal ligament. The patient was immediately placed on anticoagulant therapy postoperatively. This was maintained for several months by his family physician in his home city, where a few years later the patient underwent surgical excision of his varicosities. Recently he traveled to a major clinic, where further excisional therapy was recommended; at this time the patient decided to return to us for another opinion. He had not progressed to ulceration in the interim since 1960, and although there were some visible varicosities, it did not appear worthwhile to us for him to undergo further surgical treatment; instead, we recommended the heavyweight elastic stocking which had been prescribed 14 years earlier and which he had worn for a few years.

There are several points to be considered. First, despite a family history of thrombophlebitis and several spontaneous episodes of thrombophlebitis, no underlying cause emerged during the 30 years since his initial bout. Secondly, despite the facts that the

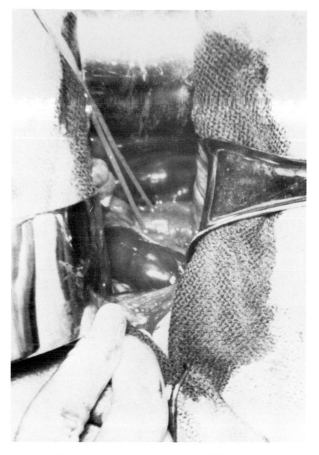

Figure 6-5. Tape is around vena cava. Vein closer to the surgeon, darker and apparently larger, is the ovarian vein.

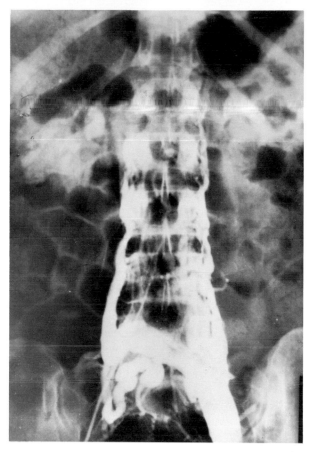

Figure 6-6. Collateral circulation around vena cava. While collateral circulation appears to be extensive, it is doubtful that an embolus small enough to pass through these collaterals would have a significant effect on the lung.

initial episode appears to have been severe and both his right saphenous and common femoral veins had been divided, he did not develop ulceration over a period of 30 years. Finally, the right limb is only slightly larger than the left (Fig. 6-4), despite the fact that the major veins were divided in the inguinal area but no surgical treatment was carried out on the deep veins of the left lower extremity.

LIGATION OF THE INFERIOR VENA CAVA

The first reported ligation of the inferior vena cava was inadvertently performed by Kocher in 1883[4, 5] during the dissection of metastatic carcinomatous retroperitoneal lymph nodes; at autopsy a ligature was found about the inferior vena cava.[5] The second case was reported in 1885 by Billroth,[4, 5] who, again accidentally, tied the vena cava, mistaking it for the renal vein, his patient died an hour postoperatively. Bottini reported the first successful case in 1893.[6] In 1937 Krotoski[7] collected 48 cases of

total ligation of the inferior vena cava, the majority of which had been carried out either inadvertently or for trauma.

In 1945 three reports[5, 8, 9] appeared on the use of ligation of the inferior vena cava for the prevention of pulmonary embolism, the first patient in each series having been operated on in 1944. In 1958 Dale[10] reviewed 468 cases reported in the literature in the United States, exclusive of all series with fewer than 5 patients. Currently the number of patients so treated is very likely incalculable since caval ligation for thromboembolic disease is widely used and well established.

Effectiveness of Vena Cava Ligation

Ligation of the inferior vena cava for thromboembolic disease was introduced as a lifesaving measure, to be resorted to as definitive therapy. In 944 reported vena cava ligations collected from the

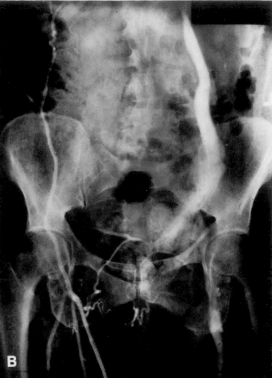

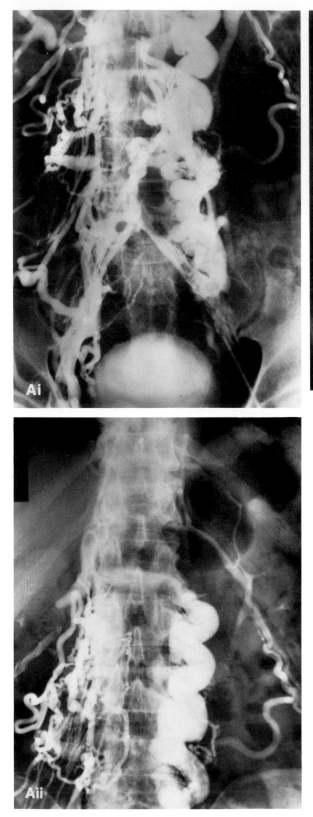

United States literature,[5, 8–10, 11–32] 4 patients were known to have died from pulmonary embolism in the postoperative period. Twenty of the reports, comprising 486 operations, reported no postoperative fatal pulmonary emboli; four reports (458 cases) indicated four instances of fatal pulmonary emboli (0.9 per cent). Taking all 944 reports together, recurrent pulmonary emboli number 0.4 per cent. Thus, the reported failure rate in the United States is less than one-half of 1 per cent. On the basis of these published results, it can be said that ligation of the inferior vena cava is highly effective in preventing fatal pulmonary emboli.

RECURRENT PULMONARY EMBOLI

When failures occur, they may be attributed to emboli arising from the right heart, to thrombus formation above the site of ligature, or to emboli passing through large veins, such as the ovarian, or through any dilated collateral vein. Indeed, we have observed the ovarian vein to be as large as the vena cava itself (Fig. 6-5); in such an instance, a large lethal embolus unquestionably could be carried to the lung. A small embolus is not likely to prove fatal, except in a patient with severe cardiopul-

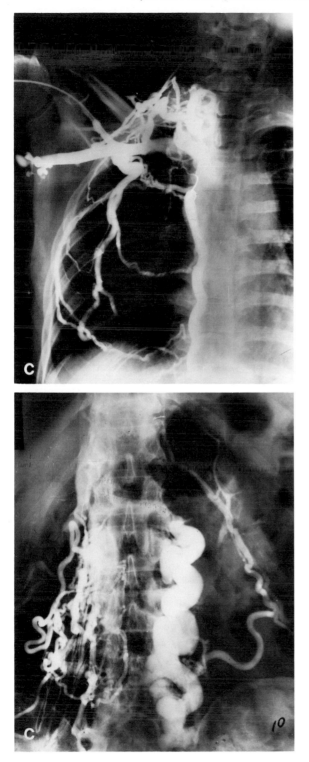

monary disease. (See Chapter 8.) Most probably, the majority of emboli that pass through the collateral channels are small (Fig. 6-6). Occasionally, however, very large collateral channels exist which could easily carry a large clot. Figure 6-7*A* shows a venocavogram taken 10 years after vena cava ligation, disclosing huge collateral veins that could well carry a clot. However, the patient's complaint was large, painful abdominal varices which were excised with relief. A second patient (Fig. 6-7*B*) with similar symptoms had relief from excision of abdominal varices which followed spontaneous thrombosis of the vena cava which was not treated surgically. A third patient (Fig 6-7*C*) with obstruction of undetermined etiology of both venae cavae is discussed in the following case report.

Case Report 6-2

This patient was first seen in the fall of 1963. On September 30, 1963 an axillary phlebogram was obtained; on the same day she underwent excisional biopsy of a mass in the neck. The phlebogram showed compression of the superior vena cava, conceivably by the mass, which proved to be malignant. On October 9, 1963, a venocavogram was obtained, which demonstrated a hugely dilated ovarian vein and obstruction of the inferior vena cava. On October 15 she underwent thyroidectomy and radical neck dissection for carcinoma of the thyroid. She was then treated with radioiodine. In May 1974 she is well. She has had no symptoms, such as swelling,

Figure 6-7. Ai. and **Aii.** Venocavogram taken 10 years after vena cava ligation. Patient's complaint was large, painful abdominal varices which were excised with relief. **Ai.** Early phase showing an enlarged vein, probably spermatic. **Aii.** Later phase. (See also Figure 6-39.) **B.** Second patient with spontaneous vena cava obstruction that was not treated surgically. Venocavogram in follow-up demonstrates large ovarian vein which could admit emboli of significant size. **C.** Patient was seen in 1963 for carcinoma of thyroid, which was surgically treated. Film demonstrates compression of superior vena cava, possibly from the thyroid mass. There was also obstruction of inferior vena cava. Inferior venocavogram visualizes a huge ovarian vein, which could be the route of a lethal embolus. **Bottom.** Patient is well 11 years after thyroidectomy, without swelling of either upper or lower extremities. No definite cause for obstruction of either superior or inferior venae cavae has been determined. She has had no symptoms referable to the cava obstructions.

TABLE 6-1. Collected Series Reporting Operative Mortality and Deaths from Recurrent Pulmonary Emboli

AUTHORS AND DATE OF PUBLICATION	NO. CASES	OPERATIVE MORTALITY	FATAL RECURRENT EMBOLI
1. O'Neil 1945	8	0	0
2. Northway and Buxton 1945	10	0	0
3. Gaston and Folsom 1945	2	0	0
4. Moses 1946	21	9	0
5. Thebaut and Ward 1947	36	2	0
6. Veal, Hussey, and Barnes 1947	30	3	0
7. Connerley and Heintzelman 1949	10	2	0
8. Shea and Robertson 1951	37	2	0
9. Collins, Norton, Nelson, Weinstein, Collins, and Webster 1952	70	8	0
10. Zollinger and Teachnor 1952	20	0	0
11. Owens 1952	12	0	0
12. Payne 1953	5	0	0
13. Madden 1954	18	0	0
14. Kirtley, Riddell, and Hamilton 1955	34	4	0
15. Bowers and Leb 1955	33	5	0
16. Dale 1958 and 1962	17	0	0
17. Zoeckler 1960	14	0	0
18. Bergan, Kinnaird, Koons, and Trippel 1965	11	1	0
19. Stevens, Fitzpatrick, Stewart, and Burdette 1965	41	8	0
20. Nabseth and Moran 1965	71	10	1
21. Mozes, Bogokowsky, Antebi, Tzur, and Penchas 1966	118	14	1
22. Amador, Li, and Crane 1968	119	18	1*
23. Pollak, Sparks, and Barker 1973	57	1	0
24. Cranley 1974	150	13	1
Totals	944	100 (10.5%)	4 (0.4%)

* One other death was caused by an embolism considered to be from thrombus found in the heart at autopsy.

of her upper or lower extremities, referable to the obstruction of the venae cavae. The exact cause of the obstruction of the cavae is still not known.

Parrish et al.[33] studied the effectiveness of vena cava ligation in dogs; in 16 of 17 instances, injection of radiopaque clot into the common femoral vein resulted in the development of pulmonary emboli. Also, in 6 patients studied by cavography after vena cava ligation, prominent collateral venous channels capable of transmitting small- and medium-sized emboli were visualized. Nevertheless, only 1 patient was believed to have had recurrent multiple pulmonary emboli after ligation of the vena cava. McIntyre et al.[34] reported a patient with nonfatal pulmonary embolus proved by lung scan and pulmonary angiography. In a patient at the Massachusetts General Hospital,[35] fatal pulmonary embolism occurred 18 days postoperatively, and a fresh, friable, granular, adherent thrombus 2 cm

in diameter was found just above the site of ligation. Reporting a large series from Jerusalem, Mozes et al.[36] described four recurrences (one fatal) of pulmonary embolism after ligation in 118 patients, a percentage of 3.4; however, the fatal embolus was shown at autopsy to have arisen from the right heart. Gurewich et al.[37] reported a pulmonary embolism recurrence rate of approximately 20 per cent following caval ligation. Their results were challenged by Moran and Nabseth[38] and by Thomas[39] for not indicating the population at risk and for failure to describe the operative techniques. A more serious criticism may be raised because these nonsurgical specialists reported on 9 cases, but in only 1 patient was the precise source of the recurrent emboli found at autopsy. In a second patient, who died of progressive cor pulmonale secondary to multiple pulmonary emboli 4 years after ligation, a recent embolus, believed to have arisen in a leg vein, was found in the lung at autopsy. Moran and Nabseth[38] corrected the actual recurrence rate from "approximately 20 per cent" to 9.2 per cent. This percentage is in line with the findings of Amador et al.,[30] who reported on 37 autopsies of patients who underwent ligation of the inferior vena cava, 3 of whom (8 per cent) showed significant recurrent pulmonary embolism. Reporting on a series in 1964, Crane[40] found a 2 per cent recurrence rate after caval ligation, including a 1 per cent recurrence of fatal pulmonary embolism. In our experience, recurrent pulmonary embolism was proved in 1 patient[32] (0.6 per cent), who died of massive embolism 5 months after ligation. He had untreated, uncontrolled polycythemia and entered the hospital with a hemoglobin of 23 gm.

The majority of reports (Table 6-1) in the United States literature seems to confirm the effectiveness of vena cava ligation in the prevention of pulmonary embolism.

OPERATIVE MORTALITY

The collective operative mortality, including all deaths from any cause during the postoperative and hospitalization period, is 10 per cent (Table 6-1). In very few of these patients, however, might the operation *per se* be considered the cause of death. Death on the operating table has occurred in 2 of our patients (1.3 per cent). Two intraoperative deaths have been reported by Thebaut and Ward[12]; in such instances the operation was performed too late, i.e., when the lungs of the patients were already filled with multiple old and new emboli. These deaths must be attributed not to the surgical procedure but rather to the inability or failure to subject the patient to operative therapy in time. The operative trauma of caval ligation is not great. On the contrary, the surgeon is relieved that the patient is being anesthetized and an endotracheal tube is being inserted, because during the operation and for up to 24 hours thereafter, as long as the endotracheal tube is in place, the patient's lungs can be fully aerated in the absence of a new embolus. Furthermore, throughout the intraoperative and postoperative periods, the patient's anxiety, effort, and strain are relieved by anesthesia and analgesics. He may have arrived in the operating room in a moribund state, however, once unconscious and intubated, his anxiety and alarm vanish and he no longer needs to strain for breath. The sometimes

dramatic improvement following vena cava ligation may be attributed, at least in part, to the interval during which the patient has been adequately ventilated while the natural processes of resolution or impaction of the emboli more distally in the lung have occurred.

OPERATIVE TECHNIQUE

In the majority of our patients the retroperitoneal muscle-splitting incision of Madden was used;[21, 41] in a few, the approach was transabdominal. In all ligations, umbilical tape was used; in every retroperitoneal approach an attempt was made to ligate

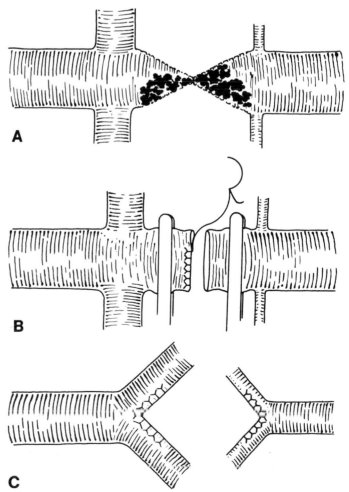

Figure 6-8. A. Ligature placed around the vena cava midway between renal and lumbar veins can produce a cul-de-sac both proximally and distally, which may contain soft clot. **B.** Preferred method in which vena cava is divided between noncrushing clamps and its ends oversewn. **C.** When clamps are released, retraction of vessel eliminates the cul-de-sac.

A

B

C

the vessel just distal to a large lumbar tributary, and in the abdominal approach, just distal to the renal vein. In a woman with pelvic thrombophlebitis, the transabdominal approach was used so that both ovarian veins could be occluded. In a desperately ill patient, it is not safe to try to get close to the renal veins through the retroperitoneal incision. In better surgical candidates, a transabdominal interruption can be performed; it is our choice to divide and ligate the vena cava just below the renal vein in order to eliminate a cul-de-sac and to improve collateral flow (Fig. 6-8). Two operative complications must be avoided: (1) *hemorrhage from a torn lumbar vein* (a helpful maneuver to protect against this mishap is simply to grasp the vena cava once with an atraumatic forceps and to draw it toward the operator; the tenting-up of the vena cava permits the operator to slip a blunt-nosed large vascular clamp around the vena cava itself under direct vision while watching out for lumbar veins); and (2) *shock on the table from trapping of the blood in the lower portions of the body* (this frequently alluded-to complication has not been encountered in our experience).

In the moribund or desperately ill patient, an extraperitoneal approach can be accomplished within 15 to 25 minutes; however, no undue haste is called for, as long as the patient is being ventilated by the anesthesiologist. (Compare the discussion in section on Operative Mortality.)

ANOMALOUS VENA CAVA

Milloy *et al.*[42] have studied the variations in the inferior caval veins and in their renal and lumbar communications; while variation is almost the rule rather than the exception, the surgically important anatomic anomalies can be divided into two major classifications: transposition of the vena cava or sinistration, and doubling. The frequency of transposition or left-sided vena cava[43] is not known exactly but has been estimated as 0.2 per cent by Reis and Esenther[44] and 0.45 per cent by Gladstone.[45] Bilateral inferior vena cava (Fig. 6-9), often quite asymmetric, is said to occur in 1 per cent of the population.[43, 46] Dardik *et al.*[47] have reported a rare type of anomalous inferior vena cava, viz., a "C-pattern" variation. They point out that recognition of anomalous venae cavae is clinically important and that recurrent pulmonary embolization following standard ligation or plication should suggest

bilaterality of the caval system. Further interruption on the left side may then be required. The C-pattern inferior vena cava may present to the unsuspecting surgeon as agenesis, leading to incompletion of his intended procedures. Radiologic study should be made during the preoperative evaluation.

PATHOPHYSIOLOGIC EFFECTS OF LIGATION OF THE INFERIOR VENA CAVA

Maraan and Taber[48] reported on the falling cardiac output in dogs following temporary occlusion of the vena cava, which returned to normal in 10 to 15 minutes. Gazzaniga *et al.*[49] studied this problem extensively in a group of patients at Peter Bent Brigham Hospital who had undergone ligation of the inferior vena cava between 1963 and 1965. Of the 71 patients, 46 had heart disease; of this subgroup, 24 (34 per cent) developed oliguria and hypotension postoperatively. In 8 of these patients with cardiac disease, death occurred from acute renal failure. Subsequently, Gazzaniga and associates studied 7 patients who were undergoing ligation of the inferior vena cava. Venous pressures in the superior and inferior venae cavae showed consistently predictable patterns. Central venous pressure in the superior vena cava fell immediately upon ligation of the inferior vena cava and remained at low levels (3 to 5 cm H_2O) for approximately 8 hours postoperatively; it gradually returned to normal in the ensuing days. The inferior caval pressure below the ligature in 3 patients rose immediately after ligation and then fell progressively toward normal in the next 8 hours. In all patients, colloid replacement was necessary after ligation, and in 3 patients, additional plasma or whole blood was needed during the remainder of the 24-hour period, an average of 730 cc of plasma and 140 cc of whole blood being administered in the first 8 hours. Diminished hourly urine output, hypotension, and tachycardia 8 hours postoperatively were findings in 1 patient; these signs were altered after a rapid infusion of 250 cc of plasma. A second patient showed prolonged oliguria and hypotension in the first 24 hours; these were reversed with whole blood (500 cc) and plasma (1500 cc). Serial hematocrit determinations showed a steady and constant fall during the first 48 hours following caval ligation but gradually rose thereafter. The total blood volume was reduced almost entirely as a function of red cell loss, since the plasma volume remained relatively stable because of parenteral fluid replacement. Urine volumes were low during the initial 8 hours postoperatively; they increased within 48 hours, approaching preoperative levels. In all, approximately one-third of the patients manifested hypotension and oliguria following ligation of the vena cava. These changes were usually most severe during the first 8 hours after surgery; they may extend for a longer time, especially in patients with cardiac disease.

Cardiac output following caval ligation may have indeed dropped in some of our patients; however, such measurements were not made. In only 1 patient was difficulty experienced.

Case Report 6-3

A 41-year-old male was initially seen in 1964 when he had been involved in an auto accident, sustaining a fracture of the right tibia. When the cast was removed, deep thrombophlebitis developed. When seen, he had deep iliofemoral thrombophlebitis of the right extremity, with a large pulmonary infarct. His vena cava was ligated on July 24, 1964. By the next day, he had developed typical bilateral phlegmasia cerulea dolens, requiring bilateral iliofemoral thrombectomy. He also had severe sinus tachycardia, believed to be secondary to the low blood volume.

Routine postoperative care, including elevation of the extremities and administration of fluids, colloid and blood, effectively restored his cardiac status to normal. Nine and a half years later he was doing well, with bilateral pigmentation and postphlebitic swelling controlled by elastic stockings, and chronic obstruction pattern was observed on phleborheography.

MORBIDITY: LONG-TERM EFFECTS OF CAVAL LIGATION

Anatomy: Collateral Circulation

The collateral circulation following ligation of the inferior vena cava has been studied in stillborn infants by Robinson[50] and in the living patient by Filler and Edwards[51] and by Ferris et al.[52] The classification used by Ferris et al. will be followed. They point out that there are many routes for return of blood after occlusion of the inferior vena cava; for descriptive convenience they divided these channels into four groups. (1) *Central channels* (Fig. 6-10A). These are composed of the ascending lumbar plexus, internal and external vertebral venous plexus, hemiazygos-azygos system, and cava above the level of occlusion. (2) *Intermediate channels* (Fig. 6-10B). These comprise the ovarian-testicular veins, the uteric veins, and the left renal-azygos system. (3) *Portal system*. As noted by Sappey and Dumontpallier,[53] the portal system may be useful as a collateral channel when the vena cava is obstructed. Filling is via the superior hemorrhoidal anastomosis with the middle and inferior hemorrhoidal plexus. Abdominal wall veins (Fig. 6-10C) may communicate with a patent umbilical vein, thus creating another means of portal vein filling. (4) *Superficial routes*. These are extensive (Fig. 6-10D). In general, the inferior epigastric veins drain superiorly into the internal mammary veins. The superficial epigastric and circumflex iliac veins drain via thoracoabdominal veins, and the lateral thoracic vein drains into the axillary vein. The lumbar veins may redirect the venous drainage into the vertebral venous plexus (Fig. 6-10E), the ascending lumbar veins, or the cava above the obstructed segment. These veins communicate freely. Robinson[50] found it necessary to ligate the azygos vein at its termination and the superior vena cava at the level of the heart to prevent a retrograde flow of the injection mass into the veins of the thorax and neck following injection into the saphenous or femoral vein. It is also necessary to ligate the ascending aorta to prevent filling of the arterial system. In our experience, greater dilatation of the superficial veins has been seen in unoperated instances of vena cava thrombosis (Fig. 6-11) than following caval ligation.

LONG-TERM RESULTS REPORTED BY OTHERS

During the 1950s a series of papers[15, 23] appeared pointing out the potential for incapacitating venous insufficiency following vena cava ligation. No paper spread more alarm than Shea and Robertson's.[15] It was widely quoted in subsequent reports; indeed, one could not discuss vena cava ligation at scientific meetings without hearing of the dire results noted by Shea and Robertson in their follow-up evaluation of 25 patients following caval ligation. Since their work is the most frequently quoted, it is profitable to review it.

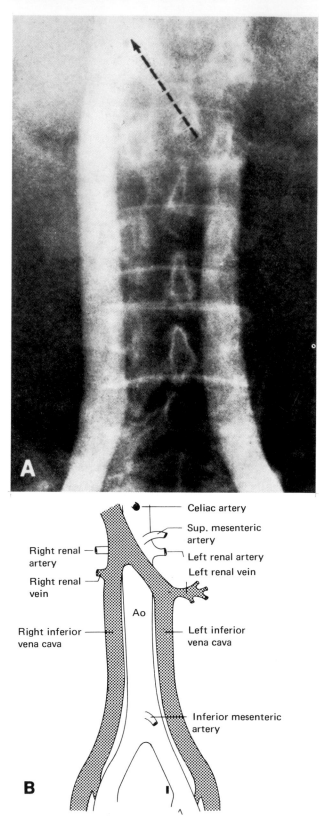

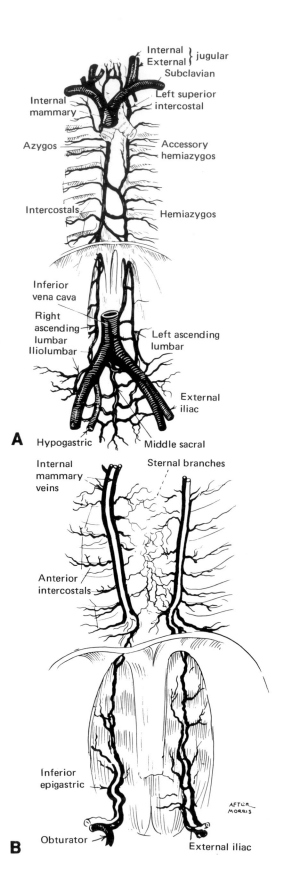

Figure 6-9. A. Phlebogram showing bilateral inferior vena cava. **B.** Gross pathologic findings at autopsy. (*From Hirsch, D. M., and Chan, K.-F. JAMA 185:729, 1963. Copyright 1963, American Medical Association.*)

150

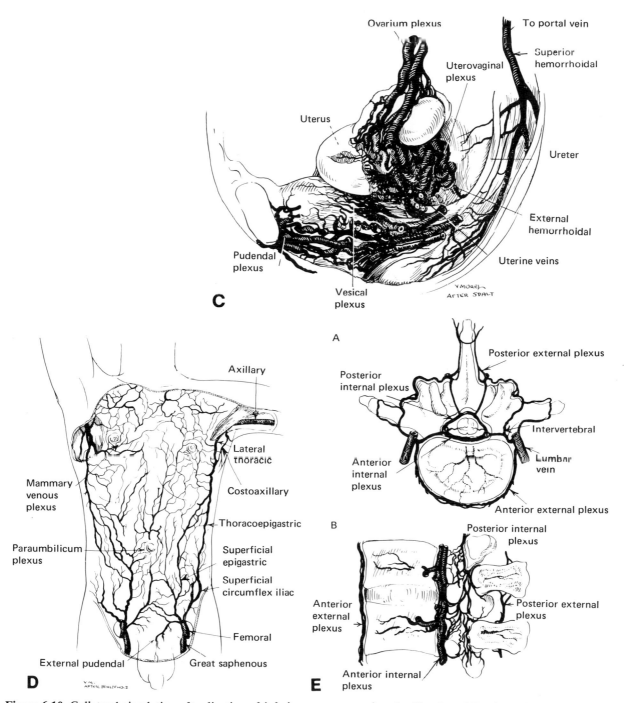

Figure 6-10. Collateral circulation after ligation of inferior vena cava, using classification of Ferris *et al.* **A.** Central channels. (*From Robinson, L. S.* Surgery 25:329, 1949.) **B.** Collateral routes on interior surface of abdominal wall. (*From Tandler,* Lehrbuch der systematischen Anatomie. *Berlin. Springer-Verlag, 1926, vol. 3, p. 151.*) **C.** Anastomosis between caval and portal system in the pelvis. **D.** Superficial routes. **E.** Vertebral vein system, name suggested by Batson for plexus described in 1832 by Breschet. It is an enormous venous lake in which blood is conducted under low pressure through a valveless venous system. (**C, D** and **E** *from Spalteholz, K. W.* Handatlas der anatomie des Menschen. *Leipzig, Hirzel, 1895–1903.*)

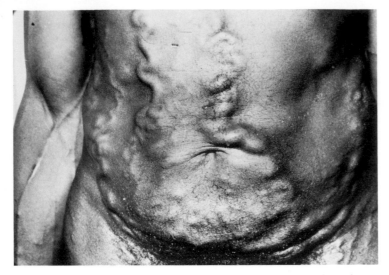

Figure 6-11. Photo shows large, superficial collateral vessels following chronic occlusion of inferior vena cava by thrombosis. In our experience, greater dilatation of superficial veins has been seen in unoperated instances of vena cava thrombosis than is seen following vena cava ligation.

First, on the positive side, Shea and Robertson emphasized that ligation of the inferior vena cava had proved to be a most effective method of preventing pulmonary infarction due to venous thrombosis of the lower extremity and pelvis; they also emphasized that none of their patients had died of recurrent pulmonary embolism. They stressed that it was the surest known method of preventing pulmonary embolism from the lower extremity and that none of their 25 patients experienced subsequent pulmonary infarction.

Secondly, although "only 1 of 25 patients questioned was free of complaints of changes in his physical well-being and the status of the lower extremities in particular," Shea and Robertson noted that in 12 patients the postoperative swelling was persistent, varying "evenly" in degree of severity from moderate to extreme, and that in the 13 remaining patients, swelling was intermittent in 7 and absent in 6. Restating these data another way, their results do not appear so alarming: Of 25 patients, 6 had extreme postligation swelling and 19 had either moderate, intermittent, or no swelling. It is pertinent that lumbar sympathectomy was performed on 4 of these patients at the time of the vena cava ligation, unilateral in 3 and bilateral in 1. It is our belief that this procedure would aggravate venous insufficiency of the lower extremity.

Thirdly, Shea and Robertson took note that "the socio-economic status of the majority of their patients was below average; many of them were indigent, suffered chronic nutritional deficiencies, and had occupational handicaps. The home care was frequently poor because of financial reasons or lack of understanding." In their opinion, for the reasons given, it is unfair to compare their series with patients seen in private practice. Indeed, this is the crux of the matter. The fact that the ligations for the most part were carried out by the resident surgical staff does have an indirect bearing on the follow-up results. The sequelae of venous insufficiency have very little to do with surgical technique or quality of hospital care; the major problem is the difficulty of obtaining prolonged follow-up care from the operating surgeon. We have fought to have high-quality rubberized bandages and heavyweight elastic stockings available for patients in the vascular clinics of local hospitals; their unavailability presents the real problem in the management of postligation edema. Today's recommended types differ drastically from the cotton wrappings that were in general use during the 1950s when Shea and Robertson's report appeared. It is no wonder that 10 of their patients (40 per cent) developed ulceration of the lower extremity, 3 of them of the intractable type.

Other investigators[10, 21, 22, 27–29, 36, 54, 55] have not found such a high incidence of disabling sequelae. For example, Nabseth and Moran[27] noted that all their patients were able to return to their occupational activities after recovery from the ligation, unlike Shea and Robertson's findings that 9 of 25 patients had limitations in their capacity to carry out either previous or adequate means of livelihood.

TABLE 6-2. Treatment for Acute Deep Venous Thrombosis

TREATMENT	NO. PATIENTS	%
Conservative	2384	89 (of total)
Surgical	307	11 (of total)
Vena cava ligation with and without thrombectomy	150	49 (of 307)
Femoroiliac ligation with and with thrombectomy	139	45 (of 307)
Vena cava clip	16	5 (of 307)
Vena cava umbrella	2	1 (of 307)

RESULTS

Between 1952 and 1973, 150 patients underwent ligation of the inferior vena cava as prophylaxis of thromboembolic disease; this represents 6 per cent of all patients seen in our private practice for acute deep venous thrombosis of the lower extremities and pelvis (Table 6-2).

Mortality

There have been 13 in-hospital deaths (8 per cent) (Table 6-3). This figure includes two deaths on the operating table, one just before the vena cava could be ligated and the other during closure. Both patients were autopsied; each had suffered multiple small pulmonary emboli, followed by a massive embolism. The remaining 11 patients died from 1 day to 6 weeks postoperatively. Four died of cardiac disease, 3 of metastatic carcinoma, 1 of massive gastrointestinal hemorrhage, 1 of clotting deficiency, 1 of chronic renal failure, and 1 of undetermined cause. This last was a patient with carcinoma of the ovary and deep venous thrombosis of the lower extremity who died 10 days after ligation of the vena cava; at autopsy, no cause of death was apparent.

Of the 137 patients (92 per cent) who left the hospital alive, 26 (22 per cent) have been lost to follow-up, all during the first 3 postoperative years. For the most part, these were residents of outlying communities or patients who were transiently in our area.

Late Mortality

The remaining 111 patients (78 per cent) have been followed to death or to date. Twenty-five (22 per cent) of this group have died, 11 during the first postoperative year and 14 from 1 to 16 years after operation (Table 6-4). Cardiac disease was the cause of death in 9 (36 per cent), of the 25 patients; carcinoma in 8 (32 per cent), stroke in 2 (8 per cent), pulmonary embolism in 1 (4 per cent), pancreatic and subphrenic abscesses in 1 (4 per cent), and alcoholism in 1 (4 per cent). In 3 (12 per cent), the cause of death was not known. The patient who died of pulmonary embolism 5 months after ligation of the vena cava was a 54-year-old male with uncontrolled polycythemia; on his admission to the hospital in the terminal state, his hemoglobin was 23 gm.

TABLE 6-4. Late Deaths Following 111 Vena Cava Ligations

CAUSE OF DEATH	MO. POSTOPERATIVE	NO. PATIENTS
Cardiac disease	2, 10, 40, 60, 84, 84, 96, 96, 120	9
Carcinoma	3, 3, 4, 12, 14, 18, 84, 192	8
Stroke	11, 60	2
Pulmonary embolus	5	1
Pancreatic and subphrenic abscesses	55	1
Alcoholism	3	1
Unknown	1½, 1½, 60	3
Total		25 (22%)

TABLE 6-3. In-Hospital Deaths Following 150 Vena Cava Ligations

Cardiac arrest on table (postmortem diagnosis of massive pulmonary emboli)	2
Cardiac death (after 3 days, 3 wks, 3 wks, 4 wks)	4
Carcinoma	
Of liver (1 day)	1
Of cervix (2 wks)	1
Metastatic (4 wks)	1
Massive gastrointestinal bleeding (10 days)	1
Clotting deficiency (3 wks)	1
Chronic renal failure (6 wks)	1
No apparent cause at postmortem examination (10 days)	1
Total	13 (8%)

TABLE 6-5. Follow-Up of Vena Cava Ligations of 111 Patients

LENGTH OF FOLLOW-UP (YR)	LATE DEATHS	PATIENTS LIVING	TOTAL PATIENTS
Less than 1	10	0	10
1–2	3	10	13
3–5	5	28	33
6–10	6	31	37
11–15	0	12	12
16–20	1	5	6
Totals	25 (22%)	86 (78%)	111 (100%)

Longterm Survival

Of those who survived beyond the first postoperative year, the average period till death was 6¼ years, with a span from 14 months to 16 years. Of these, 10 patients survived at least 5 years. Of the 86 patients still living or 62 per cent of 137 who left the hospital alive, 71 have survived at least 5 years (Table 6-5), the average being 9 years and the range from 1 to 20 years.

Morbidity

With few exceptions, postoperative swelling presented no real problem. Five patients (3.6 per cent) of those who were discharged from the hospital developed uncontrollable swelling.[32] Thrombophlebitis recurred in 22 (20 per cent); 4 are of special interest[26] because of the multiplicity of the bouts (Table 6-6). All of these episodes were separately diagnosed attacks of thrombophlebitis requiring admission to a hospital for anticoagulation therapy. The patient with eight bouts was studied by cavography, which demonstrated complete absence of visible deep venous system in the pelvis and lower extremities (Fig. 6-12). This patient died of pancreatic abscesses associated with a bleeding diathesis approximately 5 years after ligation.

Certain patients are more susceptible to venous thrombosis than others; whether this tendency is potentiated by caval ligation cannot be determined. These patients have been studied hematologically, and no cause for the hypercoagulability of the blood

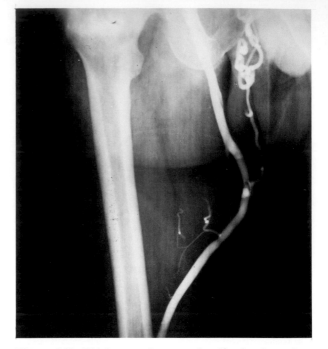

Figure 6-12. Phlebogram 2 years after ligation in patient who had had eight episodes of deep venous thrombosis, demonstrating complete absence of visible deep venous system in pelvis and lower extremities. Patient died of pancreatic abscesses associated with bleeding diathesis 5 years after ligation. At autopsy the vena cava above ligature was patent.

could be determined. Without exception, however, they have all required unusually high doses of anticoagulants for maintenance of the prothrombin level within therapeutic range.

Psychiatric complications have presented a challenge. Three of the 5 patients[32] with uncontrollable swelling have had serious psychiatric problems, and 4 others in this series have had distinct emotional imbalances predating ligation but worsening in the postoperative period. Coincidence may account for this phenomenon; however, some as yet unclarified cause and effect relationship is not entirely ruled out.

VARICOSITIES OF THE LOWER EXTREMITIES

Twenty-four patients (21.6 per cent) of 111 in this series developed varicose veins; the time of onset ranged from 3 months to 16 years postoperatively, the average being 4.5 years. In 8 patients the varices were bilateral. In 4 patients, they occurred in the thigh. Ten per cent of the patients developed varicosities of the abdominal wall, time of onset being 2 months to 16 years after ligation with the average being 6 years (Table 6-5).

TABLE 6-6. Complications Following 111 Vena Cava Ligations

COMPLICATION	NO.	%
Immediate massive swelling	2	1.4
Late uncontrollable swelling	5	4.0
Recurrent thrombophlebitis	22	20.0
6 times	1	
7 times	1	
8 times	1	
15 times	1	
Varicose veins (av time 4.5 yr)	24	20.0
Varicosities of abdominal wall (av time 6 yr)	12	10.0
Venous ulceration	4	3.6
Intractable	2	
Patient neglect	2	
Venous claudication (av onset 2 yr)	18	16.0

VENOUS ULCERATION

Intractable venous ulcers of the lower extremity occurred in 2 patients; they were not amenable to our usual conservative therapy. In 2 other patients, ulceration developed; however, in 1 it was a recurrent ulcer in an extremity with a preligation history of ulceration. A second patient omitted her heavyweight elastic stocking at her own discretion 4 and 8 years after ligation, with resultant ulceration each time. These two extremities were treated with pressure and healed easily. Both patients have remained healed by using the heavyweight stocking.

VENOUS CLAUDICATION

In 18 patients (16 per cent), venous claudication was a complaint. It occurred bilaterally in 7 patients. The average time of onset was 2 years after ligation.

CASE REPORTS OF SPECIAL INTEREST.
Uncontrollable   Swelling—Multiple   Recurrent Thrombophlebitis, Ulceration.

Case Report 6-4

This 40-year-old Caucasian male was first seen in January 1954. A diagnosis of multiple pulmonary emboli (confirmed by chest x-rays) led to a decision to ligate the inferior vena cava. At operation large clots, some fresh and some organized, were found in the vena cava, extending up to the vicinity of the renal veins. Tremendous swelling complicated his initial postoperative course. He was discharged on anticoagulant therapy phenindione (Hedulin, 2-phenyl-1,3-indandione). The patient was 6 feet 4 inches tall (193 cm) and in the next few months gained weight to 210 pounds (95.2 kg). Nevertheless, he returned to work in May 1954, wearing heavyweight elastic stockings of the recommended type.

Between January and June he had three attacks of venous thrombosis, followed by four later, totalling seven that we could document. It is believed that he had others while under the care of other physicians.

Eleven months postoperatively he developed pigmentation of the left ankle, which led to ulceration within 2 weeks. He was still on anticoagulant therapy. The ulcer healed in 3 months with pressure dressings. A phlebogram obtained in March 1955 did not demonstrate the patency of the femoral vein; therefore, exploration was carried out. The superficial and common femoral veins, the external iliac vein, and the saphenous vein in this area were all patent. A fibrous cord along the wall of the common femoral vein was interpreted as the original clot. An incision was made in the vicinity of the previous ulceration, and some superficial veins were excised. No communicating veins could be found in the lowest fourth of the leg. No visible varicosities were present in the upper three-fourths of the leg. The patient again returned to work.

Six months later he entered the Veterans Administration Hospital for recurrent thrombophlebitis and was studied in a seminar. It was decided that he should be continued on the anticoagulant therapy on which he had been maintained for approximately 2 years since his discharge after vena cava ligation.

Three months later (August 1957) he was seen again with a recurrent ulcer, which was healed with pressure after great difficulty. A second phlebogram showed patency of the vena cava up to occlusion by the ligature and a huge internal spermatic vein. At operation the long saphenous vein was removed from groin to ankle, and subfascial ligation of four large communicating veins of the leg was performed. He did well and again returned to work on a maintenance dose of anticoagulant agents, with the prothrombin concentration being kept between 20 and 35 per cent most of the time. At one time he developed venous thrombosis while taking 200 mg phenindione a day. He regulated his prothrombin concentration himself, and he was convinced that he felt better when it was around 25 per cent than when it was closer to 40 per cent.

During the next few years he was seen several times for ulceration of the lower extremity and once with multiple ulcers of the left leg, including one ulcer above the knee. All these ulcers had small engorged veins underlying them, and it was obvious that their origin, including the one on the thigh, was venous. In all our experience we have never seen another venous ulcer above the knee. His ulcers were always amenable to healing, at times with great pressures. He wore heavyweight elastic stockings plus a 4-inch rubber bandage from toes to knees and a 6-inch bandage from knee to groin. In 1959 he was admitted to the Veterans Administration Hospital, where he died of carcinoma of the lung in April 1961, 7 years after vena cava ligation.

Case Report 6-5

This 50-year-old Caucasian male was first seen in April 1956 for superficial thrombophlebitis of the left lower extremity. He gave a history of multiple bouts of superficial and deep thrombophlebitis. Arterial pulsations were absent bilaterally below the groin, and he complained of intermittent claudication and lack of sexual drive for the past 2 years. A diagnosis of bilateral Leriche's syndrome (obliteration of the terminal aorta) was made as well as superficial thrombophlebitis of the left lower extremity and postphlebitic syndrome of the right lower extremity. He was next seen in consultation in June 1956, and a diagnosis of multiple pulmonary emboli led to our decision to ligate his inferior vena cava. Postoperatively there was great swelling in the left lower extremity, even above the high-thigh heavyweight elastic stocking with which he had been fitted. Because of his concomitant bilateral aortoiliac and femoropopliteal obliterative arterial disease, he was unable to endure the pressure, and he was changed to a tensor bandage above a knee-length heavyweight elastic stocking. In November 1957 he developed ulceration of the left lower leg. He had omitted his stocking because it was painful. He was a short (67 inches), exceedingly obese (195 pounds) man who worked 16 to 18 hours daily as manager of his own restaurant, during which time he was constantly on his feet. He required short periods of bed rest to heal this ulcer and the recurrent one 1½ years later.

In January 1960 he was admitted to the hospital for study of his obliterative arterial disease; an aortic graft was inserted bilaterally from the aorta to the femoral arteries. Postoperatively the peripheral pulses were restored. However, he continued to have recurrent venous ulcers bilaterally over the next several years; he healed at least four with difficulty by pressure, using methods learned from us. He admitted that the recurrences were due to gross neglect, i.e., omitting elastic support or wrapping his legs only with worn-out bandages.

He was recalled for follow-up study in late 1966; at this time he had incipient ulcerations bilaterally for the 12th time, but his peripheral pulses were still palpable. He was still gaining weight, was short of breath, was wearing a corset, and could not stoop to put his elastic stockings on.

When last seen he was 13 years post ligation and 9 years post aortofemoral graft, still working full-time at his restaurant and still trying to heal bilateral ulcers himself, applying pressure dressings as he had been instructed. Six months later we learned of his death from a friend, also our patient. He had suffered a cerebral vascular accident and died en route to the hospital.

With the exception of the few patients with intractable swelling and multiple bouts of throm-

bophlebitis discussed above, the patients in this series have led relatively normal lives as far as their lower extremities are concerned. On the whole, complaints have been few and minor. When present, varicose veins of the extremities or abdominal region and venous claudication have not deterred these patients from carrying out their usual occupations or from resuming the activities which they participated in prior to undergoing ligation of the inferior vena cava (Fig. 6-13).

It is our belief that our results are significantly influenced by the following factors: (1) These patients are from our private practice and have been followed continuously in the postoperative period. (2) The special heavyweight elastic stocking to control edema has been available and has proved successful in most patients in preventing postphlebitic sequelae. (3) Whenever possible, anticoagulant therapy has been instituted in the immediate postoperative period. (4) These patients have benefited from our familiarity with the needs of patients with chronic venous insufficiency.

Phleborheography Following Vena Cava Ligation

Forty-seven patients were studied by bilateral phleborheography at an average of 9 years after caval ligation. Of the 94 thigh studies, 72 (77 per cent) showed a normal tracing and 22 (23 per cent) were abnormal. Twelve patients had unilateral abnormal thigh tracing, and 5 patients had bilateral abnormal thigh tracings. A normal tracing in the thigh indicates to us that there is minimal or no obstruction to the outflow of blood from the thigh through the pelvis and abdomen.

Of the leg tracings studied in 47 patients only 33 of 94 (35 per cent) were normal; 61 (65 per cent) were abnormal. Seventeen of 47 patients (18 per cent) had unilateral abnormal tracings, and 22 of 47 patients (47 per cent) had bilateral abnormal tracings. To us, the abnormal tracings indicate residual obstruction in the veins at and below the midthigh level.

In a much smaller series of patients (10) followed a short period of time (average of 19 months) following clipping of the vena cava with an Adams-DeWeese clip, the results appear to be better in the thigh tracings. Nineteen of 20 (95 per cent) of the thigh tracings were normal. In the

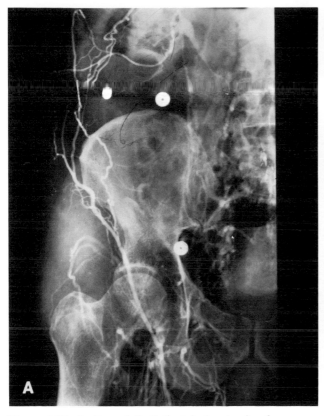

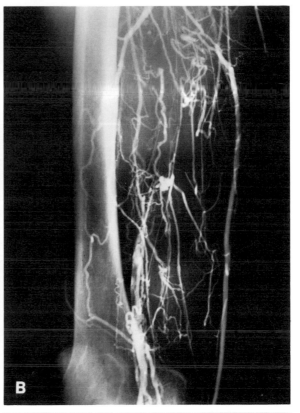

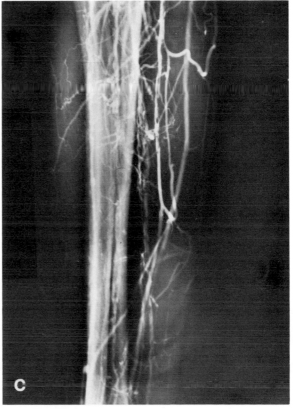

Figure 6-13. A, B, and C. Patient had extensive femoro-iliac thrombophlebitis demonstrated at operation in July 1964, when vena cava was ligated. This phlebogram was obtained November 1970, because of acute exacerbation of symptoms. There was fresh clot just above the knee in femoral vein and in one of superficial veins of the leg. This system is still controlled. When seen in May 1973, 9 years after vena cava ligation, patient was getting along well with medium-weight elastic stockings. He had not worn a heavyweight stocking for 5 years.

lower extremity the results were approximately the same as those following ligation of the vena cava: 8 of 20 (40 per cent) were normal.

The primary indication for vena cava ligation has been the hope of preventing fatal pulmonary embolism. In such a life-threatening situation, both the surgeon and the patient are willing to accept the possibility of chronic disability of the lower extremities secondary to the operation. Indeed, in our earlier years we fully expected disabling complications following this procedure. It was a pleasant surprise to find that the swelling of most patients can be controlled and that they can return to their former state of life with minimal disability. We have no intention or desire to urge any surgeon to employ this procedure nor to advocate its indiscriminate use. In a small group of our patients who have been treated by clipping rather than by ligation, the early results are favorable; should we become convinced that clipping is an equally effective procedure, we will turn to it more often (Figs. 6-14 to 6-49).

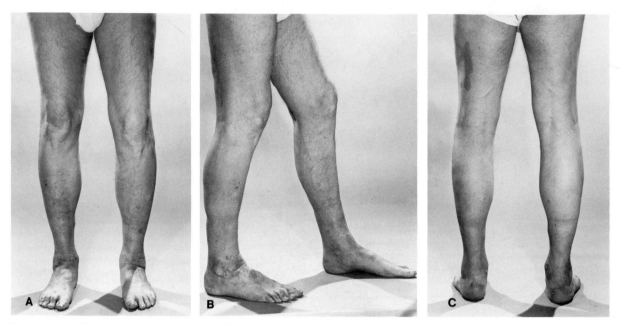

Figure 6-14. Fifty-three-year-old white male, 1⅓ years after vena cava ligation for threatened pulmonary embolism secondary to femoropopliteal thrombophlebitis of right lower extremity and 11 days following removal of apparently (not proved) infected thrombosed Mobin-Uddin filter. **A.** Frontal. **B.** Lateral. **C.** Posterior.

Figure 6-15. Sixty-two-year-old white female, 2½ years after vena cava ligation for multiple pulmonary emboli. **A.** Frontal. **B.** Lateral. **C.** Posterior.

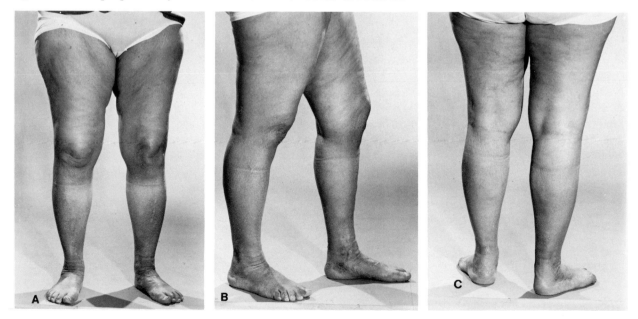

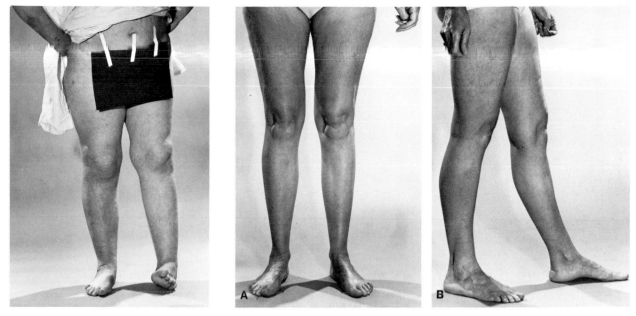

Figure 6-16. Thirty-six-year-old white female, 2 years after vena cava ligation for threatened pulmonary embolism secondary to recurrent bilateral thrombophlebitis of lower extremities.

Figure 6-17. Fifty-four-year-old white female, 3 years after vena cava ligation for massive pulmonary embolism secondary to femoropopliteal thrombophlebitis of right lower extremity occurring while patient on anticoagulant therapy. **A.** Frontal. **B.** Lateral.

Figure 6-18. Sixty-three-year-old white male 3⅔ years after vena cava ligation plus iliofemoral thrombectomy for history of multiple pulmonary emboli and recurrent iliofemoral thrombophlebitis of lower extremities. **A.** Frontal. **B.** Lateral. **C.** Posterior.

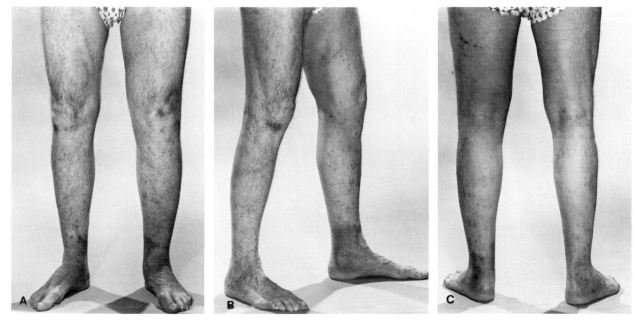

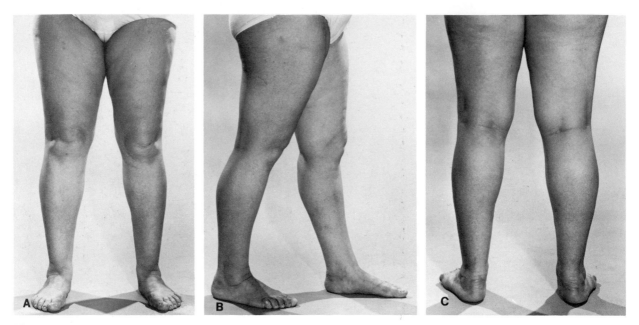

Figure 6-19. Forty-eight-year-old white female, 4 years after vena cava ligation for recurrent multiple pulmonary emboli. **A.** Frontal. **B.** Lateral. **C.** Posterior.

Figure 6-20. Fifty-three-year-old white male, 4½ years after vena cava ligation for threatened pulmonary embolism secondary to phlegmasia cerulea dolens of the left lower extremity, which was treated conservatively. **A.** Frontal. **B.** Lateral. **C.** Posterior.

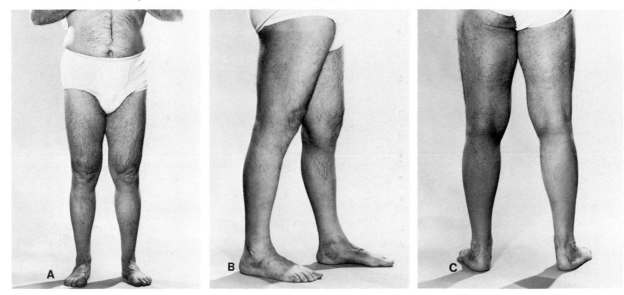

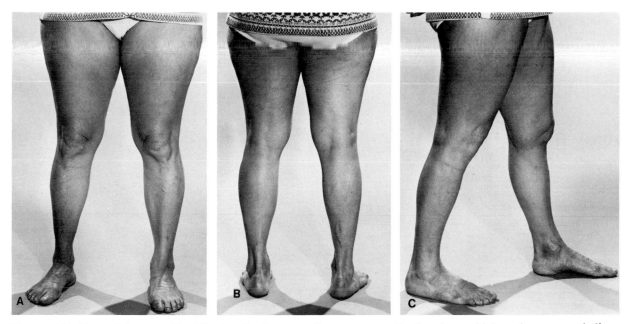

Figure 6-21. Forty-eight-year-old white female, 5 years after vena cava ligation for multiple pulmonary emboli occurring while patient was on contraceptive therapy. **A.** Frontal. **B.** Posterior. **C.** Lateral.

Figure 6-22. Fifty-eight-year-old white male, 6⅓ years after vena cava ligation for pulmonary embolism secondary to femoroiliac thrombophlebitis of left lower extremity and 8 months after removal of thrombosed venous aneurysm of right popliteal vein. **A.** Frontal. **B.** Lateral. **C.** Posterior, showing scar of surgically treated thrombosed venous aneurysm of right popliteal vein. This aneurysm was huge, filling entire popliteal space and preventing venous drainage. It was excised, with attempted unsuccessful thrombectomy of the superficial femoral vein.

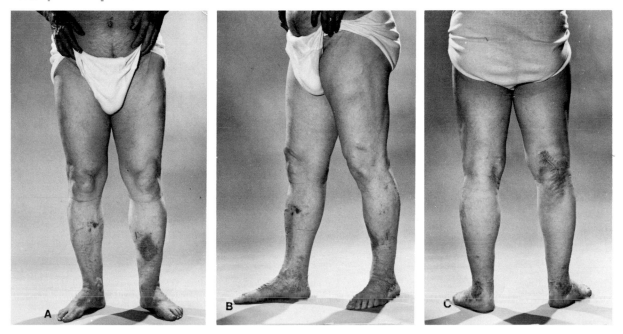

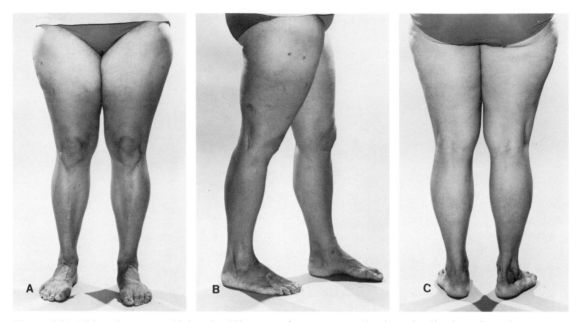

Figure 6-23. Thirty-three-year-old female, 7⅓ years after vena cava ligation, plus ligation of ovarian veins for massive pulmonary embolism 8 days post partum. **A.** Frontal. **B.** Lateral. **C.** Posterior.

Figure 6-24. Forty-two-year-old white female, 7 years after vena cava ligation for multiple pulmonary emboli secondary to femoroiliac thrombophlebitis of the right lower extremity. **A.** Frontal. **B.** Right lateral. **C.** Left lateral. **D.** Posterior.

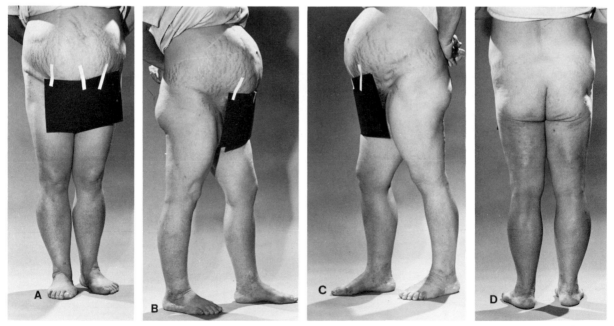

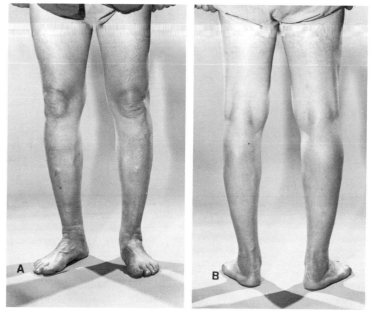

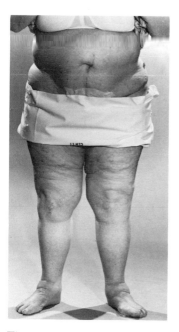

Figure 6-25. Sixty-five-year-old white male, 7 years after vena cava ligation for multiple pulmonary emboli secondary to recurrent femoroiliac thrombophlebitis. **A.** Frontal. **B.** Posterior.

Figure 6-26. Seventy-two-year-old white female, 8 years after vena cava ligation for threatened pulmonary embolism and femoroiliac thrombophlebitis of right lower extremity.

Figure 6-27. Forty-eight-year-old white male, 8½ years after vena cava ligation for recurrent multiple pulmonary emboli secondary to bilateral femoroiliac thrombophlebitis. **A.** Frontal. **B.** Lateral. **C.** Posterior.

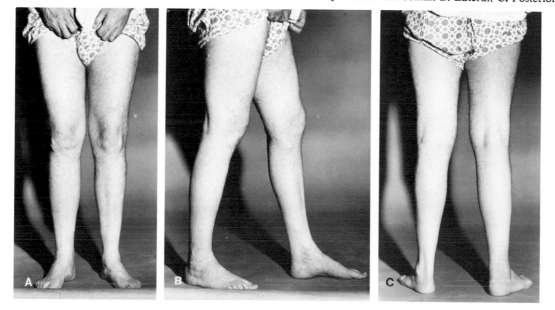

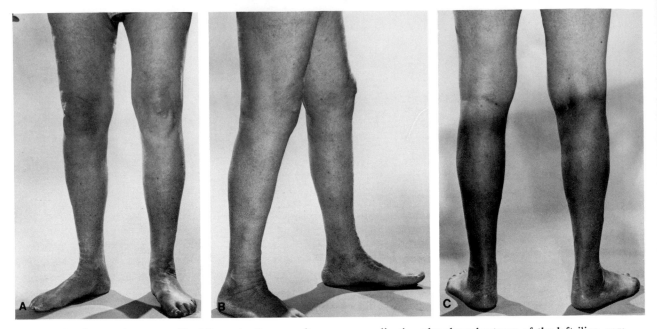

Figure 6-28. Seventy-four-year-old white male, 8 years after vena cava ligation plus thrombectomy of the left iliac, common, superficial, and deep femoral veins for threatened pulmonary embolism secondary to left femoroiliac thrombophlebitis. **A.** Frontal. **B.** Lateral. **C.** Posterior.

Figure 6-29. Fifty-year-old white female, 8½ years after vena cava ligation for threatened pulmonary embolism secondary to femoroiliac thrombophlebitis following a vaginal hysterectomy. **A.** Frontal. **B.** Lateral. **C.** Posterior.

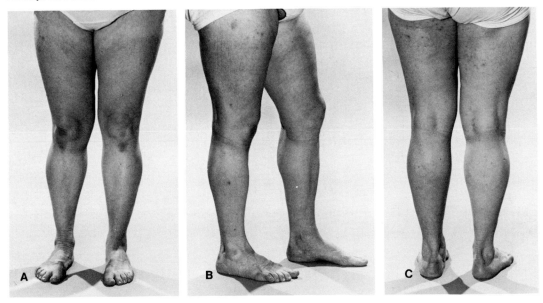

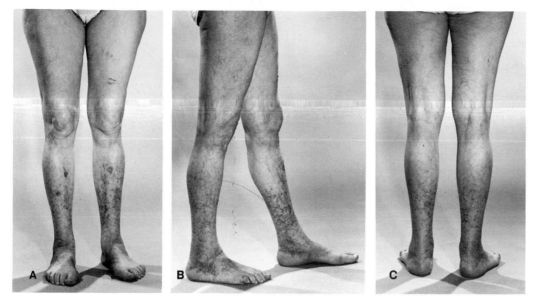

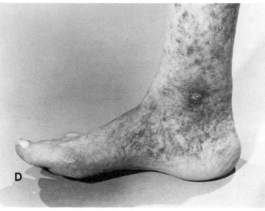

Figure 6-30. Fifty-one-year-old white female, 8⅓ years after vena cava ligation for pulmonary embolism secondary to femoropopliteal thrombophlebitis of the left lower extremity. **A.** Frontal. **B.** Lateral. **C.** Posterior. **D.** Pigmentation of distal third of left foot.

Figure 6-31. Thirty-one-year-old white male, 8½ years after vena cava ligation for pulmonary embolism secondary to superficial and deep thrombophlebitis of right lower extremity. **A.** Frontal. **B.** Lateral. **C.** Posterior.

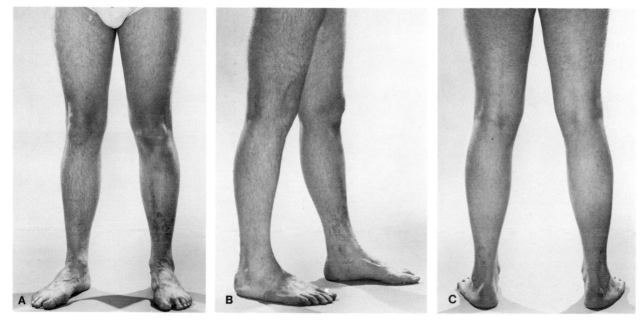

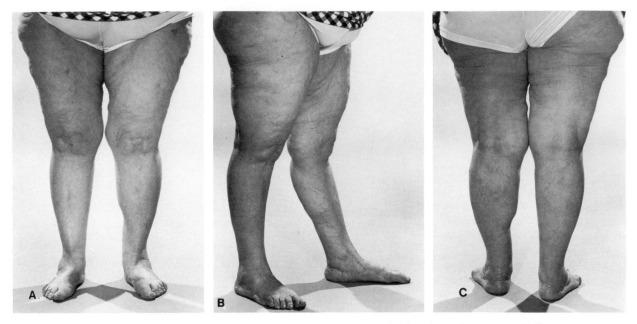

Figure 6-32. Sixty-eight-year-old white female, 10 years after vena cava ligation for pulmonary embolism secondary to femoroiliac thrombophlebitis. **A.** Frontal. **B.** Lateral. **C.** Posterior.

Figure 6-33. Seventy-three-year-old white female, 10½ years after vena cava ligation for recurrent pulmonary emboli secondary to femoropopliteal thrombophlebitis of left lower extremity. **A.** Frontal. **B.** Lateral. **C.** Posterior.

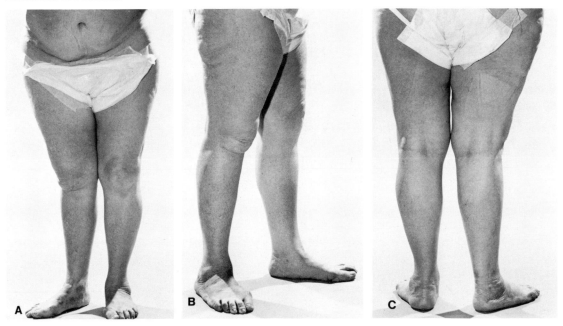

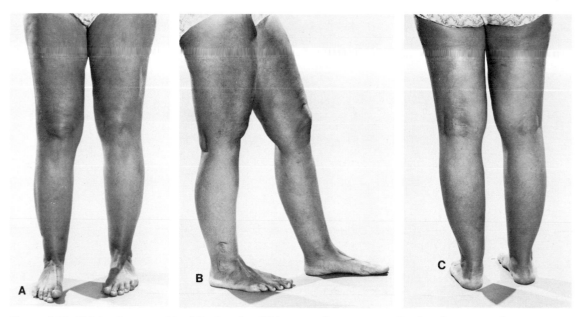

Figure 6-34. Thirty-nine-year-old white female, 10½ years after vena cava ligation for recurrent femoral thrombophlebitis of right lower extremity. **A.** Frontal. **B.** Lateral. **C.** Posterior

Figure 6-35. Seventy-five-year-old white male, 10¾ years after vena cava ligation for multiple pulmonary emboli secondary to femoropopliteal thrombophlebitis of left lower extremity. **A.** Frontal. **B.** Lateral. **C.** Posterior. **D.** Abdominal varices.

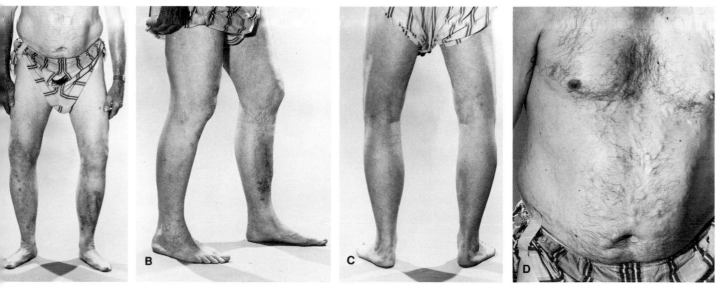

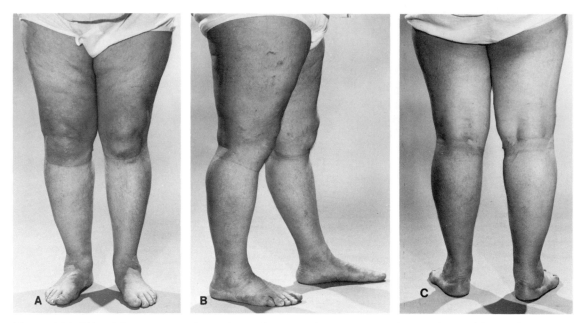

Figure 6-36. Fifty-eight-year-old white male, 11½ years after vena cava ligation for multiple pulmonary emboli secondary to iliac thrombophlebitis of the left lower extremity. **A.** Frontal. **B.** Lateral. **C.** Posterior.

Figure 6-37. Forty-nine-year-old white female, 11½ years after vena cava ligation for multiple bilateral pulmonary emboli secondary to femoropopliteal thrombophlebitis of right lower extremity. **A.** Frontal. **B.** Lateral. **C.** Posterior.

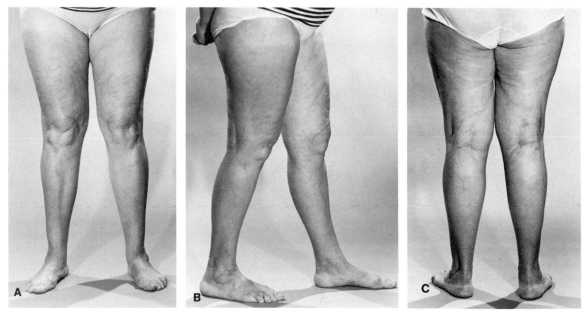

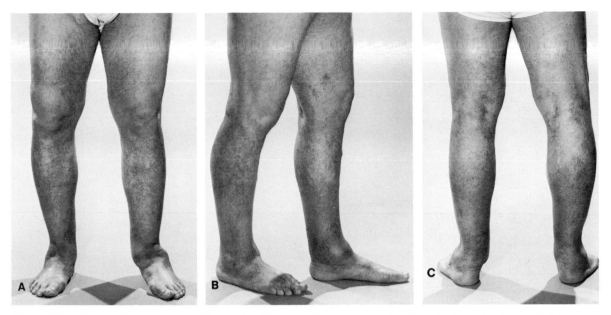

Figure 6-38. Seventy-four-year-old white male, 12 years after vena cava ligation plus thrombectomy of right superficial and deep femoral veins for multiple pulmonary emboli secondary to thrombophlebitis of right lower extremity. **A.** Frontal. **B.** Lateral. **C.** Posterior.

Figure 6-39. Fifty-year-old white male, 12 years after vena cava ligation for pulmonary embolism secondary to bilateral femoropopliteal thrombophlebitis and 7 months after excision of varicose veins bilaterally and excision of abdominal varices. **A.** Frontal. **B.** Lateral. **C.** Posterior.

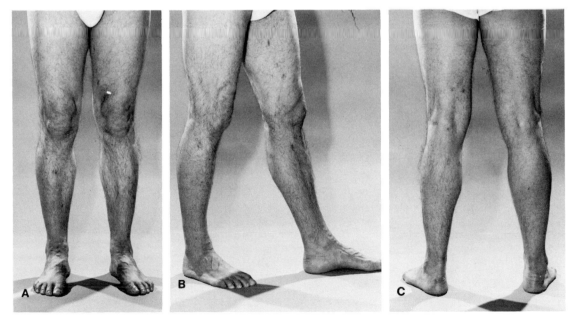

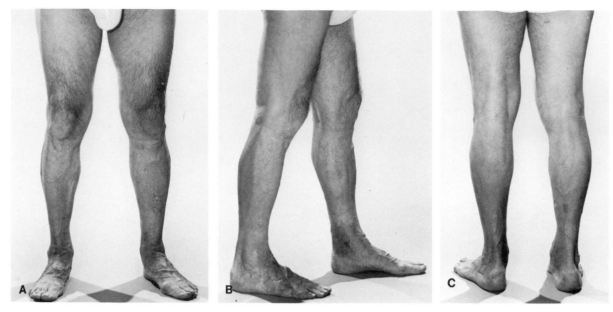

Figure 6-40. Seventy-one-year-old white male, 12 years after vena cava ligation plus thrombectomy of left common femoral, external iliac, and saphenous veins for pulmonary emboli secondary to femoroiliac thrombophlebitis of left lower extremity. **A.** Frontal. **B.** Lateral. **C.** Posterior.

Figure 6-41. Forty-five-year-old white male, 12½ years after vena cava ligation plus thrombectomy of left common femoral vein for multiple pulmonary emboli secondary to femoroiliac thrombophlebitis of left lower extremity. **A.** Frontal. **B.** Lateral. **C.** Posterior.

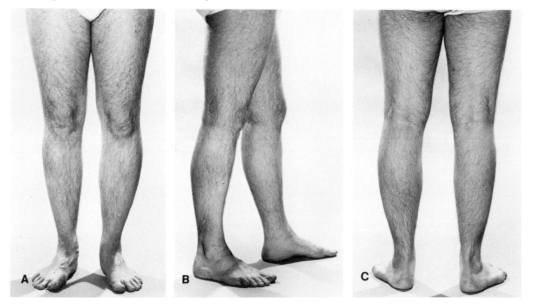

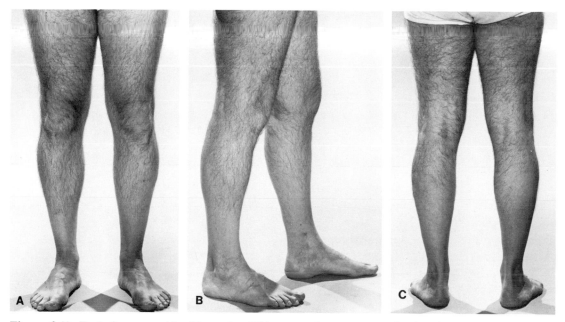

Figure 6-42. Forty-four-year-old white male, 12½ years after vena cava ligation for pulmonary embolism plus left common femoral thrombectomy. **A.** Frontal. **B.** Lateral. **C.** Posterior.

Figure 6-43. Thirty-four-year-old white female in eighth month of eighth pregnancy, 13 years after vena cava ligation for femoroiliac thrombophlebitis of right lower extremity secondary to ruptured ectopic pregnancy. Patient has never worn an elastic stocking. **A.** Profile. **B.** Frontal. **C.** Lateral. **D.** Posterior.

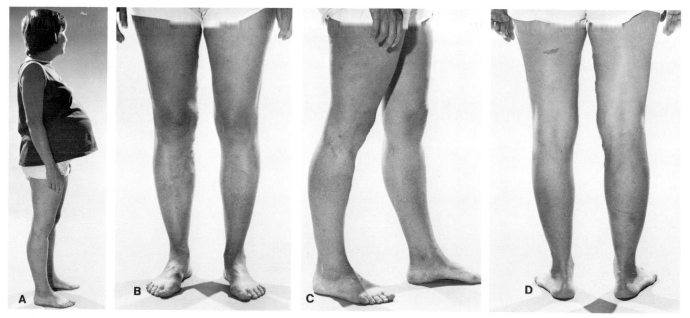

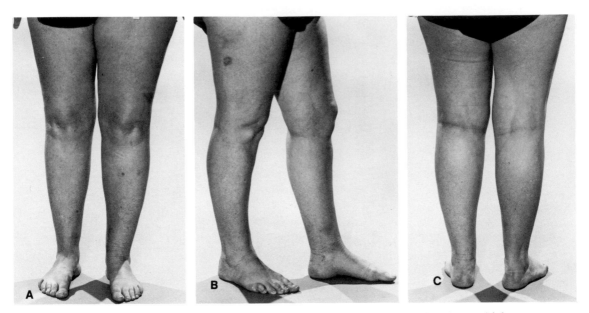

Figure 6-44. Thirty-nine-year-old white female, 13 years after vena cava ligation for multiple pulmonary emboli from pelvic thrombophlebitis secondary to ruptured uterus. **A.** Frontal. **B.** Lateral. **C.** Posterior.

Figure 6-45. Sixty-three-year-old white male, 15½ years after vena cava ligation for bilateral recurrent pulmonary emboli. **A.** Frontal. **B.** Lateral. **C.** Posterior.

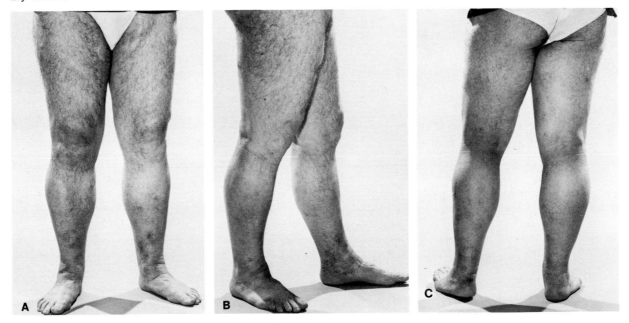

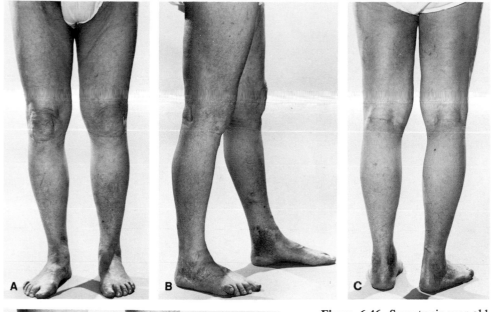

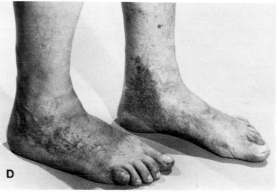

Figure 6-46. Seventy-six-year-old white male, 16 years after vena cava ligation for multiple pulmonary emboli secondary to femoroiliac thrombophlebitis of right lower extremity. **A.** Frontal. **B.** Lateral. **C.** Posterior. **D.** Pigmentation of right medial malleolus.

Figure 6-47. Forty-four-year-old white female, 18 years after vena cava ligation for bilateral femoroiliac thrombophlebitis and pulmonary embolism. Burn on thigh was secondary to application of heating pad to greatly swollen limb. **A.** Frontal. **B.** Lateral. **C.** Posterior.

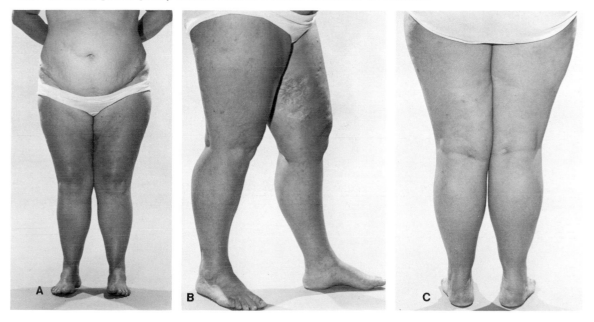

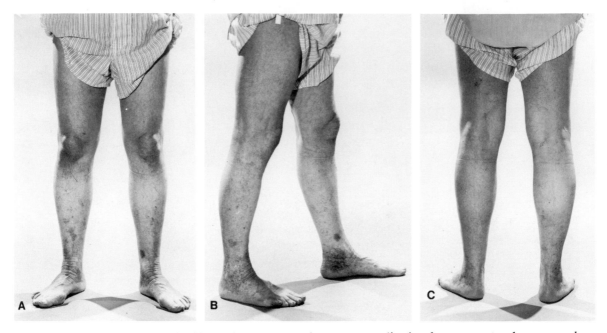

Figure 6-48. Sixty-eight-year-old white male, 19 years after vena cava ligation for recurrent pulmonary embolism secondary to deep venous thrombosis while on "adequate" anticoagulant therapy. **A.** Frontal. **B.** Lateral. **C.** Posterior.

Figure 6-49. Eighty-two-year-old white male, 20 years after vena cava ligation for pulmonary embolism secondary to right femoroiliac thrombophlebitis. **A.** Frontal. **B.** Lateral. **C.** Posterior.

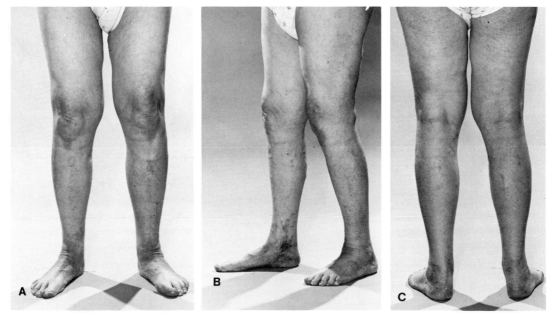

TEMPORARY AND PARTIAL CAVAL INTERRUPTION

During the 1950s and 1960s, surgical investigators sought techniques that would provide the effectiveness of caval interruption without the potential complications of lower-extremity sequelae.

Absorbable Ligatures

Streuter and Paine in 1953[56] began studies of temporary occlusion of the inferior vena cava by absorbable catgut ligatures. When 36 dogs were studied by cavogram following ligation of the inferior vena cava with catgut, reopening was demonstrated in 82 per cent at an average time of 6 weeks, with extremes of 18 to 78 days; it was concluded that it would be feasible to attempt this procedure in humans. In 1955,[57] Pualwan *et al.* carried out a similar study; recanalization of the vena cava was demonstrated in 85 per cent of the operated dogs. They later reported[58] treating 5 patients by this technique, with no mortality or further embolization in a brief follow-up period.

Clips

Moretz *et al.*[59] in 1954 reported their experiments with other methods of temporarily occluding the vena cava of dogs by a technique that could be reversed at will. The vena cava was either tied with umbilical tape, cotton, or collagen or clipped with stainless steel clips. The ties or clips were removed at a later operation. Following this the cava would reopen, and the collaterals that had formed immediately after the initial operation would then decrease in size. Eight dogs died in the immediate postoperative period from pooling of blood in the lower extremities. Having noted a similar death in 1 patient, Moretz and associates suggested the possibility of using temporary occluding devices in clinical practice so that the devices could be removed in patients in whom serious sequelae developed. They later reported[60] that when the vena cava in dogs was occluded with Lucite or Teflon clips, removal of the clips later resulted in restoration of the caval patency. This idea was further developed, resulting in Teflon clips with 1.5-mm gaps which would partially occlude the cava; partial occlusion provides a barrier to the passage of a major pulmonary embolus to the lungs but at the same time does not interfere with the flow of blood to the point of causing a significant elevation in venous pressure. Following these experiments with animals, Moretz and his group used the partially occluding clip in 10 patients. Further embolization was noted only in a patient who had known clot in the vena cava at the time the clip was applied. From this experience they concluded that partial interruption of the vena cava should be useful in clinical practice.

Serrated Clips

There have been a number of modifications of plastic clips for partial interruption of the vena cava, including the Moretz clip with a flat bar. Miles and others[61-65] reported on a clip with serrations in it to convert the caval lumen into a series of channels individually small enough to prevent the passage of a lethal-sized embolus yet large enough when combined to allow maximal bloodflow (Figs. 6-50 and 6-51). Taber *et al.*[66] in 1966 described a serrated Teflon clip. Adams and DeWeese[67, 68] placed the serrations on only one side of the clip (Fig. 6-52), thus making it easier to slip it onto the vena cava.

Intraluminal Grids

M. S. DeWeese and Hunter[69, 70] studied another approach to the problem of partial, temporary occlusion of the inferior vena cava. They constructed an intraluminal filter of thread in the vena cava, the strands placed to form a so-called harp-string grid tangentially across the lumen. The grid was composed of parallel mattress sutures of 5–0 silk placed approximately 2 mm apart; this did not constrict the lumen of the vena cava (Figs. 6-53 and 6-54). They had two objectives: that the grid would stop the passage of any potentially fatal embolus and that smaller emboli would be shunted to one side of the vena cava by the slanting grid, thus permitting easy flow of blood through the central portion of the vena cava. In 1963 they reported on 24 patients[71]; there were two postoperative deaths, one of which was unexplained and represented a possible failure of the method. During the follow-up period no patient in their study was known to have died of thromboembolism, and none showed clinical

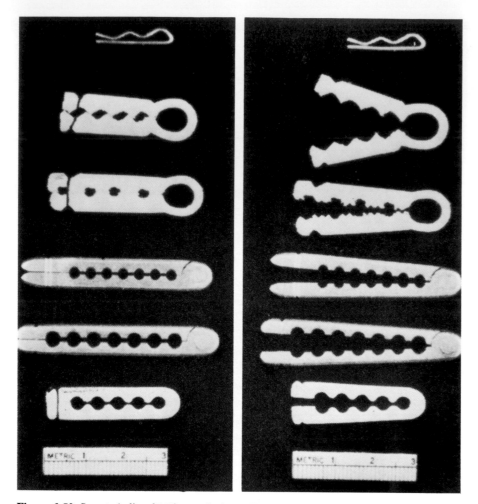

Figure 6-50. Serrated clip of *Miles* et al. Amer Surg *30:42, 1964.*

Figure 6-51. Close-up of Miles clip. (*Miles* et al. Ann Surg *169:885, 1969.*)

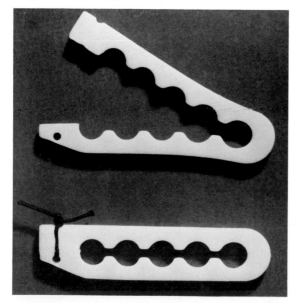

evidence of recurrent pulmonary infarction. However, a small embolus, 3 mm in diameter, was found in the lung of one autopsied patient, and in 2 other patients, interception of emboli by the filter was demonstrated.

Plication

The concept of plicating the inferior vena cava was introduced by Spencer and associates.[72–74] In this technique the walls of the vena cava are sewn together at intervals, creating small channels within the lumen that permit rapid passage of blood but obstruct the passage of a major embolus. Spencer[74] (Fig. 6-55) suggests that the lumen be occluded between two horizontally placed clamps so that the anterior and posterior walls are flattened against

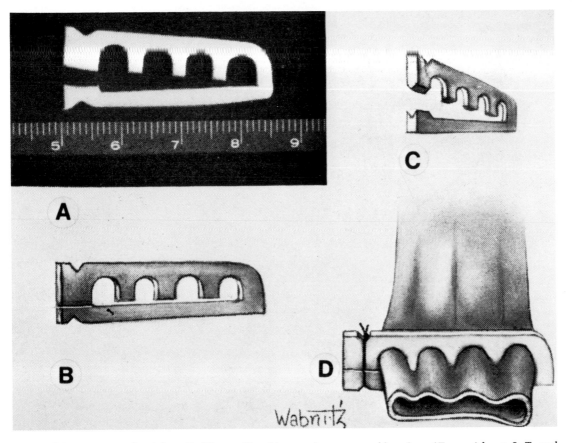

Figure 6-52. A to **D.** The Adams-DeWeese clip with serrations on one side only. (*From Adams, J. T. and De Weese, J. A. J. Surg Gynecol Obstet 123:1087, 1966. By Permission of Surgery, Gynecology & Obstetrics.*)

each other. A single row of transverse mattress sutures of 4–0 silk is inserted between the anterior and posterior walls; channels 3 to 4 mm in diameter are constructed by placing individual sutures 4 to 5 mm apart. The individual sutures are inserted from the anterior wall through the posterior wall and then in the reverse direction and are finally tied on the anterior surface. Three to five sutures are required, depending on the diameter of the vena cava.

Compartmentation

In 1966 Ravitch et al.[75] recommended compartmentation of the vena cava with a mechanical stapler. Mozes and Antibe[76] described compartmentation by placing sutures through plastic beads and tying this ligature around the vena cava.

Transvenously Placed Caval Filters

Mobin-Uddin et al.[77–81] developed an ingenious umbrella-like device that could be implanted in the inferior vena cava through the jugular vein. When first placed, this umbrella (Fig. 6-56) effectively stops migration of any major embolus and at the same time does not significantly affect the flow of blood from the lower extremities. Over a period of time fibrous tissue encases the filter with a smooth lining, so that in effect the vena cava is slowly occluded. In some patients it remains patent.

Working independently, Eichelter and Schenk[82–84] developed a plastic catheter that can be converted into a ribbed strainer which can be placed in the vena cava through the saphenous vein at the saphenofemoral junction (Fig. 6-57). Pate et al.[85] have designed a spring device which is intended to de-

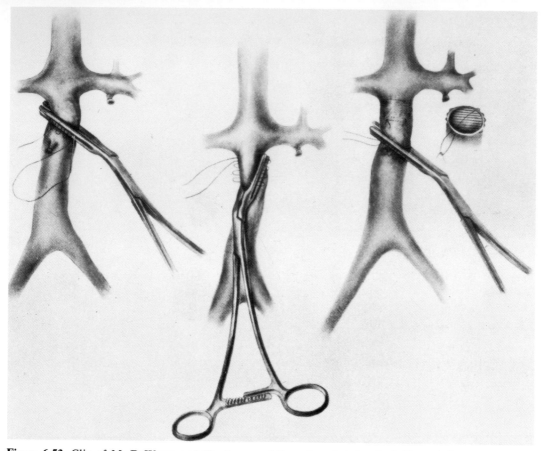

Figure 6-53. Clip of M. DeWeese and Hunter, consisting of an intraluminal filter of thread within the vena cava. (*De Weese* et al. Ann Surg 178:*249, 1973.*)

Figure 6-54. Modification of M. DeWeese's clip. (*De Weese* et al. Ann Surg 178:*249, 1973.*)

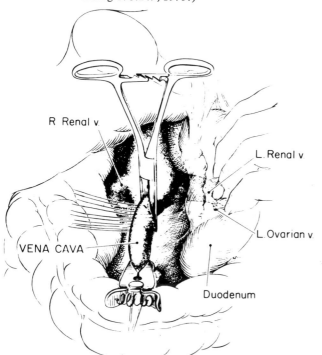

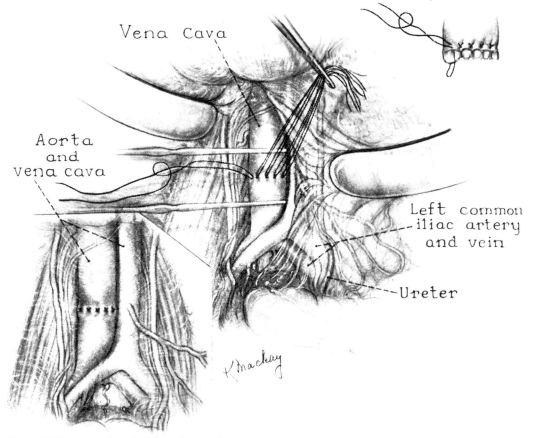

Figure 6-55. Spencer's technique of occluding lumen of vena cava between 2 horizontally placed clamps. (*Spencer* et al. Ann Surg 155:*827, 1962.*)

form the wall of the vena cava into a narrow slit and to be covered completely by neointima. Hunter et al.[86] have devised a balloon technique for interrupting the vena cava permanently transvenously through the jugular vein. The deflated balloon was placed in the vena cava of dogs and inflated by injecting 50% Hypaque solution; this permits visualization of the balloon on x ray and its gradual fibrous fixation to the walls of the vena cava. Lewis et al.,[87] using the Fogarty venous thrombectomy catheter, blockaded the inferior vena cava of a patient for 12 days and successfully controlled his thromboembolic disease. Greenfield et al.[88] have studied a cone-shaped steel-wire filter inserted into the inferior vena cava through a femoral venotomy. In the 24 dogs evaluated, none of the filters was occluded by 12 weeks; in those in which a clot was later injected, the clot was trapped in all instances with preservation of the flow around the margin of the device. They determined that the cone-shaped filter may be filled with clot to 70 per cent of its depth with blockage of only 49 per cent of the cross-sectional area.

RESULTS

Clips

In 1969 Brackney[89] reported on Moretz's behalf that they had inserted the Moretz clip into the vena cava of 70 patients in the preceding 12 years with no operative deaths and no fatal recurrent pulmonary emboli. However, there were five nonfatal recurrent emboli (7.1 per cent). During a follow-up period ranging from 3 months to 12 years, 45 patients had venacavograms: the vena cava in 39 (86.8 per cent) was patent, in 2 (4.4. per cent) was partially occluded, and in 4 (8.8 per cent) was

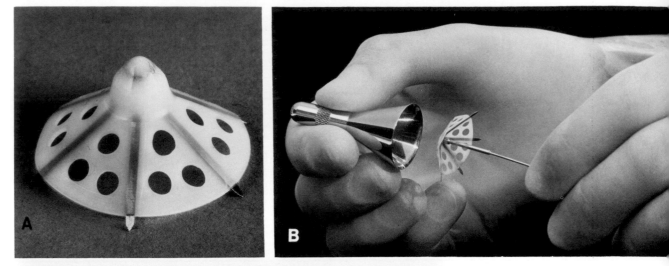

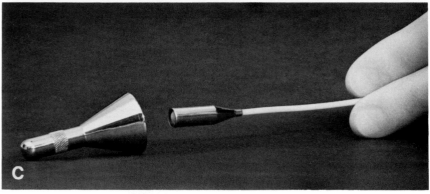

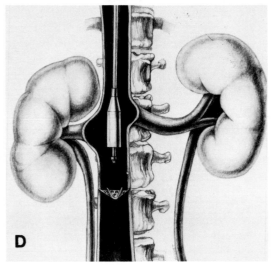

Figure 6-56. A to **D.** Umbrella-like device of Mobin-Uddin *et al.* (*Courtesy of Edwards Laboratories.*)

totally blocked. Leather *et al.*[90] in 1968 reported on a 5-year experience with the Moretz clip in 62 patients. There were four (6.4 per cent) in-hospital deaths, including one secondary to a recurrent embolus in a patient who had an open clip at autopsy. There were three nonfatal recurrent emboli, two of which were cardiogenic in origin. Forty-three cavograms were performed up to 59 months after clipping; in 36 (84 per cent) the vena cava was patent and in the remaining 7 was totally occluded. Totaling these two sets of data of 132 patients treated with the Moretz clip, the long-term patency rate was 80 per cent (71 of 88 patients studied by cavography over 12 years).

In 1971 Miles and Elsea[65] published their cumulative results with the Miles serrated clip. Of 121 patients treated, 10 (8.2 per cent) died in the hospital. There was one proved fatal postoperative

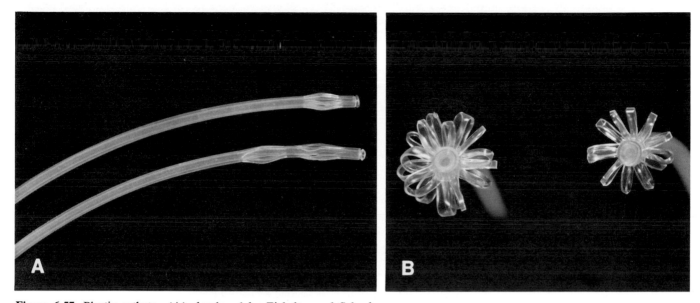

Figure 6-57. Plastic catheter (**A**) developed by Eichelter and Schenk that can be inflated into a (**B**) balloon which can be placed in the vena cava through the saphenous vein at the saphenofemoral junction. (*Eichelter & Schenk*. Arch Surg 97:348, 1968.)

embolism, which was found at autopsy to be cardiac in origin, and three nonfatal recurrent pulmonary emboli found by x ray, one of which was due to a technical error in the clipping procedure. In a follow-up period spanning 8 years, 34 of the clipped venae cavae were studied, 10 at autopsy and 24 by cavography; 26 (76 per cent) were patent and 8 (24 per cent) totally occluded. Of the 121 patients, 93 had edema of the lower extremity prior to or at clipping; 82 patients (including 19 with acute thrombophlebitis) experienced edema after clipping. In 4 of 28 patients (14.3 per cent) free from edema prior to clipping, swelling did occur postoperatively. In the 93 patients with existing edema at clipping, swelling decreased in 47 after clipping and disappeared completely in 33 of the 93.

The patency rates of the Moretz and the Miles serrated clip are 80 per cent and 76 per cent, respectively, so that generally speaking, inserting a clipping device into the vena cava has proved to be an effective means of partially interrupting the venous return. Whether the clip is superior to ligation of the cava as far as postphlebitic sequelae are concerned is hard to prove on the basis of published data. At recent seminars on pulmonary embolism, both Dalen and Crane commented on the high incidence of venous thrombosis after clipping procedures; this argues for stasis as the cause of venous thrombosis in many postoperative patients. (See Chapter 2.)

Intraluminal Grids

DeWeese *et al.*[91] have reported a 15-year clinical experience with their intraluminal grid. A total of 112 patients who had the intraluminal caval filter constructed during the years 1957 to 1972 were available for study. No deaths occurred in the operating room; the overall early postoperative mortality was 9 per cent, similar to the rate for vena cava ligation. None of these early deaths was due to pulmonary embolism. During the follow-up period extending from 1 to 153 months, 17 patients died (15.2 per cent), but, on clinical and autopsy findings, no deaths were secondary to recurrent pulmonary infarction. It is remarkable that no patient in the entire series died of pulmonary embolism; nonfatal pulmonary embolism was believed to have occurred in 7 patients (6.2 per cent).

Almost two-thirds of the patients had no clinical evidence of edema postoperatively and were not required to wear elastic support hose. Caval patency was demonstrated by phlebography in 11 (58 per cent) of 19 patients who had either unilateral or bilateral edema. Sixteen (15.7 per cent) of the patients developed recurrent thrombophlebitis postoperatively; caval patency was proved in several of these by phlebography. In the follow-up period, 4 patients (3.9 per cent) had stasis ulcers; in 2 patients the ulcers were present prior to interruption of the vena cava, and in a third the ulcer developed after trauma to the ankle. Two ulcers were healed conservatively, and two required excision and skin grafting. In this series 56.9 per cent of the patients were entirely symptom-free and did not require elastic support or other supportive measures in their postoperative management. Data regarding filter patency were obtainable in 45 (40.1 per cent) of the patients by phlebography, autopsy, or reoperation; the filter was found to be patent in 32 (71 per cent) and occluded in 13 (29 per cent).

Plications

Spencer and associates[72-74] have reported excellent results following the operation of plication. Spencer,[74] who devised the technique, has a zero recurrence rate of pulmonary embolism in patients under his personal care; the vena cava has been shown to be patent in an estimated 75 to 80 per cent of his patients. In a combined series from the hospitals at Johns Hopkins in Baltimore and at the University of Lexington, Kentucky,[73] no pulmonary emboli occurred during the first several weeks after operation in 39 patients who underwent plication. There were 6 deaths (15 per cent) in the first month: three resulted from extensive pulmonary emboli existing prior to plication, two from myocardial infarction, and one from peritonitis and shock. Extensive venous thrombosis developed in 4 (14 per cent) of 29 patients. In 3 of these, iliofemoral thrombectomy was performed with moderate success. In late results of the 33 patients surviving more than a month, 1 patient developed repeated pulmonary emboli: she underwent vena cava ligation and died of congestive heart failure 6 months after ligation. At autopsy, thrombi in the ovarian vein were thought to be the source of the emboli. Nonfatal embolus may have occurred in another patient. Venocavograms obtained in 8 patients 1 year or more after operation showed patency in all. This group included a patient whose vena cava thrombosed a few weeks after plication; by the end of the first year, recanalization had taken place. Recurrent thrombophlebitis occurred in only 2 patients. Signs of venous insufficiency were uncommon. Massive edema developed in a patient in whom the vena cava was thought to have become occluded 3 weeks postoperatively. Moderate edema occurred in 4 patients and minimal edema in 4; however, the same degree of swelling had been present preoperatively. Three patients required elastic support hose, and none developed ulceration of the leg.

De Meester et al.[92] reported on 56 patients who underwent plication of the vena cava at Johns Hopkins Hospital. There were 7 postoperative deaths (12.5 per cent). At autopsy, 5 patients had clot (believed to be antemortem) just cephalad to the plication site. Of the 49 patients who survived operation, 15 (31 per cent) developed extensive iliofemoral thrombophlebitis; massive retroperitoneal hematoma occurred in 2 patients. During the follow-up period, 35 of 56 patients had patency of the vena cava demonstrated by venocavogram or autopsy examination; 21 (60 per cent) of the plications were patent, and 14 (40 per cent) were thrombosed. Postoperative edema occurred in 10 of 10 patients with thrombosed plications and in 4 of 12 patients in whom the plication site was patent. In this series there were five proved and three suspected recurrent pulmonary embolisms after plication of the vena cava. Four of these repeated embolic episodes occurred in the early postoperative period. The source of the thromboemboli was thought to be an unligated right ovarian vein in 1 patient, the heart in 2, and the inferior vena cava in 2. In these last 2 patients, thrombus was found in the vena cava just cephalad to the plication site; thus, two of the five recurrent emboli might be attributed to failure of the operation. In discussing this paper, Spencer pointed out the importance of routine anticoagulant therapy postoperatively, the danger of plicating through clot in the lumen of the vena cava, and the technical importance of placing the sutures 5 mm apart.

The Vena Cava Umbrella Filter

Mobin-Uddin et al.[93] have summarized the results of clinical filter implants in 2215 patients as reported by physicians participating in the evaluation program (Tables 6-7 and 6-8). Omitted from the tables are 71 patients in whom the umbrella filter could not be implanted through the right internal jugular vein. In 2 of these patients the left internal jugular vein was used to implant the device, and in 1 the right common femoral vein was used. Rate of fatal recurrent pulmonary embolism was 0.8 per cent, of nonfatal, 2.2 per cent. In 3 patients, blood clot from the proximal surface of the umbrella filter was implicated as the source of recurrent pulmonary emboli. Significant clinical edema or phlebitis of the lower extremities which was not previously present occurred in 115 patients (5.1 per cent). The majority of these patients improved with standard medical treatment.

THERAPEUTIC PROCEDURES

See Chapter 2 for a discussion of excision of phlebitic veins and for a discussion of thrombectomy. For a discussion of pulmonary artery embolectomy, see Chapter 8.

Results of Excision of Phlebitic Veins

Between 1952 and 1974, 195 patients (210 extremities) were treated for acute superficial thrombophlebitis of the lower extremities by excision of phlebitic veins with or without simultaneous ligation of the long and/or short saphenous veins. This represents 21 per cent of 912 patients seen for acute superficial thrombophlebitis of the lower extremities.

Operative mortality has been zero, and morbidity has been minimal.

Results of Thrombectomy

Thrombectomy has been carried out in conjunction with ligation of the femoral or iliac veins in 21

TABLE 6-7. Summary of Clinical Results in Patients Treated with Umbrella Filter as of November 1973

	NO. PATIENTS		
	23 MM FILTER	28 MM FILTER	TOTAL
Proximal filter migration	20	2	22 (0.9%)
Distal filter migration*	6	0	6 (0.27%)
Filter dislodgement without migration	20	0	20 (0.9%)
Misplacement of filter			
Right renal vein	7	0	7 (0.3%)
Right iliac vein	20	0	20 (0.9%)
Recurrent emboli			
Fatal	18	0	18 (0.8%)
Nonfatal	47	6	53 (2.3%)
Clinical edema or phlebitis	102	13	115 (5.1%)
Total filter implants	1981	234	2215

* Following closed cardiac massage
From Mobin-Uddin et al. In *Pulmonary Thromboembolism.*
Springfield, IL, Thomas, 1975.

TABLE 6-8. Umbrella Filter Dislodgement and Proximal Migration

FILTER MIGRATED TO	NO. PATIENTS
Pulmonary artery	13
Fatal embolization with massive thrombus—3	
Removed—7 (2 died postoperatively)	
Left in place—3 (1 died few days later;	
2 died after 3 mo, death unrelated)	
Right ventricle	2
Removed on cardiopulmonary bypass—1	
Died 6 days later, no autopsy—1	
Right atrium	4
Fatal embolization with massive thrombus—1	
Found at autopsy, death unrelated—1	
Removed—2 (1 died postoperatively)	
Suprarenal inferior vena cava	3
Died of cancer after 6 wk—1	
Died of myocardial infarction after 1 yr—1	
Alive and well—1 (venogram showed patency	
of inferior vena cava)	

From Mobin-Uddin et al. In *Pulmonary Thromboembolism.*
Springfield, IL, Thomas, 1975.

extremities; our first thrombectomy was performed in August 1954 on a patient with clots in the common femoral vein, the source of his pulmonary embolism. More recently, thrombectomy has been performed in conjunction with ligation of the inferior vena cava in patients with marked edema or with phlegmasia cerulea dolens if the operation is performed within 24 to 36 hours after the onset of the massive edema. This combination of procedures was performed in 33 patients in this series, 9 for "benign" phlegmasia cerulea dolens and 24 for massive venous thrombosis of the femoroiliac system.

SWELLING AFTER CAVAL LIGATION ALONE AND WITH THROMBECTOMY

A group of 29 patients were studied[94] at least 5 years after treatment for femoroiliac thrombophlebitis, 13 patients by caval ligation and 16 by ligation plus thrombectomy. Followup averaged 10 years (extremes 5 and 15 years) after ligation alone and 9 years (extremes 5 and 14 years) after thrombectomy. In 44 per cent of thrombectomized patients swelling was absent and in 56 per cent persistent swelling was controlled by heavyweight elastic stockings. In the nonthrombectomized group, 54 per cent had no swelling, 31 per cent had edema controllable by stockings, and 15 per cent had intractable swelling.

OTHER POSTPHLEBITIC SEQUELAE

In the thrombectomized group, 12.5 per cent had varicose veins, compared with 61 per cent of those with ligation alone. Pigmentation was present in 46 per cent of the ligated group and in none of those who underwent thrombectomy. There were no ulcerations in the thrombectomized group, but 2 (15%) of 13 patients with ligation alone experienced ulceration (see case reports in preceding section). Venous claudication was reported by 2 patients after ligation and by none after thrombectomy.

Results of Conservative Treatment

Concurrently, 27 patients managed by conservative measures were studied[94] an average of 8 years after therapy (extremes of 5 and 14 years). Twenty-seven per cent were free from swelling and were not using elastic support; 54 per cent had swelling controlled by heavyweight stockings; and 15 per cent had swelling not well controlled by stockings. Varicosities appeared in 14 per cent of these patients and pigmentation in 4 per cent; none developed ulceration or venous claudication. In assessing these results, however, it must be borne in mind that patients who were treated either by ligation or by thrombectomy had more severe and more extensive venous thrombosis than those who were treated with conservative measures.

REFERENCES

1. Homans, J. Thrombosis of deep veins of lower leg, causing pulmonary embolism. *N Engl J Med 211:*993, 1934.
2. Linton, R. R. Venous interruption in thromboembolic disease, editorial. *Surgery 19:*434, 1949.
3. O'Keefe, A. F., Warren, R., and Donaldson, G. A. Venous circulation in lower extremities following femoral vein ligation. *Surgery 29:*267, 1951.
3a. Hafner, C. D., Cranley, J. J., Krause, R. J., *et al.* Venous thrombectomy: Current status. *Ann Surg 161:*411, 1965.
4. Pfaff, O. G. Ligation of the inferior vena cava. *Am J Obstet Gynec 11:*660, 1926.
5. Northway, R. P., and Buxton, R. W. Ligation of the inferior vena cava. *Surgery 18:*85, 1945.
6. Costa, G. Contributo allo studio delle ferite della vena cava inferiore. *Arch Ital di Chir 4:*339, 1921.
7. Krotoski, J. Zur Venenunterbinduung bzw. -extirpation bei der puerperalen Allgemeininfektion vom chirurgischen Standpunkt. *Chirurg 9:*425, 1937.
8. O'Neil, E. E. Ligation of the inferior vena cava in the prevention and treatment of pulmonary embolism. *N Engl J Med 232:*641, 1945.
9. Gaston, E. A., and Folsom, H. Ligation of the inferior vena cava for the prevention of pulmonary embolism: Report of two cases. *N Engl J Med 233:*229, 1945.
10. Dale, W. A. Ligation of the inferior vena cava for thromboembolism. *Surgery 43:*24, 1958.
11. Moses, W. R. Ligation of the inferior vena cava or iliac veins: A report of 36 operations. *N Engl J Med 235:*1, 1946.
12. Thebaut, B. R., and Ward, C. S. Ligation of the inferior vena cava in thromboembolism: Report of 36 cases. *Surg Gynecol Obstet 84:*385, 1947.
13. Veal, J. R., Hussey, H. H., and Barnes, E. Ligation of the inferior vena cava in thrombosis of the deep veins of the lower extremities. *Surg Gynecol Obstet 84:*605, 1947.
14. Connerley, M. L., and Heintzelman, J. H. C. Treatment and prophylaxis of pulmonary embolism by vein interruption. *N Engl J Med 240:*830, 1949.

15. Shea, P. C., and Robertson, R. L. Late sequelae of inferior vena cava ligation. *Surg Gynecol Obstet 93:* 153, 1951.

16. Collins, C. G., Norton, R. O., Nelson, L. W., Wolfstein, B. B., Collins, J. H., and Webster, H. D. Suppurative thrombophlebitis: IV. Results of study of 70 patients treated by ligation of the inferior vena cava and ovarian vessels. *Surgery 31:*528, 1952.

17. Pratt, G. H. Control of pulmonary emboli by inferior vena cava ligation. *JAMA 147:*126, 1951.

18. Zollinger, R., and Teachnor, W. H. Late results of inferior vena caval ligations. *Arch Surg 65:*31, 1952.

19. Owens, F. M. Vena caval ligation in thromboembolic disease. *Arch Surg 65:*600, 1952.

20. Payne, J. T. Indications for ligation of the inferior vena cava in venous thrombosis. *Arch Surg 67:*902, 1953.

21. Madden, J. L. Ligation of the inferior vena cava. *Ann Surg 140:*200, 1954.

22. Kirtley, J. A., Riddell, D. H., and Hamilton, E. C. Indications and late results of ligation of the inferior vena cava. *Ann Surg 141:*653, 1955.

23. Bowers, R. F., and Leb, S. M. Late results of inferior vena cava ligation. *Surgery 37:*622, 1955.

24. Zoeckler, S. J. Inferior vena cava ligation. *J Iowa Med Soc 50:*552, 1960.

25. Dale, W. A. Inferior vena caval ligation for venous thromboembolism. *Rev Surg 19:*1, 1962.

26. Krause, R. J., Cranley, J. J., Hallaba, M. A. S., Strasser, E. S., and Hafner, C. D. Caval ligation in thromboembolic disease. *Arch Surg 87:*184, 1963.

27. Nabseth, D. C., and Moran, J. M. Reassessment of the rôle of inferior-vena-cava ligation in venous thromboembolism. *N Engl J Med 273:*1250, 1965.

28. Bergan, J. J., Kinnaird, D. W., Koons, K., and Trippel, O. H. Prevention of pulmonary embolism: Comparison of vena cava ligation, plication, and filter operations. *Arch Surg 92:*605, 1965.

29. Stevens, E. L., Fitzpatrick, W. K., Stewart, G. K., and Burdette, W. J. Ligation of the inferior vena cava. *Arch Surg 90:*578, 1965.

30. Amador, E., Li, T. K., and Crane, C. Ligation of inferior vena cava for thromboembolism: Clinical and autopsy correlations in 119 cases. *JAMA 206:*1758, 1968.

31. Pollak, E. W., Sparks, F. C., and Barker, W. F. Pulmonary embolism: An appraisal of therapy in 516 cases. *Arch Surg 107:*66, 1973.

32. Cranley, J. J., Krause, R. J., Strasser, E. S., and Hafner, C. D. Results of vena cava ligation. *J Cardiov Surg 13:*403, 1972.

33. Parrish, E. H., Adams, J. T., Pories, W. J., Burget, D. E., and DeWeese, J. A. Pulmonary emboli following vena caval ligation. *Arch Surg 97:*899, 1968.

34. McIntyre, K. M., Belko, S., and Sasahara, A. A. Pulmonary embolism: Premonitory signs and recurrence after vena cava ligation. *Arch Surg 98:*671, 1969.

35. Case Records of the Massachusetts General Hospital, Case 34-1967. Weekly Clinico-pathological Exercises. B. Castleman, ed. *N Engl J Med 277:* 399, 1967.

36. Mozes, M., Bogowsky, H., Antebi, E., Tzur, N., and Penchas, S. Inferior vena cava ligation for pulmonary embolism: Review of 118 cases. *Surgery 60:*790, 1966.

37. Gurewich, V., Thomas, D. P., and Rabinov, K. R. Pulmonary embolism after ligation of the inferior vena cava. *N Engl J Med 274:*1350, 1966.

38. Moran, J. C., and Nabseth, D. C. Pulmonary embolism following vena cava ligation: Letter to editor. *N Engl J Med 275:*733, 1966.

39. Thomas, G. L. Pulmonary embolism following vena cava ligation: Letter to the editor. *N Engl J Med 275:*734, 1966.

40. Crane, C. Femoral vs. caval interruption for venous thromboembolism. *N Engl J Med 270:*819, 1964.

41. Cranley, J. J. Obliterative Arterial Diseases, Technique of Lumbar Sympathectomy. In *Peripheral Arterial Diseases.* Harper & Row, Hagerstown, 1972, p 26.

42. Milloy, F. J., Anson, B. J., and Cauldwell, E. W. Variations in the inferior caval veins and in their renal and lumbar communications. *Surg Gynecol Obstet 115:*131, 1962.

43. Gryska, P. F., and Earthrowl, F. H. Left-sided inferior vena cava. *Arch Surg 94:*363, 1967.

44. Reis, R. H., and Esenther, G. Variations in the pattern of renal vessels and their relation to the type of posterior vena cava in man. *Am J Anat 104:*295, 1959.

45. Gladstone, R. J. Development of the inferior vena cava in the light of recent research, with special reference to certain abnormalities, and current descriptions of the ascending lumbar and azygos veins. *J Anat 64:*70, 1929.

46. Hirsch, D. M., and Chan, K.-F. Bilateral inferior vena cava. *JAMA 185:*729, 1963.

47. Dardik, H., Loop, F. D., Cox, P. A., and Keshishian, J. M. "C-Pattern" inferior vena cava: Embryogenesis and clinical implications. *JAMA 200:*248, 1967.

48. Maraan, B. M., and Taber, R. E. The effects of inferior vena caval ligation on cardiac output: An experimental study. *Surgery 63:*966, 1963.

49. Gazzaniga, A. B., Cahill, J. L., Replogle, R. L., and Tilney, N. L. Changes in blood volume and renal function following ligation of the inferior vena cava. *Surgery 62:*417, 1967.

50. Robinson, L. S. Collateral circulation following ligation of the inferior vena cava: Injection studies in stillborn infants. *Surgery 25:*329, 1949.

51. Filler, R. M., and Edwards, E. A. Collaterals of the lower inferior vena cava in man revealed by venography. *Arch Surg 84:*28, 1966.

52. Ferris, E. J., Vittimberga, F. J., Byrne, J. J., Nabseth, D. C., and Shapiro, J. H. The inferior vena cava after ligation and plication: A study of collateral routes. *Radiology 89:*1, 1967.

52a. Tandler, *Lehrbuch der systematischen Anatomie.* Berlin, Springer-Verlag, 1926, vol. 3, p 151.

53. Sappey, and Dumontpallier. Physiologie pathologique: Note sur cas d'oblitération de la veine cave inférieure avec circulation collatérale; suive de faits analogues démonstrant qu'il existe trois principales variétés d'oblitération de cette veine. *Gaz Méd de Paris 17:*52–54, 66–70, 82–83, 1862.

53a. Spalteholz, K. W. *Handatlas der anatomie des Menschen.* Leipzig, Hirzel, 1895–1903.

54. Schauble, J. F., Stickel, D. I., and Anlyan, W. G. Vena caval ligation for thromboembolic disease. *Arch Surg 84:*17, 1962.

55. Moran, J. M., Kahn, P. C., and Callow, A. D. Partial versus complete caval interruption for venous thromboembolism. *Am J Surg 117:*471, 1969.

56. Streuter, M. A., and Paine, J. R. Temporary occlusion of the inferior vena cava suggested as a means of treatment in thromboembolism requiring caval ligation. *Surgery 34:*20, 1953.

57. Pualwan, F., Jones, G. E., Bruny, S. J. A., and Dale, W. A. Effects of ligation of the inferior vena cava with absorbable ligature. Surgical Forum: Proceedings 40th Clinical Congress of American College of Surgeons, Atlantic City, NJ, November 1954. Philadelphia, Saunders, 1955, pp 179–184.

58. Dale, W. A., Pualwan, F., and Bauer, F. M. Ligation of the inferior vena cava with absorbable catgut. *Surg Gynecol Obstet 102:*517, 1956.

59. Moretz, W. H., Naisbitt, P. F., and Stevenson, G. P. Experimental studies on temporary occlusion of the inferior vena cava. *Surgery 36:*384, 1954.

60. Moretz, W. H., Rhode, C. M., and Shepherd, M. H. Prevention of pulmonary embolism by partial occlusion of the inferior vena cava. *Am Surg 25:*617, 1959.

61. Miles, R. M., and Young, J. M. Recanalization of the inferior vena cava—an experimental study. *Surgery 33:*849, 1953.

62. Miles, R. M., Chappell, F., and Renner, O. A partially occluding vena cava clip for the prevention of pulmonary embolism. *Am Surg 30:*40, 1964.

63. Miles, R. M. Prevention of pulmonary embolism by the use of a plastic vena caval clip. *Ann Surg 163:*192, 1966.

64. Miles, R. M., Richardson, R. R., Wayne, L., Elsea, P. W., Stewart, S. B., and Duncan, D. Long-term results with the serrated Teflon vena caval clip in the prevention of pulmonary embolism. *Ann Surg 169:*881, 1969.

65. Miles, R. M., and Elsea, P. W. Clinical evaluation of the serrated vena caval clip. *Surg Gynecol Obstet 132:*581, 1971.

66. Taber, R. E., Zikria, E., Hershey, E. A., and Lam, C. R. Prevention of pulmonary emboli with a vena caval clip. *JAMA 195:*889, 1966.

67. Adams, J. T., and DeWeese, J. A. Experimental and clinical evaluation of partial vein interruption in the prevention of pulmonary emboli. *Surgery 57:*82, 1965.

68. Adams, J. T., and DeWeese, J. A. Partial interruption of the inferior vena cava with a new plastic clip. *Surg Gynecol Obstet 123:*1087, 1966.

69. DeWeese, M. S., and Hunter, D. C. A vena cava filter for the prevention of pulmonary emboli. *Bull Soc Int Chir 17:*17, 1958.

70. DeWeese, M. S., and Hunter, D. C. A vena cava filter for the prevention of pulmonary embolism: A five year clinical experience. *Arch Surg 86:*852, 1963.

71. Spencer, F. C. Experimental evaluation of partitioning of the inferior vena cava to prevent pulmonary embolism. *Surg Forum 10:*680, 1960.

72. Spencer, F. C., Quattlebaum, J. K., Quattlebaum, J. K., Jr., Sharp, E. H., and Jude, J. R. Plication of the inferior vena cava for pulmonary embolism: A report of 20 cases. *Ann Surg 155:*827, 1962.

73. Spencer, F. C., Jude, J., Rienhoff, W. F., and Stonesifer, G. Plication of the inferior vena cava for pulmonary embolism: Long-term results in 39 cases. *Ann Surg 161:*788, 1965.

74. Spencer, F. C. Plication of the vena cava for pulmonary embolism. *Surgery 62:*388, 1967.

75. Ravitch, M. M., Snodgrass, E., McEnany, T., and Rivarola, A. Compartmentation of the inferior vena cava with the mechanical stapler. *Surg Gynecol Obstet 122:*561, 1966.

76. Mozes, M., and Antibe, E. A simple method for plication of the inferior vena cava. *Surg Gynecol Obstet 125:*362, 1967.

77. Mobin-Uddin, K., Smith, P. E., Martinez, L. O., Lombardo, C. R., and Jude, J. R. A vena caval filter for the prevention of pulmonary embolus. *Surg Forum 18:*209, 1967.

78. Mobin-Uddin, K., McLean, R., and Jude, J. R. A new catheter technique of interruption of inferior vena cava for prevention of pulmonary embolism. *Am Surg 35:*889, 1969.

79. Mobin-Uddin, K., McLean, R., Bolooki, H., and Jude, J. R. Caval interruption for prevention of pulmonary embolism. *Arch Surg 99:*711, 1969.

80. Mobin-Uddin, K., Trinkle, J. K., and Bryant, L. R. Present status of the inferior vena cava umbrella filter. *Surgery 70:*914, 1971.

81. Mobin-Uddin, K., Callard, G. M., Bolooki, H., Robinson, R., Michie, D., and Jude, J. R. Transvenous caval interruption with umbrella filter. *N Engl J Med 286:*55, 1972.

82. Eichelter, P., and Schenk, W. G. Prophylaxis of pulmonary embolism: A new experimental approach to prophylaxis of pulmonary embolism. *Rev Surg 24:*455, 1967.

83. Eichelter, P., and Schenk, W. G. Prophylaxis of pulmonary embolism: A new experimental approach with initial results. *Arch Surg 97:*348, 1968.

84. Williams, R. W., and Schenk, W. G. A removable

intracaval filter for prevention of pulmonary embolism: Early experience with the use of the Eichelter catheter in patients. *Surgery 68:*999, 1970.

85. Pate, J. W., Melvin, D., and Cheek, R. C. A new form of vena caval interruption. *Ann Surg 169:*873, 1969.

86. Hunter, J. A., Sessions, R., and Buerger, R. Experimental balloon obstruction of inferior vena cava. *Ann Surg 171:*315, 1970.

87. Lewis, M. R., Kamat, P. V., and Dale, W. A. Balloon blockade of the inferior vena cava. *Arch Surg 102:*209, 1971.

88. Greenfield, L. J., McCurdy, J. R., Brown, P. P., and Elkins, R. C. A new intracaval filter permitting continued flow and resolution of emboli. *Surgery 73:*599, 1973.

89. Brackney, E. L., in discussion Miles *et al. Ann Surg 169:*881, 1969.

90. Leather, R. P., Clark, W. R., Powers, S. R., Parker, F. B., Bernard, H. R., and Eckert, C. Five-year experience with the Moretz vena caval clip in 62 patients. *Arch Surg 97:*357, 1968.

91. Deweese, M. S., Hunter, D. C., Kimmelstiel, W. P., Gill, H. H., and Thompson, N. W. Fifteen-year clinical experience with the vena cava filter. *Ann Surg 178:*247, 1973.

92. De Meester, T. R., Rutherford, R. B., Blazek, J. V., and Zuidema, G. D. Plication of the inferior vena cava for thromboembolism. *Surgery 62:*56, 1967.

93. Mobin-Uddin, K., Utley, J. R., and Bryant, L. R. The inferior vena cava umbrella filter. In *Pulmonary Thromboembolism.* Springfield, IL, Thomas, 1974.

94. Cranley, J. J., Krause, R. J., Strasser, E. S., and Hafner, C. D. Femoroiliac thrombophlebitis: Immediate and late results after thrombectomy, caval ligation, and conservative management. *J Cardiov Surg 10:*463, 1969.

7

Special Syndromes

I. SYNDROMES OF THE SUPERIOR VENA CAVA
Ernest H. Meese

ANATOMY OF THE SUPERIOR VENA CAVA

The superior vena cava carries to the heart the blood returning from the head, neck, and upper extremities by way of the right and left innominate (brachiocephalic) veins and their tributaries and the blood returning from the walls of the thorax through the azygos veins. The superior vena cava is formed by the junction of the two innominate veins; it has no valves. It originates behind the lower border of the first right costal cartilage, close to the sternum, descends vertically behind the first and second intercostal spaces, and ends in the upper part of the right atrium, opposite the third right costal cartilage anteriorly and the seventh thoracic vertebra posteriorly. It is 7 to 8 cm (3 inches) long. Slightly more than one-half is contained within the pericardium; the serous layer of the pericardium is reflected obliquely over the superior vena cava immediately below the spot where it is joined by the azygos vein, on a lower level than the reflection of the pericardium on the aorta. In its course it describes a slight convexity to the right (Fig. 7-1).

Relations

In front the superior vena cava is related to the anterior margins of the right lung and pleura, with the pericardium intervening below. These structures separate it from the internal mammary artery, the first and second intercostal spaces, and the second and third costal cartilages. The trachea and the right vagus nerve are posteromedial and the right lung and pleura posterolateral to its upper part. The hilum of the right lung is a direct posterior relation below. On its right courses the right phrenic nerve and right pleura. On the left it is related to the beginning of the innominate artery and the ascending aorta, the latter overlapping it.

Surface Relationships

The superior vena cava is 2 cm wide and lies partly behind the right margin of the sternum. The shadow of its lateral border is visible on most front-view radiographs of the chest.

Tributaries

The tributaries include the azygos vein and several small veins from the pericardium and other structures in the mediastinum.

DISORDERS OF THE SUPERIOR VENA CAVA

Trauma

A review of the literature regarding penetrating wounds of the heart and great vessels reveals that

189

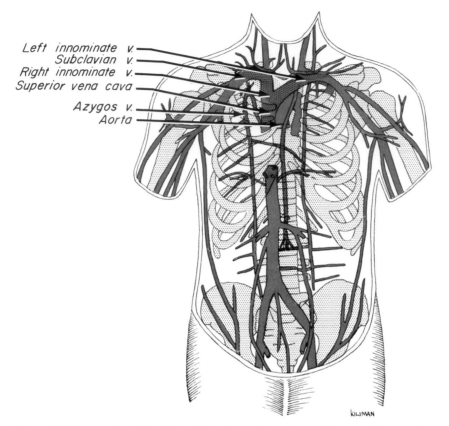

Left innominate v.
Subclavian v.
Right innominate v.
Superior vena cava

Azygos v.
Aorta

KILIMAN

Figure 7-1. Anatomic relationships of the skeletal structures of thorax with superior vena cava and its tributaries. Note venous connections with inferior vena cava, important in establishing collateral circulation.

superior vena caval injuries are extremely rare.[1-5] Few surgeons have managed more than one case of penetrating injury to the superior vena cava or innominate veins. The incidence of such wounds is low in both military and civilian practice. One reason for the low incidence is the relative protection supplied by the overlying manubrium and clavicles. Secondly, a solitary venous penetrating injury rarely occurs; it is usually combined with an arterial wound because of the close proximity of the ascending aorta and innominate artery. It is possible that most patients with combined injuries of the great vessels die before reaching the hospital; even so, a general lack of salvage in this group has been reported.

SIGNS AND SYMPTOMS

Penetrating wounds of the superior vena cava may present differently, depending on whether they in-

volve the innominate branches and the portion of the vessel above the pericardial reflection or the intrapericardial portion. The former type of wound may cause a massive mediastinal hematoma above the pericardium or (if the pleura is entered) may present as a massive hemopneumothorax. The second type of wound causes pericardial tamponade and presents as a cardiac wound. Therefore, the clinical picture is that of hemorrhagic shock, that of cardiac tamponade, or a combination of both. If there is no associated arterial injury, the wound in the low-pressure venous system may present symptoms more slowly, with increased central venous pressure as the only sign of the injury. In this type of patient, preoperative phlebography may be carried out to show the venous laceration.[5]

The management of vascular trauma to the thorax has been presented earlier. For a detailed discussion, see Volume I, Chapter 7.[6]

Most wounds of the superior vena cava or innominate vein require operative treatment. Exposure of this area is best achieved with a median sternotomy incision, which may be extended into an interspace on either side if indicated. Superior vena caval injuries are managed by direct suture repair whenever possible. A partially occluding Satinsky vascular clamp may be useful to gain control of hemorrhage while repair is performed. The patient can also tolerate a short period of total occlusion between vascular clamps if necessary.[7] A large defect in the vein may require a patch of autogenous vein or adjacent pericardium, using a temporary internal superior vena caval shunt if necessary (Fig. 7-2). Replacement with autogenous vein graft is occasionally necessary. While it is important not to totally obstruct the vena cava, ligation of one of the innominate veins, should the need arise, is carried out with little hesitation; postligation sequelae have not been observed following unilateral occlusion.

The Superior Vena Caval Syndrome

Obstruction of the superior vena cava may be produced by a variety of pathologic processes. The basic anatomy and related physiologic disturbances are essentially the same both for malignant and benign caval obstruction. There are important etiologic and prognostic differences, however. Therefore, an accurate clinical evaluation of every patient who presents with this syndrome is mandatory.

OBSTRUCTION BY MALIGNANT DISEASE

Obstruction by malignant disease in the superior mediastinum is estimated to cause 75 to 90 per cent of all cases.[8–13] The most frequent malignant

Figure 7-2. Large defect in superior vena cava repaired by an autogenous composite vein graft while continuous venous flow is maintained by temporary internal venous shunt.

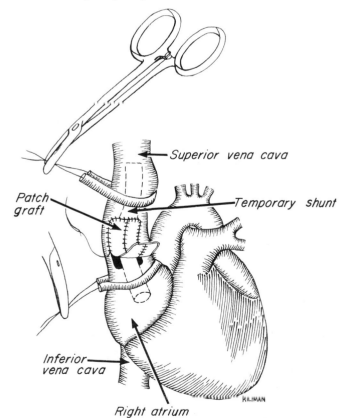

lesion is bronchiogenic carcinoma in the medial portion of the right upper lobe.[11, 12] Carcinoma arising in adjacent pulmonary tissue and encroaching on the vein may totally obstruct the cava by thrombosis, by actual invasion of the venous system, or by constriction resulting from an associated inflammatory reaction surrounding the primary bronchial carcinoma.

Malignant mediastinal tumors, particularly those of thymic origin, may produce an identical syndrome.[14, 15] Although malignant lesions which cause the superior vena caval syndrome arise primarily in the mediastinum or the adjacent lung, metastatic malignant disease may occasionally obstruct the vena cava;[11, 16] we have seen this occur from carcinoma of the breast and from seminoma. The caval block may result from localized extrinsic pressure from large neoplastic masses involving the mediastinal lymph glands, such as malignant lymphoma or Hodgkin's disease.[17]

OBSTRUCTION BY BENIGN DISEASE

NEOPLASMS. Benign lesions in the mediastinum may occasionally cause caval obstruction. Neoplastic masses such as dermoid cyst, benign thymoma, and substernal goitre ordinarily do not cause obstruction even if they grow to considerable proportions. However, an intrathoracic goitre of sufficient size may cause compression of the innominate veins at the thoracic inlet. Although this is not a true caval obstruction, it presents the same physiologic disturbances and clinical picture.[11, 18–21] Chemodectoma of the mediastinum has been reported as an infrequent cause of superior vena cava obstruction.[22]

ANEURYSMS. Aneurysms of the ascending or transverse aorta or the innominate artery are the second most frequent cause of benign vena caval obstruction. In 1757 William Hunter reported the first patient with the superior vena caval syndrome; the condition was secondary to a syphilitic aneurysm of the aorta. As late as 1949, McIntyre and Sykes[23] reported that 30 per cent of superior vena caval syndromes were caused by aortic aneurysm. Since then the incidence has decreased to approximately 4 per cent.[24] However, in view of our ever-increasing geriatric population and the recent re-

crudescence of syphilis in the general population, the incidence of thoracic aneurysm may increase.

IDIOPATHIC PRIMARY THROMBOSIS. Idiopathic primary thrombosis of the superior caval system may occasionally be seen.

CHRONIC FIBROSING MEDIASTINITIS. The most common cause of thrombosis is chronic fibrosing mediastinitis, either idiopathic or granulomatous.[25, 26] Approximately 20 per cent of superior vena caval obstructions are caused by granulomatous or fibrotic lesions of the mediastinum; this establishes these lesions as the leading cause of benign superior caval syndrome.[11, 27]

Mediastinal granuloma is a descrptive term for a lesion whose cause is unknown. Most of the patients with this lesion have immunologic evidence of previous infection with *Histoplasma capsulatum*.[27] Mediastinal granuloma originates primarily as a lymph node disease. The node enlarges and undergoes central caseation necrosis. Adjacent nodes coalesce; the integrity of the individual gland is ultimately lost after a conglomerate mass of encapsulated material develops to form the tumefaction. When the right paratracheal nodes near the azygos vein are involved, the well-circumscribed lesion is seen on chest roentgenograms. When this granuloma of the paratracheal area enters its healing phase, severe localizing fibrosis, called fibrosing mediastinitis, probably develops (Fig. 7-3).

THROMBOSIS OF IATROGENIC ORIGIN. Some rare iatrogenic causes of obstruction have been reported. Friedli et al.[28] discovered several cases of superior vena caval obstruction following surgical repair of partial anomalous pulmonary venous drainage when the procedure was used to redirect an anomalous vein draining far from the right atrium into the superior vena cava. This occurred also when the superior vena cava was enlarged with a pericardial patch, especially when there was a left superior vena cava, since then the right superior cava was already narrower than normal. Wertheimer et al.[29] reported a case of thrombosis occurring around a transvenous endocardial pacemaker electrode.

Cha[30] reviewed seven cases in which superior cavography was performed as a follow-up study of

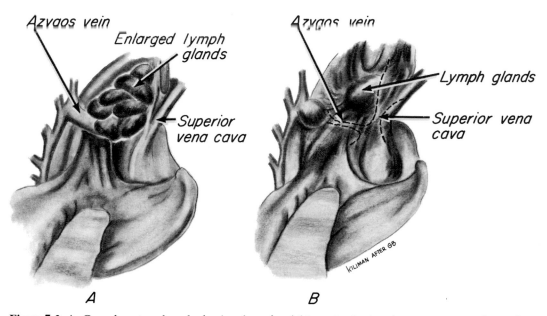

Figure 7-3. A. Granulomatous lymph glands enlarge in right paratracheal region near azygos vein, coalesce, and undergo central caseation necrosis. Conglomerate mass of encapsulated material develops to form the tumefaction. **B.** When granuloma enters its healing phase, severe localizing fibrosis develops in mediastinum, producing benign obstruction of superior vena cava.

ventriculoatrial shunt performed for treatment of hydrocephalus. Thrombosis due to the shunt produced partial or complete obstruction of the superior vena cava, with collateral circulation forming to the right heart in an effort to bypass the block.

OBSTRUCTION BY MISCELLANEOUS LESIONS. Mazzei and Mulder[31] reported the occurrence of superior vena caval syndrome due to delayed stricture of the intra-atrial pericardial baffle used in the Mustard procedure. They attributed the scarring and constricture to a subacute bacterial endocarditis on the revised portion of the baffle, as demonstrated by positive blood cultures.

A single case of superior vena caval obstruction has been reported secondary to sarcoidosis.[32] Moene *et al.*[33] reported an unusual case of obstruction caused by severe pressure of congested herniated lung on the superior vena cava through a congenital right-sided pericardial defect into the pericardial cavity.

The remainder of benign causes include pericardial calcification, chronic constrictive pericarditis (Fig. 7-4), mediastinal hematoma from closed or penetrating thoracic trauma, pyogenic infections of the mediastinum, and thrombophlebitis of the great veins.

COLLATERAL CIRCULATION

The collateral venous pathways which develop after caval obstruction are extensive. If the obstruction develops slowly, as with benign lesions, little or no symptomatic distress occurs, since the collateral circulation adapts itself to the increased venous flow from the head, neck, upper torso, and extremities. Sudden and complete caval obstruction is usually fatal; it is most often caused by technical errors made during resection of extensive malignant lesions involving the cava or by direct injury to the cava with resultant compression by a mediastinal hematoma.

In the rapidly developing caval obstruction, such as that caused by malignant infiltration or encasement from adjacent pulmonary carcinoma, the degree of distress depends not only on the rapidity of the caval obstruction but also on whether or not the azygos vein is spared. If the azygos vein remains

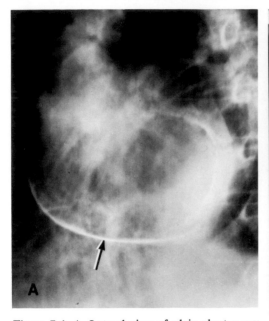

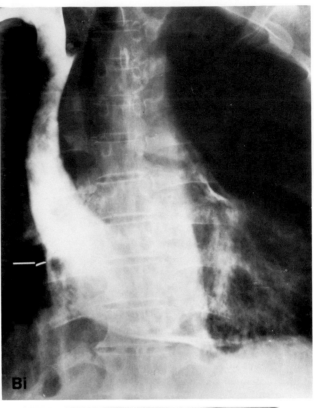

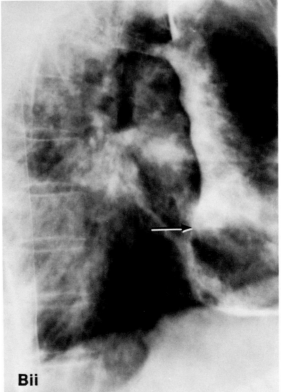

Figure 7-4. A. Lateral view of plain chest x ray demonstrating extensive pericardial calcification in patient with chronic constrictive calcific pericarditis with concurrent superior vena caval syndrome. **Bi** and **Bii.** Posteroanterior (**i.**) and lateral (**ii.**) superior cavograms demonstrating hold-up of dye in superior vena cava secondary to relative obstruction of surrounding pericardial calcification.

patent, sufficient collateral vessels may quickly develop to accommodate the increased venous load, allowing sufficient drainage into the right atrium and thereby lessening the severity of the venous hypertension so death may be averted.

Principal Collateral Pathways for Venous Return

The venous return to the heart from the upper half of the body is through five principal pathways[34] (Fig. 7-5). In addition, multiple anastomoses develop between these main alternate venous pathways. The site of obstruction and the availability of alternate venous channels dictate the most prominent pathway.

AZYGOS PATHWAY

The azygos pathway is usually found when the obstruction occurs between the entrance of the azygos vein into the superior vena cava and the right atrium. The blood flows retrograde into the hemiazygos vein, the ascending lumbar veins, and the inferior vena cava.

INTERNAL MAMMARY PATHWAY

This pathway is often prominent when the occlusion also involves the azygos vein. The blood courses through the internal mammary, superior epigastric, musculophrenic, inferior epigastric, and iliac veins and into the inferior vena cava.

LATERAL THORACIC PATHWAY

This pathway is almost inevitably used, regardless of the site of occlusion. The flow is through the lateral thoracic, thoracoepigastric, superficial epigastric, superficial circumflex, long saphenous, femoral, and iliac veins.

VERTEBRAL PATHWAY

This pathway, situated posteriorly, is less commonly used. From the vertebral vein the blood flows through the vertebral plexus down to the lumbar and sacral veins and then back to the azygos system or into the iliac system.

PORTAL PATHWAY

Esophageal varices result from the portal pathway, whose flow is caudally through the esophageal veins to the left gastric vein and the portal vein.

Venous Hypertension

Physiologically, venous hypertension develops in all tissues and organs of the upper part of the body, the neck, and the arms. Pressure in the cerebrospinal canal also increases as a result of this hypertension, so that cerebral thrombosis or hemorrhages may occur secondary to the high retrograde pressure.

CLINICAL FEATURES

Obstruction of the superior vena cava results in a syndrome that is both classic and unmistakable. If, however, the obstruction is incomplete or the progress of the disease is insidious, the clinical picture is less obvious.

Signs and Symptoms

CHEMOSIS

An early sign of obstruction is edema of the conjunctiva with suffusion (chemosis). There is notable exophthalmos and edema of the eyelids. Tearing from the eyes is an early symptom and is often wrongly attributed to other causes.

RESPIRATORY SYMPTOMS

A mild irritative or nonproductive cough, often associated with substernal distress and edema of the eyes, face, and neck, may be misinterpreted as resulting from an upper respiratory infection, a common cold, or influenza.

As the obstruction progresses, dyspnea may occur, and the initially dry cough may become productive due to the edema of the tracheobronchial tree. All of these symptoms are exaggerated as the lumen of the cava becomes progressively compromised, and the physical findings become more severe commensurate with the degree and rapidity of obstruction.

EDEMA

The head, neck, and upper extremities become swollen and edematous, as does the upper thorax, especially anteriorly. The superficial veins of these areas are distended; the tissues become progressively cyanotic from venous stasis and hypertension.

It is to be emphasized again, however, that when caval obstruction develops slowly, little or no dis-

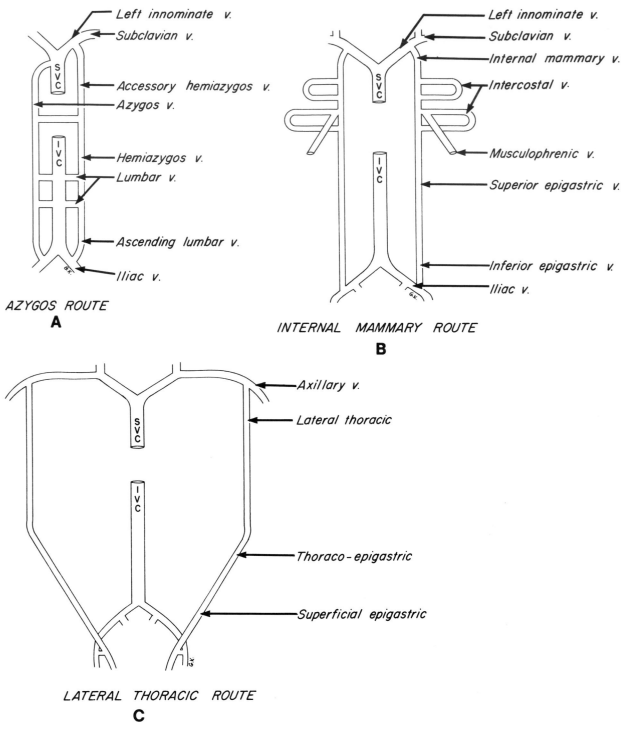

Left innominate v.
Subclavian v.
SVC
Accessory hemiazygos v.
Azygos v.
IVC
Hemiazygos v.
Lumbar v.
Ascending lumbar v.
Iliac v.

AZYGOS ROUTE

A

Left innominate v.
Subclavian v.
Internal mammary v.
SVC
Intercostal v.
Musculophrenic v.
IVC
Superior epigastric v.
Inferior epigastric v.
Iliac v.

INTERNAL MAMMARY ROUTE

B

Axillary v.
SVC
Lateral thoracic
IVC
Thoraco-epigastric
Superficial epigastric

LATERAL THORACIC ROUTE

C

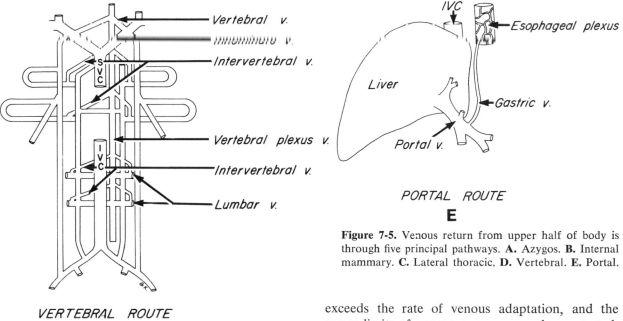

VERTEBRAL ROUTE

D

PORTAL ROUTE

E

Figure 7-5. Venous return from upper half of body is through five principal pathways. **A.** Azygos. **B.** Internal mammary. **C.** Lateral thoracic. **D.** Vertebral. **E.** Portal.

tress may be noted by the patient even though physically the venous engorgement may be remarkably demonstrable in the upper body. Facial edema, particularly of the eyelids, apparent in the morning after recumbency, may disappear later in the day if the patient remains upright. The male patient may notice a significant increase in collar size. Flushing of the face also occurs when the patient is recumbent or when he bends over to perform a simple task. In fact, stooping may so aggravate distress that some patients sleep in the sitting position to avoid dyspnea, coughing, and choking.

IMPAIRED CEREBRATION

When caval obstruction has developed rapidly, the patient may show evidence of impaired cerebration that may be attributed to venous engorgement and intracranial edema. Funduscopic examination invariably reveals venous prominence and edema of the posterior retina. The hypopharynx and larynx become edematous, and in malignant caval obstruction, vocal cord paralysis is not uncommon. Manifestations of the "wet brain syndrome" are usually encountered in patients in whom caval occlusion is rapid in onset and related to malignant intrathoracic neoplasm. In these patients the rate of occlusion

exceeds the rate of venous adaptation, and the upper limits of venous pressure are demonstrated.

Misdiagnosis

Although the clinical features of superior vena caval obstruction are striking, the incidence of misdiagnosis is high. It is not unusual for the patient to initially receive treatment for allergic blepharitis, angioneurotic edema, or congestive heart failure. Exploratory operations for diagnosis may be ill-advised. In the heavily muscled, obese patient the external venous engorgement may not be physically demonstrable. However, infrared photography easily demonstrates the extensive venous distention, collateral flow, and soft tissue edema as further evidence of venous hypertension. Both superior vena caval obstruction and chronic constrictive pericarditis are syndromes characterized by pathognomonic features well documented in the medical literature; nevertheless, many physicians seem unaware of these syndromes, and the incidence of misdiagnosis of both remains high.

Investigative Studies

CHEST X RAY

Roentgenograms of the chest almost always reveal the cause of the clinically evident superior caval syndrome by demonstrating either a tumor in the right paratracheal region adjacent to the superior vena cava (Fig. 7-6) or an aneurysm of the superior vena cava, of the ascending transverse arch of the aorta, or of the innominate artery, which compresses the vena cava as it passes through the superior mediastinum. Occasionally, however, there is only minimal mediastinal widening; in some cases of fibrosing mediastinitis, the mediastinum is of normal or near-normal width. The widened mediastinal density may be better delineated by sectional roentgenography.

ESOPHAGOGRAPHY

An esophagogram may disclose varices of the entire esophagus or, at times, varices of the upper esophagus only; these have been called "downhill" varices.[35] Varices are not inevitably present, however; they are related to the duration, location, and severity of the obstruction.

Figure 7-6. Posteroanterior roentgenogram of chest, demonstrating right paratracheal mass in patient with malignant superior vena cava obstruction.

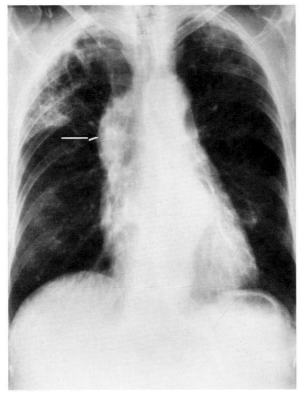

SUPERIOR CAVOGRAPHY

The most precise method for the diagnosis of superior vena caval obstruction and for delineation of collateral flow is that of superior cavography. Angiography of the superior vena cava is indicated in all malignant obstructions (Fig. 7-7) to determine the extent and location of the tumor and the extent of propagating thrombus. Benign thrombotic occlusion of the major intrathoracic veins can also be diagnosed by angiography. The procedure is simple and associated with minimal morbidity. The classic x-ray characteristics include partially or totally occluded superior vena cava with multiple dilated and tortuous venous channels proximal to the obstruction (Fig. 7-8).

INFRARED PHOTOGRAPHY

This technique demonstrates the extensive collateral network of venous pathways in the upper body in the less obvious obstruction.

Figure 7-7. Superior cavogram in patient with malignant obstruction of superior vena cava revealing extent and location of tumor.

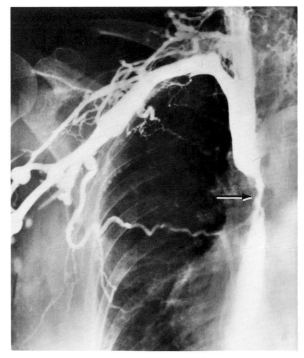

RADIOISOTOPE CAVOGRAPHY

Papadimitriou et al.[36] have advocated radioisotope cavography as a reliable method of detecting venous obstruction, displacement of the veins, and development of collaterals. It is simple to perform, results are obtained rapidly, and it is safe for the patient. They suggest that it be used as a screening test for patients in whom physical examination and clinical signs indicate possible lesions of the main venous trunks.

VENOUS BLOOD PRESSURE MEASUREMENTS

Although venous hypertension is evident from direct visualization of the enlarged and tense venous channels in the subcutaneous tissue, direct measurements of one of the enlarged tributaries may demonstrate pressure levels exceeding 100 mm H_2O. Cyanosis of the upper torso, extremities, head, and neck and the suffusion of the conjunctiva are secondary to stasis of venous blood in the enlarged, tortuous channels. As a result the hematocrit level of the blood in the upper portion of the body far exceeds that of the lower regions where there is no obstruction of the venous drainage system.

HISTOLOGIC DIAGNOSIS

CYTOLOGIC EXAMINATION. In most instances it is important to obtain a histologic diagnosis since therapy is largely, if not completely, dependent on an accurate tissue study. Salsali and Cliffton[12] reported an accurate tissue diagnosis in all of their 80 cases of malignant caval obstruction. If bronchial carcinoma is suspected, every effort should be made to detect the malignant cells in the sputum before performing a bronchoscopic examination, since this may produce severe respiratory distress and may be extremely hazardous because of the accentuation of the inflammatory reaction superimposed upon the already existing edema of the tracheobronchial tree, the hypopharynx, and the larynx. For these reasons, extreme caution should be used when bronchoscopy is performed with a rigid instrument. Endoscopic examination with the flexible fiberscope with the patient under topical anesthesia may be better tolerated by the patient and safer for him. A direct smear, washing the compressed right upper lobe orifice, or gently brushing the bronchus under fluoroscopic control may give a positive cytologic study.

Next to sputum cytology, cytologic examination of a pleural effusion (if present) is least traumatic and a simple means for obtaining a pathologic diagnosis.

BIOPSY OF LYMPH NODES. If a diagnosis of malignant disease is not obtained by the above conservative measures, palpable metastatic lymph nodes can be biopsied. Caution must be exercised, because apparent masses in the neck approached for biopsy may be found to be dilated, thrombosed veins or edematous fat pads, and control of bleeding may be difficult.

ANTERIOR SCALENE NODE DISSECTION, MEDIASTINOSCOPY, AND MEDIASTINOTOMY. These procedures are hazardous[37] because of extensive venous engorgement and because of the pressures within the venous system, which at operation appear almost at arterial levels.

Figure 7-8. Superior cavogram in patient with benign fibrosing mediastinitis revealing almost total occlusion of superior vena cava with early filling of multiple dilated and tortuous venous channels proximal to the obstruction.

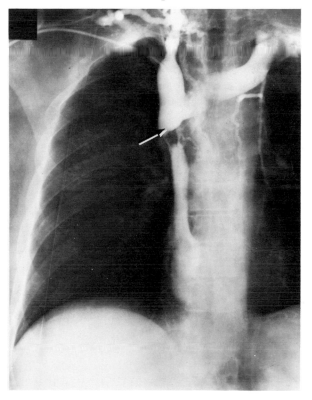

EXPLORATORY THORACOTOMY. In a few instances it may be wiser to perform a small posterolateral thoracotomy rather than to utilize mediastinoscopy, mediastinotomy, or scalene node dissection, since the vascular structures are more readily visible and more easily controlled with the greater exposure gained with a thoracotomy. On the other hand, the physician may be content to make a presumptive diagnosis of underlying malignant disease, since exploratory thoracotomy in the presence of high venous pressure may be a formidable undertaking and the information obtained may be of little help beyond satisfying academic requirements and the therapeutic radiologist.[11, 14]

TREATMENT OF SUPERIOR VENA CAVAL SYNDROMES

Malignant Obstruction

Since most malignant obstructions are due to carcinoma of the upper lobe of the right lung, treatment is directed toward the primary lesion. Bronchial carcinomas causing obstruction of the vena cava are almost always nonresectable; in these patients operation is limited to establishing a histologic diagnosis.

CONSERVATIVE MEASURES

While awaiting establishment of the diagnosis, the physician should immediately institute conservative measures, including elevation of the head of the bed and dehydration. Great benefit may be derived from diuretics and salt restriction. The symptomatic relief of fullness of the head and neck and of headache following diuresis may provide time and safety for the diagnostic procedures to be performed, thus forestalling blind irradiation without a diagnosis.

RADIATION THERAPY FOR LYMPHOMATOUS MASSES

Occasionally, however, radiation must be administered on an emergency basis for the relief of venous hypertension in the head, neck, and upper extremities; often it is administered on clinical grounds alone, without histologic verification of malignant disease. Lymphomatous masses (Hodgkin's disease, lymphosarcoma) are especially sensitive to radiation therapy, literally melting away.[38] This rapid response often indicates that a hitherto undiagnosed mass is lymphomatous rather than carcinomatous, since carcinomatous masses respond less quickly. The caval syndrome caused by malignant thymoma is often relieved by radiation therapy. Chemotherapy as an adjunctive measure is of value primarily in the lymphomas and is of little value in the other epithelial types of cancer.

RADIATION THERAPY FOR BRONCHIOGENIC CARCINOMA

In bronchiogenic carcinoma with superior vena caval syndrome, high-voltage radiation therapy is the treatment of choice and offers significant palliative benefit. The type of radiation and the treatment schedule depends on the equipment available and the experience and philosophy of the therapist. Some therapists believe that irradiation may increase edema and other symptoms, and therefore they start treatment slowly. Others believe that rapid treatment is indicated to shrink the mass quickly.[39] Holmes[40] favors a high-dose grid technique, with a tumor dose of 4500 to 5000 rads given in a single dose. His overall 6-month survival rate of 110 cases so treated was reported to be 10 per cent. Longacre and Shockman[41] reported 69 cases of malignant superior caval obstruction. In 35 cases (64 per cent), marked to excellent response was found in patients who were given 200 rads per day, 1000 rads per week, to a total of 4000 rads. They found no marked difference between the behavior of anaplastic and well-differentiated carcinomas. At Memorial Sloan-Kettering Cancer Center, Salsali and Cliffton[12] reported a 6-month survival rate of 55 per cent when patients were given 100 to 200 rads on the first and second day of treatment, the dose was increased to 250 to 300 rads per day by the third or fourth day, and administration was continued until there was improvement on clinical and x-ray examination or until a recommended total dose was reached.

ANTICOAGULANT AND/OR FIBRINOLYTIC THERAPY

Because of the high incidence of extending thrombosis with tumor,[42] the use of anticoagulant drugs or fibrinolytic agents has been suggested. It has been demonstrated that when adequate therapy is given with such agents, clinical improvement is more rapid and recanalization of the vena cava can be obtained. The survival rate also appears to be improved.

INSERTION OF BYPASS GRAFT AT THORACOTOMY

When thoracotomy is required to establish the diagnosis and an unresectable tumor is encountered, the insertion of a bypass graft often may be a simple procedure. The right atrium is usually available to receive the central end of the graft, and only a few centimeters of unobstructed innominate vein are necessary for the peripheral anastomosis. Skinner et al.[43] have reported this technique in 2 patients, with beneficial results (Fig. 7-9).

SURGICAL EXTIRPATION

The rare instances of small cancers directly invading the vena cava deserve early diagnosis and intensive therapeutic measures, combining irradiation, chemotherapy, and fibrinolysins for maximal palliative and perhaps curative results.[12] When such cancers are confined to the thoracic cavity, surgical extirpation should be considered. In such cases the superior vena cava may be resected and replaced with a graft. Since such grafting procedures in malignant disease are the exception, they are discussed in greater detail in the section on treatment

of benign caval obstruction (see below). In general, however, direct surgical intervention is to be avoided in the treatment of malignant caval obstruction, as there is usually no chance for surgical relief of malignant obstruction.

Benign Obstruction

OPERATIVE TREATMENT OF THYMOMA OR SUBSTERNAL GOITER

Benign lesions causing the vena caval syndrome, such as thymoma or substernal goiter,[19, 20] are completely relieved by surgical removal of the obstructing mass of tissue. The substernal goiter may be removed through a cervical incision. Other benign lesions, such as thymomas, may be removed either through a sternal-splitting incision or through a formal posterolateral thoracotomy. Careful hemostasis is mandatory, since invariably there is venous congestion of the thoracic wall and intrathoracic contents. The obvious venous congestion is often immediately and visibly relieved by excision of the large benign mass that is held tightly in the confines of the superior mediastinum. Edema of the face and neck extends to involve the hypopharynx, vocal cords, and larynx, so that extreme care and gentleness must be exercised in using endotracheal anesthesia.

Figure 7-9. In unresectable cases, relief of obstruction may be attempted by simple insertion of a bypass graft of autogenous vein between right atrial appendage and left innominate vein.

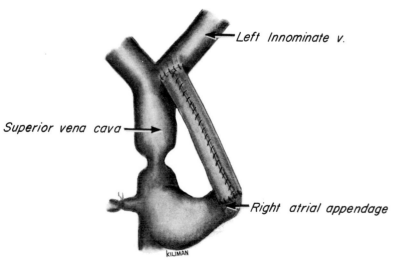

Left Innominate v.

Superior vena cava

Right atrial appendage

KILIMAN

EXTRACORPOREAL HEART-LUNG BYPASS PROCEDURES FOR AORTIC ANEURYSMS

Since the development of the extracorporeal heart-lung bypass apparatus, aneurysms of the ascending aorta or innominate artery may be successfully treated to relieve not only the caval obstruction but also often the respiratory distress due to encroachment on the tracheobronchial tree. (For a detailed discussion of the surgical technique, see Volume I, Chapter 6.[6])

ANTICOAGULANT THERAPY FOR OBSTRUCTION DUE TO INFECTION

In the rare instances of caval obstruction caused by infection in the neighboring mediastinum or lung, in which thrombosis of the vena cava is either present or imminent, anticoagulant therapy for a prolonged period is necessary, along with appropriate antibiotic therapy.

MEDIASTINAL GRANULOMA

One of the most common causes of benign superior vena caval obstruction is mediastinal granuloma. Effler and Groves[11] suggest that when this lesion heals, intense fibrosis occurs, producing the obstruction called fibrosing mediastinitis. They further suggest that the paratracheal granuloma found on chest roentgenogram should be removed from the asymptomatic patient as prophylaxis against future benign caval obstruction. When caval obstruction is present in this disease, operation is usually not required, since in time the development of collateral venous channels affords considerable relief of symptoms. It is unlikely that in such a patient any form of graft bypass can offer the long-term result ultimately achieved by the patient's own venous collateral replacement if the azygos vein is patent.

SURGICAL PROCEDURES. However, in the rare instance of a patient with obstruction from benign causes in whom the azygos vein may be compromised or whose symptoms are persistent and disabling, surgical reconstruction of the vena cava can be an effective procedure. Treatment of benign idiopathic fibrosing mediastinitis is directed toward verification of the diagnosis of the benign disease, usually by performing a limited thoracotomy. In the unusual case in which a bypass graft is indicated, the choice of prosthesis is difficult. Autologous,

homologous, and prosthetic conduits have been less than satisfactory, since thrombosis of the channel almost invariably develops.[14, 42-62]

Cooley and Hallman[63] described an original technique for relief of benign superior vena caval syndrome in which the dilated, tortuous azygos vein is mobilized from the chest wall and a side-to-side anastomosis performed between it, and the inferior vena cava just above the diaphragm. Garcia et al.[64] presented a case of 90 per cent stenosis of the superior vena cava and almost complete obstruction of the azygos vein in a patient with fibrosing mediastinitis. A good long-term result was achieved by reconstructing the superior vena cava with a patch of autologous saphenous vein, using a temporary internal shunt during the grafting procedure (see Fig. 7-2). They concluded that the long-term patency of the graft in their case may have been due to the stenosis of the azygos vein, which would tend to increase bloodflow and the vena cava-atrial pressure gradient, as shown by Gerbode et al.[65] The internal shunt was necessary because any total, sudden occlusion of the superior vena cava for longer than 10 minutes is not well tolerated, as we have found in superior vena cava-right pulmonary artery anastomosis for tricuspid atresia.[7]

Vasko et al.[66] used homologous trachea successfully in an animal for experimental vena caval replacement; Fadhli[67] suggested that the physician attempt endvenectomy and thrombectomy before resorting to graft bypass or replacement procedures. He reported a successful case of benign fibrosing mediastinitis in which this technique was used by starting the dissection from the intrapericardial free portion of the superior vena cava.

AUTOGENOUS COMPOSITE VEIN GRAFT

At this time the best choice for superior vena caval replacement or bypass appears to be the autogenous composite vein graft. It has the highest patency rate, particularly when combined with an arteriovenous fistula.[62, 68-74] The success in maintaining patency of such grafts has been attributed to an increase in bloodflow through the graft and to an increase in pressure within the graft.[75]

Miller and associates[70, 71] showed, first experimentally and then clinically, that an excellent prognosis could be expected in replacement of maximally resected superior vena cava when the autogenous vein graft was protected by an arteriovenous shunt near the cephalad suture line. During the operative procedure to replace the obstructed superior vena cava, the fibrotic mass should not be totally excised because of the possibility of transecting the right phrenic nerve. An attempt should be made to provide adequate space for the vein autograft to lie free of the aorta, the inflammatory mass, and the manubrium. An adequate length of autogenous vein may be harvested from noncritical vessels, such as the cephalic or saphenous veins. A small tributary of the saphenous vein affords an adequate-sized vessel for use as a shunt. The internal mammary artery may also be of appropriate size; however, the difficult dissection of this vessel from a fibrotic mediastinum is time-consuming.

TECHNIQUE. Reconstruction of the obstructed vena cava requires isolation of the vessel above and below the inflammatory mass. An autogenous venous cylinder of appropriate diameter and length is fashioned by sewing longitudinally opened venous segments together with a continuous over-and-over everting suture, using 6–0 or 7–0 cardiovascular Teflon-impregnated braided polyester fiber. Anastomosis to the vena cava and creation of arteriovenous fistulas are done with the same suture and same technique. Magnifying loupes are useful with the finer sutures, especially in creating the fistula.

Suturing the venous autograft end-to-end with the complementary cephalad fistula then provides successful anatomic and functional results. The internal mammary artery is sutured approximately 4 mm cephalad to the autogenous vein graft. (Fig. 7-10). If this is not available, a small reversed saphenous tributary is sutured between the ascending aorta and the innominate vein or vena cava just proximal to the graft. Reconstruction for an obstruction involving the caudal portions of both innominate veins requires dissection of the free segments and interposition of a Y-shaped venous autograft complemented with two cephalad fistulas. When the graft is excessively long, there is the possibility of stricture occurring at the caudal suture line. Two fistulas, then, one at each suture line, are required. Flow measurements are obtained to insure that cardiac output is not increased beyond the compensatory ability of the patient. The arteriove-

Figure 7-10. Reconstruction of obstructed superior vena cava by composite venous autograft with complementary cephalad internal mammary arteriovenous fistula maintains good flow and reduces incidence of postoperative thrombosis in the graft.

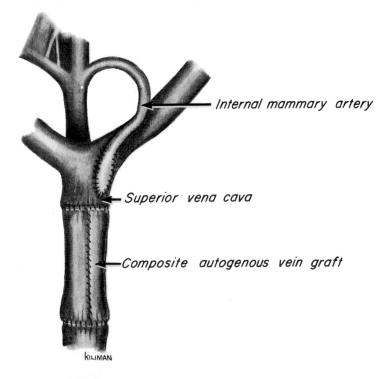

Internal mammary artery

Superior vena cava

Composite autogenous vein graft

KILIMAN

nous fistula usually closes spontaneously; if this has not occurred within 2 years or if the shunt becomes enlarged after the 3- or 4-week critical period, surgical closure is indicated. Anticoagulant agents are unnecessary when a complementary fistula is used. However, prophylactic antibiotics should be administered to patients having upper respiratory disease, dental work, or other surgical procedures, to prevent bacterial vasculitis in the region of the fistula.[71]

DEXTRAN AS PROPHYLAXIS OF THROMBOSIS OF THE VENA CAVAL PROSTHESIS. Barnes et al.[76] reported the use of dextran as an adjunct in maintaining the patency of synthetic grafts of the superior vena cava. They believed that the dextran infusion in the postoperative period provided adequate hydration and hemodilution, thereby preventing thrombosis of the caval prosthesis. Similar results with dextran infusion were found in experimentally maintaining long-term patency of pericardial tubular grafts in dogs by Brais et al.[77]

ANEURYSMS OF THE SUPERIOR VENA CAVA

Prior to the use of autogenous vein grafts to span defects of the arterial system produced by surgical excision, the term "aneurysm" was seldom, if ever, applied to veins. True or pure primary venous aneurysms were not described in textbooks of pathology or surgery prior to 1962.[78] Abbott and Leigh[79] presented evidence from the literature and their own personal experience proving that venous aneurysms are a true entity. They studied 32 of their own cases and presented a useful classification (Table 7-1). Bell[80] reported a single case of venous aneurysm presenting as a right superior mediastinal mass and proven by phlebography. Gallucci et al.[81] reported a single case of true aneurysm in a young woman diagnosed at thoracotomy performed for an unexplained mediastinal mass. They reemphasized the importance of more complete preoperative investigations, especially contrast-injection studies, in patients with undiagnosed mediastinal shadows.

X-RAY DIAGNOSTIC PROCEDURES

Aneurysms of the superior vena cava appear as smooth, rounded structures on plain posteroanterior chest roentgenograms. There may be significant change in their size and shape on inspiration-expiration studies. Fluoroscopic examination reveals pulsations which are paradoxic in timing relative to ventricular contraction in the pure fusiform lesion without associated anomalies. There is lack of pulsation in the simple saccular or diverticular type, in aneurysmal dilatation of the superior vena cava secondary to total anomalous pulmonary venous drainage, and in the pseudoaneurysm due to

combined cardiac failure and high inferior vena caval thrombosis. Aneurysms of the superior vena cava tend to enlarge when the patient is in the supine position; the enlargement is accentuated by the Mueller or Valsalva maneuvers. Final diagnosis is ultimately verified by phlebography. The contrast media should be injected at a site that does not require entrance of the catheter into the lumen of the aneurysm, to avoid perforation of the extremely thin wall.[79]

CLINICAL CHARACTERISTICS

The clinical characteristics vary markedly according to the type, location, and size of the lesion. Symptoms vary from dyspnea and localized pain to no symptoms at all. The manifestations of secondary congenital aneurysms associated with causative anomalies are due to the underlying cardiovascular abnormality. Similarly, acquired lesions relate their symptoms to the underlying disease state. Solitary false aneurysms are asymptomatic, whereas pseudoaneurysms relate their complaints to the predisposing cause. Arteriovenous aneurysms are the only ones which produce a continuous murmur or bruit.

Treatment

Treatment varies according to the type of venous aneurysm. If the involved vein may be sacrificed, local excision is preferable. Treatment is excisional or reparative in pure primary false venous aneurysms and in arteriovenous fistulas. Lesions involving the superior vena cava require reinforcement, reconstruction, or graft replacement. In congenital venous aneurysms, those resulting from associated anomalies are controlled by correction of the causative abnormality; this is also the basis of therapy of acquired lesions and of pseudoaneurysms. Complete excision, with or without graft replacement, is indicated for the arteriovenous fistulas.

II. UPPER EXTREMITY OBSTRUCTION SYNDROME

The venous outflow syndromes of the upper extremity are analogous to iliofemoral thrombophlebitis. The similarities include the frequency of initial absence of severe pain; the character of the pain when it is present, viz., a dull, aching variety; swelling of the entire extremity that is characteristically less pitting than cardiac or nutritional edema; and an elevated venous pressure causing venous distention which decreases with the passage of time and with elevation and rest of the part and which is accentuated by dependency and active movement. The syndromes differ from iliofemoral thrombophlebitis in incidence, being much less frequent; in the complication of pulmonary embolism, which is extremely rare; and in the absence of long-term effects of the postphlebitic syndrome, presumably attributable to the lesser degree of elevation of the venous pressure.

ETIOLOGY

The etiologic factors[82-85] are the same as those of thrombophlebitis in other areas of the body, the differences in our opinion being that the greater mobility of the shoulder joint favors trauma to the vein wall as the most common proximate mechanism, whereas in the lower extremity, low flow states most frequently initiate venous thrombosis. The high incidence of thrombosis secondary to injury to the vein wall probably accounts for the more adherent type of thrombus; this has a direct bearing on the lower incidence of pulmonary embolism[82, 86-90] associated with upper extremity thrombophlebitis. Another difference between the two syndromes may likewise be ascribed to the greater mobility of the shoulder, together with the narrowness of the thoracic inlet or outlet: the axillary and subclavian veins are far more susceptible to intermittent external compression[91-97] than are the femoral and iliac veins.

TABLE 7-1. Proposed Classification of Aneurysmal Disease Superior Vena Caval Systems

I. Congenital lesions
   A. Primary or simple
      1. Fusiform
      2. Saccular or *diverticular*
   B. Secondary or complex (resulting from associated anomalies)
      1. Total anomalous pulmonary venous return
      2. Anomalous venae cavae
         a. Hypoplasia or agenesis inferior vena cava
         b. Persistent levoatrial cava
         c. Complete transposition one or both cavae
   C. Obstructive anomalies (intravenous diaphragms, etc.)
   D. Miscellaneous
II. Acquired lesions
   A. Primary
      1. Fusiform—unsupported vein graft arterial replacement
   B. Secondary
      1. Trauma (*false* type)
      2. Obstruction (mediastinitis, cirrhosis): varices
      3. Associated neoplastic
III. Pseudoaneurysms
   A. Transient
      1. Cardiac failure (numerous)
      2. Cardiac failure plus Budd-Chiari Syndrome
   B. Venous neoplasms (angiomata)
IV. Arteriovenous aneurysms
   A. Congenital
      1. Systemic vessels
      2. Systemic and pulmonary vessels
      3. Cirsoid
   B. Acquired
      1. Trauma
      2. Surgical—purposeful, non-purposeful
      3. Associated disease (lues)

From Abbott, O. A. and Leigh, T. F. Aneurysmal dilatations of the superior vena caval system. *Ann Surg 159:* 859, 1964. (By permission of authors and Lippincott.)

INCIDENCE

In analyzing the case material at Charity Hospital in New Orleans over a 12-year period, Ochsner et al.[86] found only 2 per cent of 871 instances of peripheral vein thrombosis localized in the upper extremities. At the Mayo Clinic, Barker and associates[87] found 24 instances of postoperative venous thrombosis in the veins of the upper extremities, an incidence of 1.7 per cent of 1401 locations in 938 patients. Although no incidence is cited by Adams et al.,[98] the 25 cases of primary axillary or subclavian vein thrombosis which they reviewed at the University of Rochester Medical Center seems to be a relatively small number of instances,[99] as does the 48 cases of thrombosis of the major veins of the upper extremity collected by Tilney and associates[85] from hospitals in the Boston area over the past 25 years. In our practice in Cincinnati in a period of approximately 20 years, 52 patients were seen with deep venous thrombosis of the upper extremity, whereas over 2000 instances of this disease were observed in the lower extremities; this is an incidence of 2.7 per cent for acute obstructive venous disease of the arm.

HISTORICAL REVIEW

Sir James Paget in 1875[100] described two examples of venous obstruction of the upper extremity, having observed his first patient in 1855. In 1884 von Schrötter[101] reported a similar syndrome in the right arm of a healthy painter who was at work at the time of onset. Hughes made an exhaustive review of the extant literature up to 1949 and collected reports of 320 cases.[82] It was his suggestion that the disease be called the Paget-Schrötter syndrome.

In the United States, Matas in 1934[83] reviewed the literature and, after describing in great detail a patient with primary thrombosis of the axillary vein, alluded to another patient seen 12 years earlier with the same syndrome. There can be little doubt that Matas was reporting two instances of thrombosis of the subclavian vein secondary to the strain of trauma. Since his review, many excellent reports have appeared in the American literature.[84, 85, 98, 102–104]

The fact that compression of the axillary-subclavian veins can occur without thrombosis is well established.[91–96] Cucci et al.[105] reported venous obstruction caused by a malformed valve of the subclavian vein. Wilder et al.[106] described subclavian vein obstruction secondary to hypertrophy of the terminal valve. Most physicians who write on this subject are aware that the vein can be thrombosed by direct trauma, such as a fracture of the clavicle, and by extrinsic compression caused by cancer. Such cases, however, are usually excluded[98] from discussion.

"Primary" when used to describe thrombosis of the subclavian vein must be assumed to be interchangeable with "idiopathic." Therefore, as more and more causes of thrombosis are discovered, the number of cases so designated will shrink. For a classification to be comprehensive, it should include all known causes of this syndrome.

CLASSIFICATION

I. Extraluminal Compression
   A. Intermittent compression (costoclavicular syndromes)
      1. By subclavius muscle, first rib, pectoralis minor muscle, costocoracoid ligament
      2. Positional, as during sleep
   B. Constant external compression, usually with associated thrombosis
      1. By surgical trauma, scar tissue, hematoma, or fracture of clavicle
      2. By carcinoma of axilla
II. Intraluminal Thrombosis
   A. Primary or idiopathic secondary to stretching of the vein (probably a true effort thrombosis)
   B. Rupture of a valve of subclavian vein, causing thrombosis
   C. Chemical, secondary to intravenous therapy

DIAGNOSIS

Symptoms and Signs

If the symptoms caused by the direct trauma on the surrounding tissues can be separated from those caused by the intravenous thrombosis, the onset of symptoms is found to be somewhat insidious, just as in thrombosis of the veins of the pelvis and the lower extremities. A patient may simply awaken to find his arm swelling gradually or swollen, without any apparent reason. The patient who has suffered trauma (e.g., Matas'[83] telephone lineman who suddenly wrenched his arm or our patient who started to fall off the roof and managed to hook his right arm over a ladder, thus supporting his full body weight in his axilla) may experience the sharp pain of the initial injury. This is true of any kind of major trauma, e.g., swinging a golf club, throwing a stone, pitching a baseball. A period follows when the initial pain subsides and becomes minimal, only to be replaced by rapid or gradual swelling of the entire extremity. This sequence of events is basically identical to the swelling of the lower extremity following iliofemoral thrombophlebitis. Usually the temperature remains normal; no systemic effects or neurologic symptoms and signs are present. As the swelling increases, it becomes increasingly difficult to use the extremity. The symptoms resemble those complained of in the lower extremity: tiredness, heaviness, fullness, a "bursting sensation." The patient may notice the hand turning blue and the veins distending. Swelling is frequently detectable on inspection. If swelling is not visible, a tape measure can be used to compare the two arms. The hand may appear slightly bluish or reddish purple due to engorgement with blood. The veins are distended. If the arms are raised gradually, the veins of the involved arm remain distended longer. If the occlusion has been present for several days or weeks, large, engorged veins are visible about the shoulder; they can be demonstrated easily by infrared photography or by thermography.

On palpation, diffuse tenseness can be felt in the extremity. As a rule, little pitting is present. The radial and ulnar pulses are normal; if they are difficult to palpate because of swelling, oscillometric examination is helpful. Blood pressure in each extremity is normal. The diagnosis can be confirmed by measuring the venous pressure both at rest and after exercise as suggested by Veal and Hussey,[107] who demonstrated the marked elevation of pressure upon intermittent clenching of the fist in patients with venous obstruction of the upper extremity.

Phleborheography

From a hemodynamic standpoint, Veal and Hussey's[107] maneuver is similar to the intermittent compression of the calf in the diagnosis of thrombophle-

bitis by the phleborheographic technique described in Chapter 4. Our experience, however, is presently too limited in patients with deep venous thrombosis of the upper extremity to enable us to predict that phleborheography will be as reliable in that area as it has proven itself to be in the lower extremities. Preliminary data suggest, however, that axillary-subclavian venous obstruction is detectable by the phleborheographic technique.

Phlebography

Hughes discounted the value of phlebography in the detection of venous obstructions of the upper extremity.[82] However, he was writing in the early days of phlebographic development before improved instruments and contrast media enabled investigators to perfect visualization techniques. Nevertheless, neither the diagnosis nor the selection of the correct treatment can be influenced by a phlebogram[82] unless the entire brachial-axillary-subclavian trunks are visualized. Of great interest in this regard is the phenomenon described by Tagariello[108] and by Garusi and Cresti,[109] viz., "pseudostenosis." The subclavian vein, a direct continuation of the axillary trunk, in normal circulatory conditions may appear to be pseudostenosed or completely blocked in its terminal tract. These false appearances of obstruction and pseudostenosis seem to be attributable to the varying position of the terminal valve in correlation with right atrium activity. In the brief period of atrial systole, a momentary stoppage occurs in the outflow from the superior vena cava, with temporary venous blockage and possible reflux in the subclavian vein, which is checked by its terminal valve. Tagariello confirmed this hemodynamic mechanism by making phlebographic exposures during Valsalva's maneuver. In addition to the apparent obstruction caused by the valve, pseudostenosis is frequently seen at the level of the proximal end of the subclavian vein. This phenomenon originates first from the deep breathing that occurs during the injection and secondly from the massive injection of contrast medium. Coon and Willis[110] restrict their use of phlebography to those patients in whom the diagnosis is in question; they refer to a patient who experienced exacerbation of symptoms and signs requiring an extra week of anticoagulant therapy after a phlebogram was performed to rule out the "thoracic inlet" syndrome.

Differential Diagnostic Points

MODE OF ONSET

The term "acute onset" requires further definition. A patient with an acute arterial embolus, a pulmonary embolus, a ruptured plantaris tendon, or hemorrhage into a muscle has an instantaneous onset of pain that occurs as suddenly as the click of a trigger, comes on in one stroke, and happens in an instant of time that is imprinted on the memory of the patient. "Sudden onset" to some patients may mean that the discomfort comes on over a period of hours. For example, a patient may be normal when he falls asleep and have a numb or swollen limb when he awakens, or he may note that throughout the day his hand, arm, or leg is gradually becoming more and more swollen. Looking back a few weeks later, he may call this a "sudden onset." If an effort is made to distinguish between these two sharply contrasted degrees of suddenness, a distinction can be made between an arterial embolus and thrombosis, a pulmonary embolus and pneumonitis, and hemorrhage into a muscle and thrombophlebitis.

THE SITE OF PAIN

The initial episode of trauma or strain may be the source of pain in the entire area that has been traumatized, because of stretching or injury to all the involved tissues. This distress is not necessarily indicative of pain in a particular structure within that area, such as in a vein. For example, the patient who twists his arm or strains it while hanging on parallel bars may experience pain from the very strain of the muscles and ligaments and, possibly (although less likely), of the veins.

SWELLING

As the initial pain subsides over a period of hours or days, the limb swells; this is attributed to thrombosis of the vein. This is no proof that the initial pain was caused by stretching of the vein. For example, the edema may be secondary to venous obstruction which in turn is secondary to external compression of the vein by perivenous hemorrhage from the initial trauma plus a fibrous reaction,[111] such as was confirmed at operation in one of our patients. (See Case Report 7-2.)

COMPLICATIONS

Pulmonary Embolism

Pulmonary emboli are rarely associated with deep venous thrombosis of the upper extremity;[82] that they do occur, however, is well documented.[88-90, 98, 99] Barnett and Levitt[88] reported a case of "effort" thrombosis of the axillary vein with pulmonary embolism, occurring 6 days after the original trauma. The patient was hospitalized for heparin and dicoumarin (Dicumarol) therapy; at 4 months later and again at 20 months, she was asymptomatic. Adams et al.[98] reported a 12 per cent incidence of embolism in their series of 25 patients; at the time the embolism occurred, their 3 patients had x-ray proof of axillary or subclavian vein thrombosis and absence of signs or symptoms of venous thrombosis in the lower extremities. Claggett et al.[99] reported a patient with a hypercoagulable blood state and a history of probable left axillary-subclavian vein thrombosis who, after excretory urography with injection of iothalamate sodium, developed left axillary-subclavian vein thrombosis with pulmonary embolism; this was documented by chest x ray showing decreased vascularity in the left lower lung and by ventilation perfusion lung scan showing multiple areas of decreased perfusion which were more severe on the left. Physical examination of the lower extremities showed no evidence of venous thrombosis. None of the reported pulmonary emboli proved fatal.

Venous Gangrene

This rare complication has been reported twice, the first case being that seen by Fountain and Taverner in 1954;[112] their patient was under treatment with an anticoagulant drug (ethyl biscoumacetate [Tromexan]) for bilateral iliofemoral venous thrombosis (proved at autopsy) when painful cyanotic edema of the right upper extremity developed overnight. Gangrene developed in the three extremities. Postmortem examination demonstrated a patent arterial system. The widespread thrombosis was attributed to venous stasis from prolonged bed rest and low grade pelvic infections from cervical erosion. Adams et al.[98] described a patient who developed venous gangrene of the right arm secondary to subclavian vein thrombosis following a scalene fat pad biopsy. There was also similar gangrene of both lower legs, so that the subsequent fatal pulmonary embolus may have been from either the legs or the arm.

Postphlebitic Sequelae

Despite the fact that the physical disability may be prolonged and annoying to the patient, the swelling is not major. Nevertheless, the edema is not easily controlled by an elastic sleeve or other type of rubberized support. Use of the extremity causes some patients varying degrees of aggravation of their symptoms. This added discomfort on effort should be considered as "venous claudication," in that muscular use of the arm causes greater venous engorgement. The abnormal brownish pigmentation, induration of the subcutaneous tissue, scaling of the skin, and ulceration that are typical of the postphlebitic syndrome in the lower extremity have never been observed in the postthrombotic upper extremity.

TREATMENT

Intermittent Compression Syndrome

CONSERVATIVE THERAPY

Many patients with intermittent venous congestion of the upper extremity caused by external compression need only to be instructed about the nature of their condition and to follow the physician's advice to avoid positions of the arm that cause the intermittent obstruction, e.g., sleeping with the head resting on the arm or with the arm hyperabducted and sitting with the arm laid over the back of a chair. The patient whose symptoms are related to lifting heavy objects should refrain from such exertions. Physiotherapy has sometimes been found to be helpful in providing relief.[113-115]

Perhaps the most unique instance of intermittent venous obstruction in our experience is that of the young patient described in the following case history.

Case Report 7-1

A young girl of 13 was seen in January 1965. She gave a history of injury to her right shoulder under the armpit while swinging on some bars in October 1964; the next day the entire right arm was swollen. On physical examination, puffiness of the skin of the knuckles was present, with no swelling. There was no pitting, discoloration of the skin, or tenderness in the axilla. There was no evidence of peripheral nerve involvement. A diagnosis was made of recent axillary vein thrombosis of the right upper extremity.

In March 1970, now 18 years old, she returned with multiple complaints, including that her right arm swelled, her hand became swollen and bluish, and frequently her veins became distended.

On physical examination a very slight swelling was visible in her right arm. There was slight discoloration, a very faint violaceous tinge, typical of venous distention. No other physical abnormalities could be noted.

Because of her history, a presumptive diagnosis was made of venous obstruction of the right upper extremity secondary to a thrombosed subclavian vein, traceable to her original injury 6 years earlier. Bilateral phlebograms were obtained with the arms extended laterally at shoulder level. Normal venous trees were visualized (Fig. 7-11A and B). This came as a surprise since the diagnosis of right subclavian vein thrombosis had been considered a virtual certainty. Unable to accept these contradictory findings, the phlebograms were repeated with the patient's arms at her sides (Fig. 7-11C and D). These films showed obvious compression of both the right and left brachial veins by her very large breasts.

Further investigation and observation brought out the following significant information. Embarrassed by her large physique, the patient had formed the habit of standing with her arms compressed tightly against her sides. Furthermore, she habitually stood with her left arm lying across her abdomen while her left hand held her right arm just above the elbow; she maintained this position even when seated and writing. It now seemed reasonably certain that the patient's symptoms of venous obstruction at age 18 were attributable to a combination of factors, i.e., the self-consciousness which motivated her to hold her arms close to her sides and the resultant compression of both brachial veins by her breasts. She was advised to alter this pattern of behavior and discharged without further treatment.

SURGICAL TREATMENT

With few exceptions, in compression syndromes of the shoulder girdle, whether the arteries, veins, or nerves are involved, the area of compression lies between the clavicle and the first or cervical rib.[116]

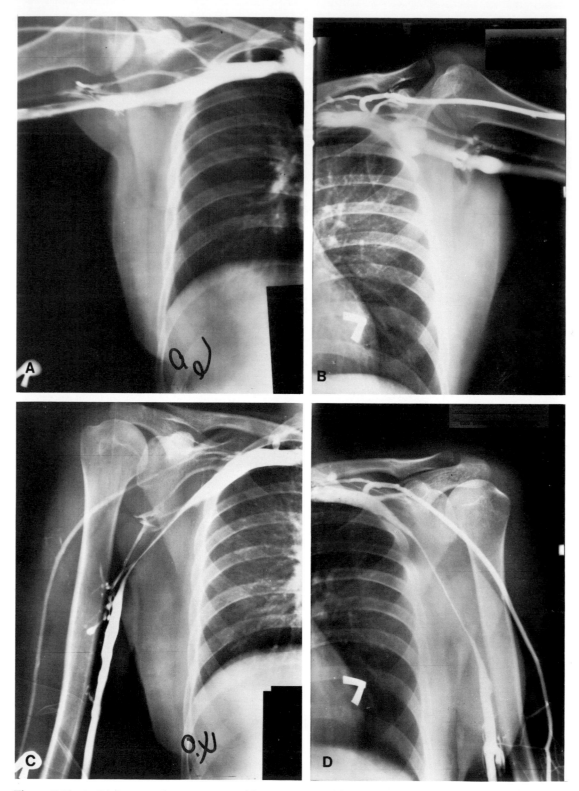

Figure 7-11. A. Right normal venous tree with upper extremities abducted. **B. Left** normal venous tree with upper extremities abducted. **C.** Right compression of brachial vein by large breast tissue. **D.** Left compression of brachial vein by large breast tissue.

When one of these variants is removed the surgical treatment is most efficacious. Lord and Rosati[97] recommend that the clavicle be removed. In our experience, removal of the first rib along with the cervical rib (if one is present) has been the most effective treatment. We have used the transaxillary approach described by Roos[117-119] rather than the posterior route or the techniques of resecting the first rib anteriorly by a subclavicular incision, described by Gol and associates.[120]

Intraluminal Thrombosis

CONSERVATIVE TREATMENT

Patients with venous thrombosis of the upper extremities are treated initially with heparin followed by coumadin (see Chapter 2, section on conservative treatment of thrombophlebitis of the lower extremities). The patient's arm is kept in an elevated position (using a pillow) during sleep, even though such positioning is difficult to maintain. Occasionally elastic sleeves have been prescribed, but they are rarely comfortable. In patients with extreme swelling, intermittent external venous compression is applied by means of a Jobst pump.

As in thrombosis of the lower extremities, the majority of patients with thrombosis of the subclavian or axillary veins can be managed by anticoagulant therapy. Enzyme therapy may soon be available and have a place in the treatment of venous thrombosis; the main problem undoubtedly will again be to identify cases sufficiently early for effective solution of the clots.

SURGICAL TREATMENT OF SUBCLAVIAN VEIN THROMBOSIS

If acute thrombosis of the subclavian vein can be treated early enough, thrombectomy is the treatment of choice. The problem, however, as in pelvic thrombosis, is that it is rare that the patient presents early for operative treatment when the clots are easily removable. In many instances the thrombus does not cause pain initially; as the clot propagates and obstructs more collateral veins of the arm, it produces symptoms. By this time, however, the thrombus is well organized and not easily removed. The more acute and more massive the swelling, the better the chance for immediate thrombectomy. It is our policy to begin heparin therapy as soon as the patient enters the hospital, order phlebograms, and make arrangements for the earliest possible operative treatment.

Our files contain 13 cases of deep venous thrombosis of the subclavian and axillary veins. Four were demonstrated by phlebography; in the rest the clinical syndrome seemed to us to be certain. Five patients (38 per cent) gave a history of trauma: breaking a fall from a roof by catching an arm around a ladder, working out in a gymnasium (i.e., using a punching bag), vigorously raking a lawn and then playing golf and billiards, strenuously twisting the arms with weights, and lifting the arms in a ballet class. Two patients gave a history of lifting heavy objects. One patient had been playing the organ. Another attributed the swelling to a crutch she was using; however, metastatic carcinoma of the breast was found on the same side at work-up, and it is probable that the axillary metastases caused the thrombosis. Two patients, one a deaf-mute, gave no history pertinent to the swelling of the upper extremity. In two instances the swelling appeared overnight following trauma. Seven patients gave a history of what could be considered a gradual onset, i.e., over a period of days. Only 1 patient related what can be called a truly sudden or instantaneous onset (Case Report 7-2).

Case Report 7-2

A 54-year-old white married female was seen in January 1973. She enrolled in a ballet class in September 1972. The particular ballet maneuver involved in the present illness was new to her. She was facing a large wall clock with a sweep-second hand and so was able to pinpoint the exact moment of onset and timing of events.

While standing on her right leg with her left leg high on a barre, the maneuver called for her to move her extended left arm gradually upward from her side at right angles to the body until it passed her head toward the right side. While in this highly stretched position, she noted a peculiar "tingling" or "runny" feeling in her forearm and arm. This was at exactly 10:10 A.M. Approximately 2 minutes later, while continuing her exercises in a sitting position, she noted that her left wrist felt full; when she looked down at it, she noted that it was changing color, becoming a diffuse pink as contrasted with the whiter color of her right arm. As the minutes went by the pink became accentuated, so much so that her classmates stopped to look at the change in the color of her hand. The veins were distended and the whole forearm and arm began to feel tight. She became aware of a sense of fullness in her axilla, causing her tight-fitting jersey dress, and her brassiere to feel tight in the underarm. From then on, her symptoms were totally typical of venous obstruction of the upper extremity: swelling and slight discomfort with no real pain (a point that she reemphasized to us).

She was treated by two physicians, the second of whom referred her to our service.

Physical examination on admission 2 days later showed swelling of the entire extremity, particularly about the elbow. The veins were very prominent and distended, not only in the arm but also in the shoulder and left side of the chest. The skin color was slightly hyperemic but not cyanotic. All peripheral pulses were present.

Phleborheography confirmed venous obstruction. By this time the diagnosis was so certain that no phlebogram was obtained. The patient was treated with partial elevation of the upper extremities and heparin and warfarin (Coumadin) therapy.

Eleven patients were treated conservatively. Management consisted of elevation of the extremity and application of bandages or a rubberized sleeve. Seven of these also received anticoagulant therapy. Two patients were treated surgically. Case Report 7-3 illuminates the advantages of early intervention; Case Report 7-4 demonstrates posttraumatic constant subclavian vein stenosis with fibrous tissue reaction, which has been reported[29] in association with intermittent obstruction.

Case Report 7-3

A 57-year-old Caucasian male was seen in January 1966 in the emergency room of the hospital with massive swelling of the left upper extremity from fingertips to shoulder. He gave a history of being at work 2 days earlier when he felt a twinge of pain in his left forearm while doing heavy lifting on a construction job. The following day he noted some swelling of his left arm. The next day the swelling, and the arm generally, was much worse. He came to the emergency room.

On physical examination, massive swelling of the entire left upper extremity was seen. There was no ecchymosis and no recent hemorrhage. A diagnosis of left subclavian vein thrombosis was made; the patient was admitted to the hospital and taken to the operating room immediately, and thrombectomy was performed. Postoperatively, his left arm was entirely

normal. He continued to do well; in 1971 he was readmitted for basilar artery disease. In regard to his arm, he had experienced no further trouble, and the result was excellent 5 years postthrombectomy.

Case Report 7-4

A 38-year-old Caucasian male was seen in May 1971, for swelling of his right upper extremity. He gave a history of 5 months earlier having broken his fall off a roof by catching hold of a ladder in such a way that he was bearing the full weight of his heavy body in right axilla. This caused him great pain, which gradually subsided. He was now noticing swelling of his right arm associated with minimal discomfort.

On physical examination the superficial veins were distended, the right arm was 3 cm larger than the left and a phlebogram showed obstruction of the right subclavian vein at the level of the scalenus anticus muscle. He was admitted to the hospital for operative treatment. An extremely hypertrophied scalenus anticus muscle was found pressing the subclavian vein at its distal termination. The internal jugular vein was traced forward down to its junction with the subclavian vein, where the subclavian was completely flattened by fibrous tissue. Actually, despite multiple lysis of adhesions, indentation of the subclavian vein persisted as it joined with the internal jugular vein. A tubular structure containing clear fluid and no blood and assumed to be a lymphatic came straight up and across the indentation. After all the adhesions and obstructions were removed, the vein filled out and began transporting blood. A portion of the scalenus anticus muscle was also removed.

Postoperatively, this patient became asymptomatic. It is assumed that at the time of trauma, perivenous hemorrhage occurred, followed by a fibrous reaction. Two years after scalenotomy and lysis of perivascular adhesions, he continues to be free of all symptoms and signs.

Recurrent Venous Obstruction of the Upper Extremity

Recurrence of symptoms has been reported by Matas[83] and many others. According to Hughes,[82] recurrences are to be attributed to inability of the venous collaterals to respond to the increased flow of blood through the arm rather than to further injury to a vein which has been incompletely occluded by the initial trauma. A patient in our series has been followed for 9 years, during which time four episodes of venous obstruction of the upper extremities have occurred, three in the right and one in the left.

Case Report 7-5

A 24-year-old Caucasian male was seen in February 1964 for pain and tenderness of the right arm which had been present for 12 days. He gave a history of awakening early in the morning with a numb right arm. The arm became severely painful so that he was unable to use it. Numbness and pain persisted. It also became swollen and tight, and his symptoms grew worse with use of the arm.

On physical examination the right arm was fairly tense and tight, with distention of the superficial veins which did not collapse with elevation. The right arm had a circumference of 1.5 cm more than the left arm. Tenderness was present along the medial aspect of the entire arm and along the course of the deep veins. There was relative absence of tenderness in the axillary region. A diagnosis of right axillary-subclavian vein thrombosis was made.

The patient was immediately admitted to the hospital for heparin therapy, phlebography, and x rays of the cervical spine to determine the presence of a cervical rib. The phlebogram showed obstruction of the deep venous system of the right arm, with some filling of the cephalic vein.

He was treated with heparin therapy and was discharged using no anticoagulant drugs. He did well and was advised not to return to his job as a construction worker, in which he used an air hammer and did heavy lifting. He was asymptomatic a month after discharge from the hospital. It was assumed that the vein had reopened.

Five months after discharge from the hospital he was seen again in the emergency room with recurrent pain and tenderness of the right arm that set in while he was back at work using the air hammer.

Tenderness was present, but there was no edema and no venous distention. He was treated conservatively with heat and advised not to do heavy work.

In December 1964, he was seen in consultation in the hospital. He had been admitted by his family physician with another episode of brachial or axillary vein thrombosis of the right arm with severe tenderness and swelling. He was on warfarin (Coumadin) therapy, and heparin was advised. This episode occurred while he was using the air hammer. He improved and was discharged on anticoagulants; he remained relatively asymptomatic until January 1965, when he was readmitted for suspected pulmonary embolus and thrombophlebitis and was treated with anticoagulant drugs and enzyme therapy. Since then he has been maintained on anticoagulants and has continued to work occasionally with a pneumatic air hammer.

In July 1971 he was seen by his physician for a swollen, tender and inflamed left upper arm, at which time he gave a history of pain in the left deltoid region. There was no history of trauma this time. He was hospitalized, and a left subclavian phlebogram was carried out, which demonstrated a well-formed thrombus completely occluding the left subclavian vein for a distance of approximately 8 cm, from the apex of the axilla to the junction of the subclavian and jugular veins. Several smaller thrombi were noted in the axillary portion of the brachial and the cephalic vein. He was managed with bed rest and anticoagulant therapy. He did well and after discharge returned to work.

He was last seen in March 1972 and was doing well.

Although all the patients in our series recovered from their axillary-subclavian vein thromboses and all had significant improvement, none of the limbs could be considered to be entirely normal, with the possible exception of the two which were treated surgically.

REFERENCES

1. Sauer, P. E., and Murdock, C. E. Immediate surgery for cardiac and great vessel wounds. *Arch Surg* 95:7, 1967.
2. Bricker, D. L., Noon, G. P., Beall, A. C., and DeBakey, M. E. Vascular injuries of the thoracic outlet. *J Trauma 10:*1, 1970.
3. Jones, E. W., and Helmsworth, J. A. Penetrating wounds of the heart. 30 years experience. *Arch Surg* 96:671, 1968.
4. Steichen, F. M., Dargan, E. L., Efron, G., Pearlman,

D. M., and Weil, P. H. A graded approach to the management of penetrating wounds of the heart. *Arch Surg 103:*574, 1971.
5. Flint, L. M., Synder, W. H., Perry, M. O., and Shires, G. T. Management of major vascular injuries in the base of the neck. *Arch Surg 106:*407, 1973.
6. Cranley, J. J. Vascular Surgery. Vol I: Peripheral Arterial Diseases. Hagerstown, Harper & Row, 1972, pp 198–204.
7. Meese, E. H., Delaney, T. B., Doohen, D. J., and

Timmes, J. J. End-to-end superior vena cava-right pulmonary shunt in tricuspid atresia. *J Thorac Cardiov Surg 47:*261, 1964.

8. Roswit, B., Kaplan, G., and Jacobson, H. G. The superior vena cava obstruction syndrome in bronchiogenic carcinoma. *Radiology 61:*722, 1953.

9. Szur, L., and Bromley, L. L. Obstruction of the superior vena cava in carcinoma of the bronchus. *Br Med J 2:*1273, 1956.

10. Failor, H. J., Edwards, J. E., and Hodgson, C. H. Etiologic factors in obstruction of the superior vena cava: A pathologic study. *Proc Staff Meet Mayo Clin 33:*671, 1958.

11. Effler, D. B., and Groves, L. K. Superior vena caval obstruction. *J Thorac Cardiov Surg 43:*574, 1962.

12. Salsali, M., and Cliffton, E. E. Superior vena caval obstruction with lung cancer. *Ann Thorac Surg 6:*437, 1968.

13. Okay, N., and Bryk, D. Collateral pathways in occlusion of the superior vena cava and its tributaries. *Radiology 92:*1493, 1969.

14. Hanlon, C. R., and Davis, R. K. Superior vena caval obstruction: indications for diagnostic thoracotomy. *Ann Surg 161:*771, 1965.

15. Marshall, R. J., Hughes, J. T., and Gilbert, E. F. Obstruction of superior vena cava and pulmonary artery by malignant thymoma. *Dis Chest 52:*251, 1967.

16. Kim, D. H., Mautner, L., Henning, J., and Volpe, R. An unusual case of thyroid carcinoma with direct extension to great veins, right heart and pulmonary arteries. *Canad Med Assoc J 94:*238, 1966.

17. Meese, E. H., Doohen, D. J., Elliott, R. C., and Timmes, J. J. Primary organ involvement in intrathoracic Hodgkin's disease. *Dis Chest 46:*699, 1964.

18. Calkins, E. A. The superior vena caval syndrome: Report of 21 cases. *Dis Chest 30:*404, 1956.

19. Sherman, P. H., and Shahbahrami, F. Mediastinal goitre: Review of ten cases. *Am Surg 32:*137, 1966.

20. Silverstein, G. E., Burke, G., Goldberg, D., and Halko, A. Superior vena caval obstruction caused by benign endothoracic goiter. *Dis Chest 56:*519, 1969.

21. Shah-Mirany, J., Mirhosini, M., and Head, L. R. Fatal pulmonary embolism from jugular veins following benign superior vena cava syndrome. *Ann Thorac Surg 11:*238, 1971.

22. Tama, L., Ellis, F. H., Hodgson, C. H., and Dockerty, M. B. Chemodectoma of the mediastinum: Report on a patient with superior vena caval obstruction treated by a shunt from the right innominate vein to the right atrium. *J Thorac Cardiov Surg 43:*585, 1962.

23. McIntyre, F. T., and Sykes, E. M. Obstruction of the superior vena cava: Review of the literature and report of 2 personal cases. *Ann Int Med 30:*925, 1949.

24. Banker, V. P., and Maddison, F. E. Superior vena cava syndrome secondary to aortic disease: Report of two cases and review of the literature. *Dis Chest 51:*656, 1967.

25. Barrett, N. R. Idiopathic mediastinal fibrosis. *Br J Surg 46:*207, 1958.

26. King, R. L. Idiopathic mediastinal fibrosis. *Bull Mason Clin 17:*1, 1963.

27. Pate, J. W., and Hammon, J. Superior vena cava syndrome due to histoplasmosis in children. *Ann Surg 161:*778, 1965.

28. Friedli, B., Guerin, R., Davignon, A., Fouron, J. C., and Stanley, P. Surgical treatment of partial anomalous pulmonary venous drainage: A long-term follow-up study. *Circulation 45:*159, 1972.

29. Wertheimer, M., Hughes, R. K., and Castle, C. H. Superior vena cava syndrome: Complication of permanent transvenous endocardial cardiac pacing. *JAMA 224:*1172, 1973.

30. Cha, E. M. Collateral circulation in superior vena caval obstruction following ventriculoatrial shunt catheterization in hydrocephalus. *Radiology 102:*605, 1972.

31. Mazzei, E. A., and Mulder, D. G. Superior vena cava syndrome following complete correction (Mustard repair) of transposition of the great vessels. *Ann Thorac Surg 11:*243, 1971.

32. Gordonson, J., Trachtenberg, S., and Sargent, E. N. Superior vena cava obstruction due to sarcoidosis. *Chest 63:*292, 1973.

33. Moene, R. J., Dekker, A., and Van der Harten, H. J. Congenital right-sided pericardial defect with herniation of part of the lung into the pericardial cavity. *Am J Cardiol 31:*519, 1973.

34. Steinberg, I. Superior vena caval obstruction. In Abrams, H. L. (ed.) *Angiography.* Boston, Little Brown, 1961, vol. 1.

35. Mikkelsen, W. J. Varices of the upper esophagus in superior vena caval obstruction. *Radiology 87:*945, 1963.

36. Papadimitriou, J., Kapelakis, G., Constandinidis, C., Kelekis, D., and Tountas, C. Radioisotope cavography. *Ann Thorac Surg 17:*36, 1974.

37. Elliott, R. C., Boyd, A. D., Snyder, W., and Meese, E. H. Mediastinoscopy. *Am Rev Res Dis 96:*981, 1967.

38. Oh, K. S. Superior mediastinal syndrome in a young child. *JAMA 208:*1177, 1969.

39. Rubin, P., Green, J., Holzwasser, G., and Gerle, R. Superior vena caval syndrome: Slow low-dose versus rapid high-dose schedule. *Radiology 81:*388, 1963.

40. Holmes, K. S. The treatment of superior vena caval syndrome by high dose grid technique. *Radiology 81:*402, 1963.

41. Longacre, A. M., and Shockman, A. T. The superior vena cava syndrome and radiation therapy: Clinical response, survival, and postmortem findings. *Radiology 91:*713, 1968.

42. Salsali, M., and Cliffton, E. E. Superior vena caval obstruction with carcinoma of the lung. *Surg Gynecol Obstet 121:*783, 1965.

43. Skinner, D. B., Salzman, E. W., and Scannell, J. G. The challenge of superior vena caval obstruction. *J Thorac Cardiov Surg* 49:824, 1965.

44. Salsali, M. A safe technique for resection of the nonobstructed superior vena cava. *Surg Gynecol Obstet* 123:91, 1966.

45. Scannell, J. G. Etiology and surgical approaches in superior vena caval obstruction. *Radiology 81:*378, 1963.

46. Peter, M. Y., Hering, A. C., and Watkins, E. Experimental Teflon replacement of the superior vena cava and atriocaval junction. *J Thorac Cardiov Surg* 40:224, 1960.

47. Allansmith, R., and Richards, V. Superior vena caval obstruction. *Am J Surg* 96:353, 1958.

48. Allansmith, R. Surgical treatment of superior vena cava obstruction due to malignant tumor. *J Thorac Cardiov Surg 44:*258, 1962.

49. Benvenuto, R., Rodman, F. S. B., Gilmour, J., Phillips, A. F., and Callaghan, J. C. Composite venous graft for replacement of the superior vena cava. *Arch Surg* 84:570, 1962.

50. Higginson, J. F. Aortic homograft substitution and bypass in superior vena caval obstruction. *J Thorac Surg 32:*684, 1956.

51. Holman, C. W., and Steinberg, I. W. Treatment of superior vena caval occlusion by arterial graft. *JAMA 155:*1403, 1954.

52. Jensen, N. K., Garamella, J. J., Schmidt, W. R., Hoffman, G. L., and Scharf, G. Vena caval replacement in man by Teflon graft. *J. Thorac Cardiov Surg 44:*56, 1962.

53. Moore, T. C., and Riberi, A. Superior vena caval replacement: III. Successful use of fresh autologous aorta. *Surgery* 44:898, 1958.

54. Moore, T. C., Teramoto, S., and Heimburger, I. L. Successful use of Teflon grafts superior vena caval replacement. *Surg Gynecol Obstet 111:*475, 1960.

55. Onodera, R., Watanabe, H., Onuma, K., Shibota, V., and Shibota, A. Obstruction of the superior vana cava treated by resection and Dacron graft: Report of a case. *J Int Coll Surg 34:*615, 1960.

56. Riberi, A., and Moore, T. C. Superior vena caval replacement: I. Unsuitability of free tubes of autogenous pericardium. *Arch Surg 76:*384, 1958.

57. Scannell, J. G., and Shaw, R. S. Surgical reconstruction of the superior vena cava. *J Thorac Surg 28:*163, 1954.

58. Whiffen, J. D., and Gott, V. L. Prosthetic thoracic vena cava grafts. *J Thorac Cardiov Surg 50:*31, 1965.

59. Fraser, R. E., Halseth, W. L., Johnson B., and Paton, B. C. Experimental replacement of the superior vena cava. *Arch Surg* 96:378, 1968.

60. Deterling, R. A., and Bhonsley, S. S. Use of vessel graft and plastic prosthesis for relief of superior vena caval obstruction. *Surgery* 38:1008, 1955.

61. Dale, W. A., and Scott, A. W. Grafts of the venous systems. *Surgery 53:*52, 1963.

62. Scheinin, T. M., and Jude, J. R. Experimental replacement of the superior vena cava: Effect of temporary increase in blood flow. *J Thorac Cardiov Surg 48:*781, 1964.

63. Cooley, D. A., and Hallman, G. L. Superior vena caval syndrome treated by azygos vein-inferior vena cava anastomosis. *J Thorac Cardiov Surg 14:* 325, 1964.

64. Garcia, J. M., Ramirez, R., Bacos, J., and Absolon, K. B. Technique for reconstruction of superior vena cava in fibrosing mediastinitis. *J Thorac Cardiov Surg 65:*547, 1973.

65. Gerbode, F. L., as cited by Haimovici, Hoffert, Zinicola *et al. Surg Gynecol Obstet 131:*1173, 1970.

66. Vasko, J. S., Kilman, J. W., and Ahn, C. Superior vena caval replacement with homologous trachea. *Ann Thorac Surg 5:*429, 1968.

67. Fadhli, H. A. Endvenectomy and decompression in fibrosing mediastinitis causing obstruction of the superior vena cava. *J Thorac Cardiov Surg 53:* 881, 1967.

68. Ellis, P. R., and del Rosario, V. C. Internal mammary artery-superior vena caval replacement. *Ann Thorac Surg 4:*74, 1967.

69. Gopalrao, T., Zikria, E., Miller, W., Samadani, S., and Ford, W. Surgical treatment of obstruction of the superior vena cava and right pulmonary artery. *J Thorac Cardiov Surg 63:*394, 1972.

70. Miller, R. E., Corneil, N. J., and Sullivan, F. J. Replacement of superior vena cava with autogenous tissue: An experimental study. *Ann Thorac Surg 15:*474, 1973.

71. Miller, R. E., and Sullivan, F. J. Superior vena caval obstruction secondary to fibrosing mediastinitis. *Ann Thorac Surg 15:*483, 1973.

72. Moore, T. C., and Yong, N. K. Experimental replacement and bypass of the large veins. *Bull Soc Int Chir 23:*274, 1964.

73. Holt, M. H., and Lewis, F. J. Experimental grafts of the superior vena cava with temporary arteriovenous shunts. *J Thorac Cardiov Surg 49:*818, 1965.

74. Mitsouoka, H., Vega, R. E., and Howard, J. M. Experimental venous replacement with a temporary arteriovenous fistula. *Arch Surg* 93:382, 1966.

75. Bryant, M. F., Lazenby, W. D., and Howard, J. M. Experimental replacement of short segments of veins. *Arch Surg* 76:289, 1958.

76. Barnes, R. W., Mohri, H., Nelson, R. J., and Merendino, K. A. The use of low molecular weight dextran in superior vena caval replacement. *Dis Chest 53:* 390, 1968.

77. Brais, M., Bertranou, E., Brassard, A., Stanley, P., and Chartrand, C. Effect of dextran on patency of pericardial tubular graft of the superior vena cava in the dog. *J Thorac Cardiov Surg 65:*296, 1973.

78. Lindskog, G. E., Liebow, A. A., and Glenn, W. W. L. *Thoracic and Cardiovascular Surgery with Related Pathology.* New York, Appleton-Century-Crofts, 1962.

79. Abbott, O. A., and Leigh, T. F. Aneurysmal dilatation of the superior vena caval system. *Ann Surg 159:*858, 1964.

80. Bell, M. J. Aneurysm of the superior vena cava. *Radiology 95:*317, 1970.

81. Gallucci, V., Sanger, P. W., Robiczek, F., and Daugherty, H. K. Aneurysm of the superior caval vein. *Vasc Surg 1:*158, 1967.

82. Hughes, E. S. R. Collective review: Venous obstruction in the upper extremity (Paget-Schroetter's syndrome). *Int Abst Surg 88:*89, 1949.

83. Matas, R. So-called primary thrombosis of axillary vein caused by strain: Report of case, diagnosis, pathogony, and treatment. *Am J Surg 24:*642, 1934.

84. Veal, J. R., and McFetridge, E. M. Primary thrombosis of the axillary vein: An anatomic and roentgenologic study of certain etiologic factors and a consideration of venography as a diagnostic measure. *Arch Surg 31:*271, 1935.

85. Tilney, N. L., Griffiths, H. J. G., and Edwards, E. A. Natural history of major venous thrombosis of the upper extremity. *Arch Surg 101:*792, 1970.

86. Ochsner, A., DeBakey, M. E., DeCamp, P. T., and Da Rocha, E. Thrombo-embolism: An analysis of cases at the Charity Hospital in New Orleans over a 12-year period. *Ann Surg 134:*405, 1951.

87. Barker, N. W., Nygaard, K. K., Walters, W., and Priestley, J. T. A statistical study of postoperative venous thrombosis and pulmonary embolism: IV. Location of thrombosis: Relation of thrombosis and embolism. *Proc Staff Meet Mayo Clin 16:*33, 1941.

88. Barnett, T., and Levitt, L. M. "Effort" thrombosis of the axillary vein with pulmonary embolism. *JAMA 146:*1412, 1951.

89. Aufsis, A. H. Venous thrombosis of upper extremity complicated by pulmonary embolism. *Surgery 35:* 957, 1954.

90. Tomlin, C. E. Pulmonary infarction complicating thrombophlebitis of upper extremity. *Am J Med 12:*411, 1952.

91. Adams, J. T., DeWeese, J. A., Mahoney, E. B., and Rob, C. G. Intermittent subclavian vein obstruction without thrombosis. *Surgery 63:*147, 1968.

92. McLaughlin, C. W., and Popma, A. M. Intermittent obstruction of the subclavian vein. *JAMA 133:*1960, 1939.

93. Falconer, M. A., and Weddell, G. L. Costoclavicular compression of subclavian artery and vein. *Lancet 2:*539, 1943.

94. Horwitz, O., and Zinnser, H. F. Subclavian vein obstruction: Report of a case studied by venography and relieved by surgery. *JAMA 151:*997, 1953.

95. Jackson, N. J., and Nanson, E. M. Intermittent subclavian vein obstruction. *Br J Surg 49:*303, 1961.

96. McCleery, R. S., Kesterson, J. E., Kirtley, J. A., and Love, R. B. Subclavius and anterior scalene muscle compression as cause of intermittent obstruction of subclavian vein. *Ann Surg 133:*588, 1951.

97. Lord, J. W., and Rosati, L. M. Neurovascular compression syndromes of the upper extremity. *Clin Symp 10:*35, 1958.

98. Adams, J. T., McEvoy, R. K., and DeWeese, J. A. Primary deep venous thrombosis of upper extremity. *Arch Surg 91:*29, 1965.

99. Claggett, G. P., Thornbury, J. R., and Penner, J. A. Upper extremity venous thrombosis with pulmonary embolism. *JAMA 227:*187, 1974.

100. Paget, J. *Clinical Lectures and Essays.* London, Longmans, Green & Co., 1875.

101. von Schroetter, L. Erkränkungen der Gefässe. In: *Nothnagel C; Handbuch der Pathologie und Therapie.* Wien, Holder, 1884.

102. Kleinsasser, L. "Effort" thrombosis of axillary and subclavian veins: Analysis of 16 personal cases and 56 cases from the literature. *Arch Surg 59:* 258, 1949.

103. Horton, B. T. Primary thrombosis of the axillary vein. *JAMA 96:*2194, 1931.

104. Swinton, N. W., Edgett, J. W., and Hall, R. J. Primary subclavian-axillary vein thrombosis. *Circulation 38:*737, 1968.

105. Cucci, C. E., Bottino, C. G., and Ciampa, V. Venous obstruction of the upper extremity caused by a malformed valve of the subclavian vein. *Circulation 27:*275, 1963.

106. Wilder, J. R., Habermann, E. T., and Nach, R. L. Subclavian vein obstruction secondary to hypertrophy of the terminal valve. *Surgery 55:*214, 1964.

107. Veal, J. R., and Hussey, H. H. The use of "exercise tests" in connection with venous pressure measurements for the detection of venous obstruction in the upper and lower extremities. *Am Heart J 20:*308, 1940.

108. Tagariello, P. Immagini flebografiche normali e patologiche dell'arto superiore. *Atti Riun Intern Angiocardiochirurgia,* 1951.

109. Garusi, G. F., and Cresti, M. Obstructed venous discharge syndromes of the superior limb. *Angiology 14:*209, 1963.

110. Coon, W. W., and Willis, P. W. Thrombosis of axillary and subclavian veins. *Arch Surg 94:*657, 1967.

111. Bedsole, D. O., and Hamrick, L. C. Bilateral intermittent obstruction of the subclavian veins. *Ann Surg 158:*1039, 1963.

112. Fountain, J. R., and Taverner, D. Gangrene of three limbs from venous occlusion. *Ann Int Med 44:*549, 1957.

113. Haggard, G. E. Value of conservative management in cervico-brachial pain. *JAMA 137:*508, 1948.

114. Peet, R. M., Henriksen, J. D., Anderson, T. P., and Martin, G. M. Thoracic-outlet syndrome: Evaluation of a therapeutic exercise program. *Proc Staff Meet Mayo Clin 31:*281, 1956.

115. Nelson, P. A. Treatment of patients with cervico-dorsal outlet syndrome. *JAMA 163:*1570, 1957.

116. Cranley, J. J. Neurovascular Compression Syn-

dromes. In Vascular Surgery: Vol. I. Peripheral Arterial Diseases. Hagerstown, MD, Harper & Row, 1972.

117. Roos, D. B., and Owens J. C. Thoracic outlet syndrome. Arch Surg 93:71, 1966.

118. Roos, D. B. Transaxillary approach for first rib resection to relieve thoracic outlet syndrome. *Ann Surg 163:*354, 1966.

119. Roos, D. B. Experience with first rib resection for thoracic outlet syndrome. *Ann Surg 173:*429, 1971

120. Gol, A., Patrick, D. W., and McNeal, D. P. Relief of costoclavicular syndrome by infraclavicular removal of first rib. *J Neurosurg 28:*81, 1968.

8

Pulmonary Embolism

INTRODUCTION

In the early years of the 19th century, hemorrhagic infarction of the lung was identified by Laënnec,[1] who called it "pulmonary apoplexy." Cruveilhier[2] noted that in a patient with pulmonary infarction "all the arterial branches which lead to the region were filled with clot that branched according to the vascular tree." Virchow[3] not only identified the thrombus but also understood that clot in the veins of the lower extremity might be swept away by the bloodstream and lodge in the lung as a pulmonary embolus.

Much has been learned about pulmonary embolus in the 125 years since Virchow's investigations, but much still remains to be clarified. The true incidence and morbidity have yet to be established. The pathologic physiology is still in doubt. The accuracy of the clinical diagnosis is said to be little more than 50 per cent, approximately equal to the tossing of a coin. Treatment is far from standardized. Methods of prophylaxis remain eclectic, unproven, and, at times, contradictory. Despite all these shortcomings, however, in recent years there are many indications that we are coming closer to improved diagnosis and treatment of this disease: there has been an incremental acquisition of knowledge anatomic and functional pathology; the development of and improvements in pulmonary scanning techniques and pulmonary angiography, and widespread use of them; the development of better methods of diagnosing deep venous thrombosis; and significant advances in the treatment of pulmonary embolism.

DEFINITION

Pulmonary embolism has been succinctly defined by Gray[4] as the "intravascular movement of an object, the embolus, from a point of origin or entry into a systemic vein to a pulmonary artery, where it produces obstruction." Any object carried by the venous current to the lung is a pulmonary embolus: fat, amniotic fluid, bacteria, and foreign bodies are all recognized as emboli. In this discussion, however, "embolus" is restricted to mean blood clot. Pulmonary emboli are defined in terms of size: massive, major, minor, miliary, or microscopic. A massive embolus is one that occludes the pulmonary artery itself or its primary branches. A major embolus occludes any major branch of the pulmonary artery. A minor embolus occludes medium-sized branches of the pulmonary tree. Beyond this, individual emboli are not recognized; one speaks collectively of miliary emboli, the small and numerous blood clots that lodge primarily in the arterioles, and of microemboli, which are platelet clumps that lodge in the capillaries.

INCIDENCE

Until it is possible to diagnose pulmonary embolism with certainty, it is impossible to determine its incidence. Many attempts have been made to determine the frequency of fatal pulmonary embolism from death certificates, hospital statistics, and autopsy reports. This type of source material contains basic defects.

Death Certificates

Clinical diagnosis without autopsy confirmation is not to be trusted. The law compels the attending physician to record a cause of death, however unaware he is of the existing condition. The diagnosis of myocardial infarction or pulmonary embolism is not likely to be questioned. Therefore, compilations of such data have little statistical value. For example, Towbin,[5] analyzing the causes of death in the population in the vicinity of Columbus, Ohio, found that pulmonary embolism was listed as the cause of death only one-fourth as often for people who died at home as for those who died in hospitals.

A second objection is raised by Hume et al.[6]: By international agreement, only one cause of death is singled out for official purposes, although two or more causes are noted on the death certificate. Several pulmonary emboli may have occurred prior to death in a patient with myocardial infarction; nevertheless, the death is considered to be due to myocardial infarction. Hume attempted to make corrections and estimated that pulmonary embolism was mentioned as the cause of death in at least 21,000 death certificates in England and Wales in 1967.

Hospital Statistics

By reviewing the data from the Commission of Professional and Hospital Activities, Hume and his associates[6] analyzed the diagnoses of venous thrombosis and pulmonary embolism made in the United States in 1966. These figures must be suspect if, as is generally agreed, the clinical diagnosis is correct in only 50 per cent of the cases. Nevertheless, these statistics suggest that a quarter of a million patients with the diagnosis of venous thrombosis and pulmonary embolism were in United States hospitals in 1966. These estimates exclude persons at home and those in nursing homes or custodial care institutions. Using another technique, these researchers estimated that a reasonable estimate of

overall incidence of fatal embolism, based on autopsy reports, is approximately 5/1000 inpatients, and the incidence of nonfatal embolism is approximately 10/1000 inpatients. For England and Wales, where 4.2 million patients were hospitalized, this yields approximately 21,000 fatal and an additional 285,000 nonfatal cases of pulmonary embolism. Although these figures exceed the estimates made by Coon and Willis in 1959,[7] i.e., approximately 47,000 deaths annually in which pulmonary embolism was the sole cause and 141,000 deaths in which it was a contributing cause, evidence seems to be accumulating that the more pulmonary embolism is looked for, the more it is found. Also, as life expectancy increases, a rising incidence of thromboembolism is to be expected, due to advancing age being a predisposing factor.

Since there is overwhelming evidence that the clinical diagnosis of thrombophlebitis and pulmonary embolism is hardly more accurate than the tossing of a coin (50-50), hospital statistics are certainly of questionable value, especially if the data were accumulated prior to the era of wide use of objective means of determining the presence of the disease, i.e., pulmonary scans, pulmonary angiogram, and phlebograms.

Autopsy Reports

It is to be presumed that autopsy reports provide sound statistics on the incidence of pulmonary embolism. The data per se are certainly accurate; however, certain variables prejudice the evidence. Foremost, the number of autopsies varies from hospital to hospital and rarely (if ever) approaches the ideal of 100 per cent. Secondly, the experience and interest of the prosector affects the number of pulmonary emboli discovered. It has been the practice to assign routine autopsies to the least experienced pathologists, e.g., to the surgical resident fulfilling his requirements or to the first-year pathology resident. Pulmonary embolus may be missed in the cadaver just as completely as in the living patient if the pathologist lacks special interest in thromboembolic phenomena. The difficulty experienced by some pathologists in distinguishing between antemortem and postmortem clot is another inconstant factor in autopsy data.

The specialized interest of the hospital itself is a

prime determinant in the variability of autopsy data. Wide variance exists in the incidence of pulmonary embolism recorded in the files of different institutions providing care for children, for maternity patients, for the aged and bedridden, or for the general population. The percentage of autopsies performed in children's hospitals is usually very high; the percentage of children with pulmonary embolism is extremely low. Jones and Sabiston[8] found only 73 instances of pulmonary embolism in children in the world literature and also 73 in the combined files of Johns Hopkins and Duke University Hospitals, for a negligible total of less than 150. It also has become evident that intravenous thrombosis in infants is basically a different disease from that in adults. Infantile thrombosis occurs primarily in the large veins of the body cavities, not in the peripheral veins of the extremities. And although the correlation between advancing age and the incidence of thrombophlebitis and/or pulmonary embolism is obvious, concomitant diseases (such as heart disease, cancer, and debility, all of which also increase with advancing age) still complicate the extrication of pulmonary embolism as the sole cause or a contributing cause of death in autopsies at individual institutions; these concomitant diseases interfere even more certainly when the goal is a combined percentage of the incidence on a national or worldwide basis.

In his attempt to get a panoramic view of the incidence, DeBakey[9] reviewed all the literature for the 50 years prior to 1954, i.e., the era before the prevalence of objective methods of diagnosis. His reports totaled almost 335,000 postmortem examinations and over 3,000,000 operations. He divided the results into four periods (Table 8-1). The average incidence of fatal pulmonary embolism given in the reports invalidates the statistics, which can have little relation to the actual incidence of fatal pulmonary embolism. In view of the enumerated difficulties, Matas,[10] DeBakey,[9] and Hume et al.[6] concluded that it is impossible to determine a reasonable estimate of the incidence of thromboembolic disease. Hume et al. reviewed major autopsy series of pulmonary embolism since the time of Virchow, in which the overall incidence showed a variance of 10 to 30 per cent and fatal embolism exhibited a range of 3 to 10 per cent. More recent reports seem to suggest that if emboli are carefully searched for, they can be found in approximately 25 per cent of autopsies on adults.[11-15]

CLASSIFICATION

It is difficult to classify pulmonary emboli by any single criterion, because the anatomic size and the location of the embolus do not correlate well with the physiologic disturbances in a living patient. Anatomically, emboli can be considered to be massive, major, minor, miliary, or microemboli. In the living patient, however, the only concern is whether the patient will die immediately or will survive, without or with chronic pulmonary disability.

Survival is a function of the residual capacity of the cardiopulmonary system, which is determined not only by the percentage of pulmonary function eliminated by the pulmonary embolus but also by the efficiency of the lung and the heart prior to embolization. Thus, an embolus blocking the right pulmonary artery might cause few symptoms in the

TABLE 8-1. Incidence of Fatal Postoperative Pulmonary Embolism Based Upon Collected Series

PERIOD	NO. OPERATIONS	NO. FATAL EMBOLISMS	% FATAL EMBOLISMS	RANGE IN % FATAL EMBOLISM
Prior to 1920	361,881	481	0.13	0.02–0.87
1921–1930	919,972	1,899	0.21	0.01–0.65
1931–1940	871,063	1,428	0.16	0.01–0.54
Since 1941	924,579	759	0.08	0.03–0.16
Total	3,077,495	4,567	0.14	0.01–0.87

From DeBakey, M. E. *Surg Gynecol Obstet* 98:1, 1954. By permission of SURGERY, GYNECOLOGY & OBSTETRICS.

normal individual but cause immediate death in a patient who has undergone left pneumonectomy or who has severe emphysema or cardiac decompensation. Similarly, a major embolus blocking off an entire lobe might cause no symptoms in a previously normal patient but cause immediate death in a patient who is a pulmonary or cardiac cripple. It it not uncommon to see a massive embolism proved by pulmonary scan or arteriogram in an asymptomatic patient or in a patient whose only symptom or sign is slight dyspnea on rolling over in bed. Thus, a single minor embolus could easily go unnoticed by a patient or his physician, even in the presence of emphysema or poor cardiac reserve. However, if they are multiple, such minor emboli can cause death. Furthermore, if they occur in overwhelming numbers, minor emboli can prove fatal to a person who has previously normal lungs. Pulmonary microemboli probably occur many times during normal life without causing symptoms or signs of pulmonary insufficiency. However, if the number is large enough and/or the pulmonary reserve low enough, such microemboli can cause the same total degree of pulmonary hypertension as occurs in a patient with massive pulmonary embolus.

Walsh et al.[16] developed an objective anatomic method of classifying pulmonary emboli by pulmonary arteriography which enabled them to categorize the severity of the disease quite accurately. This is a step forward and may well become a standard guide for the anatomic description of pulmonary emboli in a living patient. However, since the anatomic details do not always correlate well with the clinical picture, it is necessary to describe an embolus both in anatomic and functional terms, as is done with coronary artery disease, e.g., "an embolus to the right lower lobe, without or with pleural pain, cough, or hemoptysis" or "multiple emboli without or with cyanosis, hypoxemia, and elevation of pulmonary artery pressure." At present the physician must employ physiologic and anatomic descriptions alternately, as best fits the patient. Thus, the most informative description of "massive embolus" is that suggested by Bryant et al.[17]: "Acute massive pulmonary embolism is a clinical syndrome, characterized by severe respiratory distress, with sustained hypotension or

shock." Similarly, major or minor emboli should be classified according to whether or not infarction is present. Miliary emboli and microemboli may best be categorized by their effect on pulmonary artery pressure and the partial pressure of oxygen.

PATHOLOGY

Anatomic or morbid pathology may be discussed under three headings: the nature of the embolus itself; its point of origin; and the anatomic effect it has on the site of lodgment, i.e., the lung.

The Embolus

All thrombi found in the lung are presumed to be embolic. Nonembolic thrombosis rarely occurs, and

Figure 8-1. Clot filling main pulmonary artery. (*Courtesy of Dr. J. C. Parker, Lexington, Ky.*)

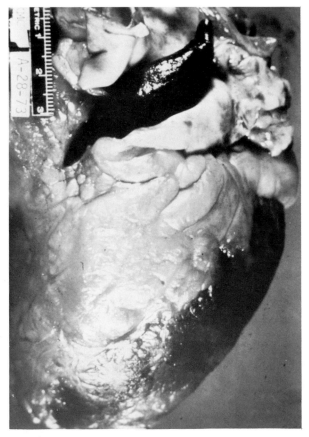

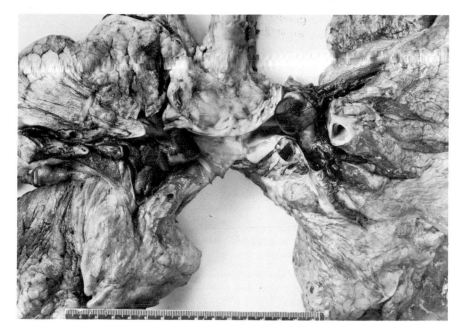

Figure 8-2. Emboli filling both major divisions of pulmonary artery.

if it does, it is in association with underlying pulmonary pathology, outside the scope of this discussion.

MAJOR EMBOLI

If an embolus that occludes the pulmonary artery (Fig. 8-1; 8-2) and causes sudden death can be extracted in one piece, it is frequently noted to be of a size that could come only from the major venous trunk of the thigh or pelvis. The diameter may be 1 to 1.5 cm and the length may be 50 cm or more. Frequently, emboli are fragmented (Fig. 8-3) in passing through the heart. If the patient survives, it may be due to the fact that large portions of the clot have been pumped away to the periphery of the lung, where they interfere less with oxygenation.

MINOR EMBOLI

Multiple small emboli in the central and peripheral arteries of both lungs are usually short and narrow, 2 to 5 mm in diameter and 1 to 3 cm in length. Occasionally, a short, thick embolus is encountered, which makes one conjecture that its site of origin is most likely the deep femoral or hypogastric vein.

MILIARY EMBOLI

Clots found in the arterioles of the lungs appear to be of the same character as major emboli but smaller in size ("miliary" is derived from the Latin

Figure 8-3. Large and small (probably fragmented) pieces of pulmonary embolism lodged in major divisions of pulmonary artery.

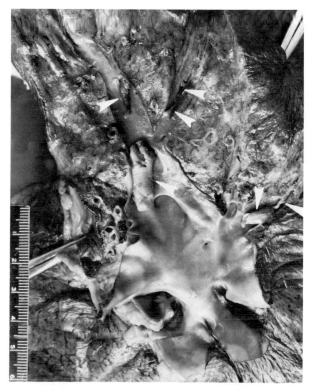

word for "millet seed"). They may represent emboli from very small veins or possibly fragments of a large embolus broken up as it passes through the heart. Eeles and Sevitt[18] described them as 0.25 to 1.0 mm in size. They do not cause infarction; however, when myriads of them block the arterioles, they may cause acute or chronic pulmonary hypertension.

MICROEMBOLI

Capillary microthrombi differ from most arterial microthrombi in appearance.[6] Some are granular, resembling aggregated platelets; others resemble a mixture of fibrin and platelets; and some have a predominantly fibrinous structure. Microemboli are found in interstitial vessels believed to be arterioles, in muscular arterioles, and in the capillaries of the alveoli. Some are attached to the wall; other are free in the vessel. Most appear to be recent; others are old enough to demonstrate invasion by fibroblasts and endothelial cells and some evidence of fibrinolysis. Eeles and Sevitt[18] determined that they consist mostly of platelet clumps that may be surrounded by fibrin and that they measure from 20μ to 100μ in diameter. Microemboli were seen histologically in lungs of 67 of 100 patients without gross embolism, as reported by Braconier.[19] Smith and associates[20, 21] found microemboli in many subjects who also had emboli in larger arteries of the lungs.

SITES OF ORIGIN

The Lower Extremities

The source of major pulmonary emboli is controversial and is being clarified as new knowledge develops. Since Virchow, it has been believed that pulmonary emboli are derived from deep veins of the leg; on this basis some surgeons recommended bilateral femoral vein ligation for patients with thromboembolic disease. Recognizing that the major veins of the pelvis might be involved frequently, physicians have widely advocated ligation, plication, or filtering of the inferior vena cava or blockage with an umbrella-like device as prophylaxis against embolization of pelvic or leg clot to the lung. The fact that the veins of the leg are not routinely dissected at autopsy is a great obstacle to the development of knowledge in this area. The

evidence in studies in which these veins have been dissected is that nearly all patients dying of pulmonary embolism have the potential source of their lung clots in the major venous trunks of the lower extremities and pelvis.

The Right Heart

Another possible source of embolus is the right heart, particularly in patients with auricular fibrillation. Coon and Coller,[12] Pollak et al.,[22] and Modan et al.[23] concluded that the major source of emboli was still the veins of the lower limb, even in patients with cardiac disease. If all of Coon and Coller's patients dying of pulmonary emboli who also had right-heart thrombi (9.2 per cent) actually did die of right-heart emboli, then a maximum of less than 10 per cent of all pulmonary emboli were derived from a cardiac source. In Pollak's[22] series, only 7 per cent of 516 patients had emboli that arose in the chest; Modan et al.[23] report the right heart as the source in 8 per cent of their autopsy subjects. In an earlier study at the Massachusetts General Hospital, Carlotti et al.[24] found that leg-vein thrombosis was the main source of pulmonary emboli, even in cardiac patients.

Our clinical experience with vena cava ligation for thromboembolic disease confirms a lower-extremity origin of pulmonary embolism. In 150 patients with caval ligation and in an additional 16 patients with clipping devices, only one death was caused by a fresh postoperative pulmonary embolism, and that occurred in a patient with untreated polycythemia vera 5 months after ligation of the vena cava.

The Hypogastric Veins

These have been reported as a possible source of pulmonary embolism, but most thrombi arising from the hypogastric vein probably are not large enough to prove fatal unless the patient has advanced cardiopulmonary disease. Other smaller veins may indeed give rise to emboli, but because of their size, chances are against their proving fatal.

Veins of the Upper Extremity

Death from pulmonary embolus of the upper extremity is rarely proven. For a discussion of upper extremity emboli, see the section on upper extremity obstruction syndromes in Chapter 7.

Central Veins and the Dural Sinuses

In children, fatal pulmonary embolism may arise from the large veins of the body cavities or from veins of the dural sinuses. In adults, such emboli are rarely, if ever, encountered.

EXOGENOUS MICROEMBOLI

Cardiopulmonary Bypass Procedures

Microemboli have been identified with venovenous bypass experiments and also with venoaortic bypass procedures in patients.[25] In the laboratory, capillary microemboli have been found in abundance in the lungs of dogs, the source being debris from blood damaged by the oxygenator. Venoarterial perfusion with cardiopulmonary bypass in patients is now less hazardous; nevertheless, the heart and brain may be affected because the blood returned from the oxygenator is perfused through the systemic capillary bed.

Stored Blood and Transfusions

In 1965 Moore et al.[26] raised the possibility of pulmonary microemboli from transfused blood; Swank and associates[27-29] have demonstrated that blood stored for future transfusions is an important source of emboli to the lungs. Reuel et al.[30] studied 29 patients with severe trauma; all were treated by standard methods except that a control group of 16 patients received 10 to 40 units of blood through a standard 170μ blood filter and the remaining[13] patients received 10 to 63 units of blood through a fine screen filter with a uniform pore size of 40μ. Of the 16 patients in the control group, 8 (50 per cent) developed posttraumatic pulmonary insufficiency; in the treated group, 2 of 13 (15.4 per cent) showed this finding. Furthermore, these 2 patients had sustained chest injuries. Thus, evidence is accumulating that pulmonary microembolism from stored blood is a true entity and that its incidence can be reduced by the use of newer, more effective filters.

Autopsy evidence[31] confirmed the presence of microemboli in systemic arterioles and capillaries of patients dying within 4 days after cardiopulmonary bypass procedures. Such small emboli were composed, at least in part, of platelet substance. The finding of similar particles in the pulmonary arterioles and capillaries of patients receiving large amounts of blood intravenously and the presence of platelet aggregates in stored blood suggested that the emboli originated in banked blood.

EFFECT OF THE EMBOLUS ON THE LUNG

Blockage of a pulmonary artery by an embolus has a much less drastic effect on the lung tissue itself than does blockage of a systemic artery by an embolus. The stoppage of bloodflow through the pulmonary arteries, which are end-arteries and have no collateral pathways, is more complete than stoppage in a systemic artery; nevertheless, it is venous blood that is being halted, and the lung parenchyma receives most of its nourishment from the bronchial arteries. Therefore, a pulmonary embolism does not necessarily cause ischemia of the lung, as does blockage of a systemic artery in the area distal to the occlusion. Thus, a patient with a massive pulmonary embolus who dies within several hours has a radiographically normal and an anatomically non-infarcted lung; in the patient who survives, the lung distal to the embolus remains anatomically normal and recovers its function after final lysis of the clot. During the period of absence of pulmonary arterial flow, the lung is nourished by the bronchial circulation. Gorham[32] demonstrated in dogs that pulmonary infarction could not be produced unless the bronchial arteries were ligated prior to the pulmonary embolism.

Pulmonary Infarction

The terms "pulmonary infarction" and "pulmonary embolism" are not synonymous. A pulmonary infarct is an area of hemorrhagic necrosis produced by pulmonary artery occlusion, almost always by an embolus. Grossly, pulmonary infarcts are always red and always involve the pleural surface. On microscopic section early after development, the alveoli are "stuffed" with red cells and there is edema of the septums. The precise cause of the alveolar hemorrhage and the edema of the septums is not fully understood, but they appear to stem from increased capillary permeability that is either secondary to a change in pressure relationships between the systemic and pulmonary circulations within the capillaries or a result of damage to the capillary walls from the loss of whatever nourishment the pulmonary arterial flow had been providing.

The early stage when the alveoli are stuffed with red cells and there is edema of the septa is referred to by pathologists as "intra-alveolar hemorrhage." Hampton and Castleman[33] use the term "incomplete infarction" to describe this stage. Pathologically, it is not an "infarction" unless there is necrosis of the septa. If a patient with an early lesion such as this survives, clinically and radiologically he is considered to have had a "pulmonary infarct" that has healed. If he dies, the same lesion is not considered to be a true pulmonary infarction. This difference in terminology is one of the basic causes of the apparent discrepancies in the reported incidence of pulmonary infarction in man.

Pathologically, if the area of intra-alveolar hemorrhage develops necrosis of the septa, it is considered an infarct; such infarcts heal by organization and finally appear as a small fibrous streak. Rarely, the infarcted area proceeds to massive necrosis and cavitation. From autopsy studies, pathologists[11–15, 33] have concluded that infarcts occur in approximately 10 per cent of patients with pulmonary embolism. This estimate would undoubtedly shrink if it were possible to count all minor emboli that go unnoticed. However, even if we accept that 10 per cent of pathologically demonstrated pulmonary emboli produce infarction, this figure is in sharp contrast to the clinical experience. The dilemma is as follows: It has previously been generally accepted that 10 per cent of patients with pulmonary embolism have an infarction pathologically. Only pulmonary infarction can produce pleurisy and pleuritic pain. Clinically, however, pleuritic pain occurs in approximately 50 per cent of patients with pulmonary emboli proved by angiography.[34] Tenable explanations include the following: the possibility that the patient with intra-alveolar hemorrhage may develop pleuritic pain as noted above; the fact that approximately 90 per cent of patients with major or minor pulmonary embolism survive, leaving only 10 per cent of the diagnosable sample for postmortem analysis; and Coon's opinion[35] that most patients who die of pulmonary embolism have multiple separate embolic episodes and the frequency of infarction in any given patient is higher than the estimated 10 per cent (indeed, at the University of Michigan, it becomes 40 per cent, which approximates the clinical experience).

Infarction is not a complication of either massive or miliary microembolism; infarctions are observed following some major and minor pulmonary emboli. Usually they occur at the junction of one or more pleural surfaces, such as at the costophrenic angles, at the anterior and posterior lung margins near the mediastinum, or at the margin of the middle lobe. Like pulmonary emboli, they occur more often in the lower lobes and in the right more often than in the left. In Hampton and Castleman's series,[33] 74 per cent were found in the lower lobes: 43 per cent in the right and 31 per cent in the left. The remainder were distributed almost equally among the other three lobes.

Pulmonary Insufficiency Secondary to Microemboli

Embolization of platelet clumps and debris of white cells is a relatively new concept that may explain some instances of acute pulmonary insufficiency, pulmonary hypertension, and death in the patient with no angiographic evidence of embolism or the death of a patient from pulmonary insufficiency with a seemingly small clot in the lung demonstrated angiographically or at autopsy.

Eeles and Sevitt[18] distinguished two types of microthrombi: (1) arterial, which are found in the pulmonary vessels 0.25 to 1.0 mm in diameter, and (2) capillary-arteriolar, found mostly in vessels 20μ to 100μ in diameter. Arterial microthrombi are considered to be similar to clot found in the peripheral veins, whereas the arteriolar-capillary microthrombi appear to be platelets. In Hardaway's view,[36] during periods of hypoperfusion of the capillaries there is stagnation of the blood, a fall in pH on the venous side, diffuse intravascular coagulation, aggregation of erythrocytes and platelets, and the formation of small thromboemboli. Robb,[37, 38] using cinephotomicroscopic techniques, observed the bowel, mesentery, lung, and liver of rabbits and identified platelet aggregations that embolized. He noted that whenever the blood pressure dropped and bloodflow slowed, blood elements separated so that like adhered to like, i.e., red cells to red cells and platelets to platelets. He observed that this phenomenon occurred most commonly on the venous side. Moore et al.[26] suggested that such microemboli might possibly be a cause of postraumatic pulmonary insufficiency, although not a common one. Blaisdell et al.[39, 40] reported on a group of patients believed to have died of microembolic phenomena following aortic aneurysmal operations. In the laboratory they were able to reproduce the same phenomena in dogs by cross clamping the aorta for 3 hours.[41, 42] Furthermore, if one pulmonary artery was clamped before the aortic clamp was released, that lung remained normal while the opposite lung showed microemboli. Finally, drainage of the vena cava of these animals disclosed microaggregates in the blood. In 1973, reporting on a series of several hundred patients with respiratory insufficiency, Blaisdell[43] concluded that this represents a specific syndrome, best termed the *respiratory insufficiency syndrome*. Some of these patients also showed microemboli in the small pulmonary blood vessels when lung biopsy was carried out early.

> If the patient survives, in the first 18 hours following the clinical insult, the gross appearance of the lungs may be relatively unremarkable except for a few scattered areas of congestion and atelectasis in the dependent portions of the lower and middle lobes. Microscopic examination shows thromboemboli in small pulmonary blood vessels, pulmonary venous and capillary engorgement, atelectasis, and interstitial edema. Between 18 and 72 hours after the episode of shock, gross inspection reveals hemorrhagic consolidation of entire lobes associated with microscopic changes of severe pulmonary congestion, scattered thromboemboli, interstitial edema, peribronchial and perivascular hemorrhage, and intra-alveolar hemorrhage. After 72 hours, hyalin membranes can be seen, and bronchopneumonia is developing, which increases in severity, and which is the predominant lesion in patients who survive more than 5 days [43].

AFTERMATH OF PULMONARY EMBOLUS

Clinically, recovery from multiple small emboli or even multiple major emboli is the rule following anticoagulant therapy and conservative measures.

Most emboli are gradually lysed, resulting in a normal-appearing lung both on x ray and by anatomic study. If, however, a careful search is made for evidence of old emboli, pulmonary bands or webs or small plaques in the pulmonary tree are discovered. The completeness of the recovery demonstrated on clinical, pathologic, and radiologic examination has long convinced physicians that there must be some natural mechanism for dissolution of clot. The premise that an inherent lytic agent circulates in the bloodstream has given impetus to the use of enzymatic therapy with urokinase. It has been reported[44, 45] that some clot and pulmonary emboli disappear following urokinase therapy.

Infarcts likewise usually heal. In other parts of the body, an infarct is an area of ischemic necrosis, and the ultimate damage is greater than that occurring in the lung, where infarcts are of the hemorrhagic type and heal with minimal scar tissue.

PATHOLOGIC PHYSIOLOGY

The lung may be considered as a nonrenewable filter.[4] The very small pulmonary vessels have been described as peculiarly endowed with sphincter-like mechanisms, designed to catch all particulate matter.[46, 47] Knisely and Knisely called these sphincters "catch-traps."[48] Krahl[49, 51] stated that it would be difficult to visualize a mechanism more suited for the removal of thromboemboli or other circulating masses from the bloodstream than the lung. This filtering undoubtedly occurs throughout life and serves to protect organs, such as the brain, kidney, and heart, which have less ability to recuperate from embolic particulate matter. In this regard, the action of the lung may be analogous to the strainer-like function of gills in fish.

The normal lung has enormous reserve capacity, a fact confirmed by the insignificant effect produced on the pulmonary artery pressure by doubling or tripling the cardiac output.[52] It has long been known[52–54] that occlusion of one pulmonary artery causes no significant rise in pulmonary artery pressure, the opposite lung merely opening up its available unperfused areas and accepting the doubled amount of flow with no increase in resistance. It is estimated that the pulmonary circulation must be constricted or reduced more than 60 per cent before a rise in pulmonary artery pressure can be recorded.[55-58] It has been also estimated that 70 to 80 per cent of the pulmonary circulation must be obstructed before signs of severe pulmonary hypertension and shock become apparent in the patient.[59] Contrariwise, it can be generally assumed that the patient who is cyanotic and severely dyspneic following pulmonary embolism has an obstruction of at least 65 per cent of normal pulmonary blood-flow.[59] When obstruction reaches approximately 85 per cent, survival is unlikely.

The status of the lung at the time of embolic lodgment is vital to the outcome. The bronchial circulation of the normal lung is so efficient that when the status of the heart is also normal, many authorities have considered it impossible to infarct the normal lung with a pulmonary embolus. At times, however, this has been known to occur.[60] In the autopsy reports of our hospital one such instance has been encountered. However, in a patient who is severely emphysematous or who has congestive heart failure, a small embolus may indeed prove fatal. A current clinical truism advises the physician to suspect pulmonary embolism when a previously controlled cardiac patient slips in and out of congestive failure.

Mechanism of Death

MASSIVE PULMONARY EMBOLI

Massive pulmonary embolus can cause complete obstruction with immediate death. Churchill[61] has given a classic account of the sequence of events:

> A large thrombus that completely blocks the outflow from the right heart will cause immediate but not instantaneous death from complete cessation of the circulation. The left ventricle continues for a moment to discharge blood that is already present in the pulmonary circuit and then its output abruptly ceases. There is a loss of consciousness due to cerebral anaemia and after a few asphyxial gasps, the respiratory center fails completely. The lack of coronary blood supply resulting from the fall of pressure in the aorta increases the dilatation of the right heart already precipitated by the obstruction of the outflow of blood.

When a patient lives a few minutes or perhaps an hour or two following massive pulmonary embolism, it can be concluded that the occlusion is not total. The increased pressure may force the embolus more distally, or in an enlarged pulmonary artery, some blood circumvents the embolus and reaches the alveoli to maintain life. During this time the following dynamic changes can be identified:[61, 62] A rise in pulmonary artery pressure is transferred immediately as a rise in pressure of the right ventricle with or without right ventricular failure, depending on the degree of resistance of the flow of blood into the pulmonary tree. This is immediately reflected by a rise in peripheral venous pressure, as evidenced by distention of the neck veins and enlargement of the liver. A deficient flow of blood from the lungs to the left ventricle results in a fall in blood pressure, cerebral ischemia, and, depending on the degree, possible coronary artery insufficiency.

MAJOR AND MINOR PULMONARY EMBOLI

The primary cause of death in pulmonary embolism is mechanical blockage of the pulmonary arterial tree, causing hypoxemia. This is easy to visualize in the case of a massive pulmonary embolus blocking the pulmonary artery, a major clot blocking an entire lobe in a patient with poor pulmonary or cardiac reserve, several major emboli in a patient with normal lungs ,or multiple minor emboli occurring repeatedly and blocking off more and more of the pulmonary arterial tree. The difficulty is to explain the cause of death in a patient with mechanical blockage of a major pulmonary artery or of a few medium-sized pulmonary arteries when at autopsy the total amount of blockage appears to be minimal or moderate, not enough to explain death by purely mechanical blockage. Clinicians were led to postulate the involvement of a reflex spasm of the pulmonary arterioles and bronchioles to explain this course of events. This is reminiscent of the invocation of reflex spasm to explain some of the signs, symptoms, and complications of peripheral arterial embolism, venous thrombosis of the lower extremity, the postphlebitic syndrome, cardiac and intestinal angina, and even certain strokes. In recent years, other possibilities have become apparent that seem to provide a more likely explanation of this syndrome than does vasoconstriction.

Humoral Substances

Comroe et al. in 1953[63] suggested that serotonin (5-hydroxytryptamine) might be instrumental in producing some of the cardiac and pulmonary changes that follow pulmonary embolism. An embolus lodged in the lung may be covered with massive numbers of platelets which either become attached to the clot as it passes up the venous tree or accumulate by accretion as blood in the pulmonary tree flows by a partially occluding clot. The breakdown of these platelets causes the release of many substances, including serotonin. Furthermore, since a fresh thrombus probably would cause a much greater adherence of platelets than one that is partially organized, another variable would be introduced. This might explain some of the great variances that occur in the response of the lung to pulmonary embolism. Thomas and co-workers[64] found evidence of humoral influences that could account for such bronchoconstriction and vasoconstriction after experimental lung embolism by microthrombi and large thrombi secondary to the release of serotonin and other active amines from platelets. It is plausible that microemboli to the lungs after injury, burns, and other agents could produce spasm of bronchi and lung vessels.[65, 66, 67] This would not be inconsistent with bronchospasm after extensive burning, especially in children, and with other ventilation-perfusion anomalies in the lungs of trauma patients. In a carefully controlled study, Puckett et al.[68] found that the alterations in the pulmonary circulation and airways that accompany pulmonary embolism do not depend on the presence of platelets or serotonin. Their study was conducted on dogs, which, as they point out, are more susceptible to the effect of serotonin than is man and which have more serotonin in their platelets than does man.

Another possibility is that a patient may have one minor embolus plus simultaneous microemboli, and the additive blocking of the pulmonary circulation causes death. The microemboli may not have been recognized in the pathologic specimen in the past, so that the patient seemingly died of a small pulmonary embolus.

CLINICAL DIAGNOSIS OF PULMONARY EMBOLISM

The accuracy of the clinical diagnosis of pulmonary embolism is usually considered to be 50 per cent.[9, 22, 69-73] Indeed, as late as 1972, Modan et al.[23] in a study of 2107 consecutive patients on

whom autopsy was performed at a major medical center found that the false-negative diagnosis of pulmonary embolism wase 66.6 per cent and the false-positive diagnosis was 61.9 per cent. In attempting to ferret out the clinical clues for diagnosis of this condition, the physician is faced with the fact that many small pulmonary emboli produce no symptoms or signs whatever; that furthermore, when emboli are proved by angiography, the correlation between the degree of pulmonary artery obstruction and the clinical signs and symptoms is far from exact.[34] The more frequent use of pulmonary scans and angiography offers hope of increasing the diagnostic accuracy, which in turn will permit analysis of the symptoms and signs to a greater degree than before. The recently completed urokinase pulmonary embolism trial and national cooperative study[34] of patients with proved massive and submassive pulmonary embolism has provided abundant data on the correlation of clinical findings in patients with proven pulmonary emboli. Since this study was prospective in nature and carefully controlled, its findings can be relied upon, and it is used freely in the forthcoming discussion.

Predisposing Factors

As with all potentially obscure diseases pulmonary embolism is most readily diagnosed if the physician maintains a high interest in and awareness of this kind of lesion and the factors that predispose to its development. The underlying etiologic factors of thrombophlebitis and pulmonary embolism, however, are so numerous that it is best to subdivide them into general categories. Virchow's triad affords a starting point. *Injury to a vein wall,* his first factor, however, is moved to third place because the clot that forms on an injured vein is usually adherent. Although some thrombus may form distal to the firm clot, in our experience this type of thrombophlebitis rarely causes pulmonary embolism. *Low venous flow states,* the third of Virchow's factors, is believed to be the primary cause, while *abnormalities of the blood* retains the second place in importance in bringing about pulmonary embolism. A summary of predisposing factors is presented in Table 8-2. A common cause of low venous flow states is inactivity following trauma (Table 8-3).

Symptoms

The absence of symptoms in a patient with multiple minor or even major pulmonary emboli may strike the physician as incredible until he is convinced by repeated interrogation of intelligent patients whose multiple emboli have been proved by pulmonary scanning and angiography. The lack of pain is due to the fact that the lung tissue contains no sensory nerves, and therefore, unless there is pleural involvement or massive pulmonary artery distention, no pain is experienced.

When present, symptoms vary in intensity and degree in correspondence with the tremendous variations that exist in the size and the number of pulmonary emboli involved in thromboembolic

TABLE 8-2. Factors That Predispose to Pulmonary Embolism

Anything that causes a decrease in rate of venous blood-flow.
   A decrease in effectiveness of the cardiac pump by any cardiac disease, particularly cardiac failure
   Any decrease in the effectiveness of the muscular pump, e.g., immobility, casting, traction, splinting, paralysis
   Any venous obstruction, such as caused by an old thrombus or extraluminal compression
   Venous dilatation due to varicose veins; decrease in tone secondary to warmth followed by inactivity
   Gravitational force, prolonged pendency without muscular activity
   Increased blood viscosity secondary to dehydration, polycythemia vera, erythrocytosis, or decrease in velocity of bloodflow
Any increase in tendency of blood to clot
   Venous thrombosis
   Increased number and/or adhesiveness of platelets; polycythemia vera; visceral neoplasia; postpartum state, particularly over age 35; contraceptive pill
General factors
   General and still not clearly defined factors, such as a history of pulmonary embolism; history of deep venous thrombosis; advancing age; obesity; trauma by violence or surgical procedures, particularly of pelvis and lower extremity
Injury to a vein wall
   Compression
   Contusion
   Laceration
   Severance
   Stretching
   Chemical irritation

episodes. Were it not for overlapping of symptoms and signs, it might be more practical to approach the subject as if five different disease entities were being discussed, viz., massive embolism, major embolism, minor embolism, military embolism, and microembolism.

DYSPNEA

Dyspnea (Table 8-4) is the most frequent symptom. In acute cor pulmonale, it is universally present. It may be found only by carefully questioning a patient with minor emboli. Dyspnea was present in all of Sasahara's patients, and in his series,[71] the larger the embolus, the more certain the dyspnea. It was present in 80 per cent of all patients in the national cooperative study with massive and submassive pulmonary emboli.[34] The fact that it is absent in some patients and that its presence did not correlate well with the degree of radiologic and hemodynamic abnormalities noted during the national cooperative study serve to underscore the fact that the degree of dyspnea is related not only to the amount of remaining functioning pulmonary tissue but also to the degree of exertion and to the cardiac status. It is not uncommon to encounter patients lying quietly in bed who deny the presence of dyspnea but become markedly dyspneic simply by rolling over in bed.

PAIN

Pain is absent in patients with small pulmonary emboli. When pain occurs, it falls into three broad

TABLE 8-3. Day of Onset of Fatal Embolism: A Clinico-Necropsy Analysis of 87 Fatal Cases

DAYS FROM INJURY TO PULMONARY EMBOLISM	PATIENTS WITH FATAL EMBOLISM
0–4	4
5–7	14
8–11	9
12–14	13
15–21	16
22–28	11
29–42	9
57–70	4
70	3
Not datable	4
Total	87

From Sevitt, S. *Am J Med 33:*705, 1962.

categories: vague chest discomfort of sudden onset, pleuritic pain, and severe chest pain similar to that observed in myocardial infarction. When vague chest discomfort is followed by dyspnea or pleuritic pain, it is highly suggestive of pulmonary embolism.

Gorham[32] in a large autopsy study of patients with massive pulmonary embolism found that 20 per cent experienced the severe type of chest pain but 80 per cent complained of neither substernal nor pleural pain before suddenly dying in dyspnea and shock. The mechanism of such pain is uncertain. Churchill[61] was of the opinion that it was secondary to tremendous distention of the pulmonary artery caused by the massive pulmonary embolus. He did not exclude the now-popular possibility that the pain might be caused by coronary artery insufficiency due to complete arrest of blood flowing into the left auricle and ventricle.

Gorham[32] attributed the pain to a remarkably dilated pulmonary artery rubbing against the pericardium.

Pleuritic pain indicates involvement of the parietal pleura, since the visceral pleura is devoid of nerve endings. Many physicians consider pleuritic pain to be caused by rubbing of one pleural surface against the other. In 1926 Bray[74] offered some pertinent comments in regard to this. While it is true that the pain occurs on deep inspiration when the pleura are moving against each other, nevertheless the pain continues while the breath is held and the pleura are no longer rubbing against each other. Despite similar motion in each maneuver, the pain is felt on inspiration and not on expiration. Strapping the chest relieves the pain despite the continued movement of the diaphragm as observed by fluoroscopy, with its consequent increased move-

TABLE 8-4. Frequency of Symptoms and Physical Signs by Angiographic Massiveness of Pulmonary Embolism

	PREVALENCE (%)		
	ALL PATIENTS (N = 160)	MASSIVENESS OF PULMONARY EMBOLISM	
		MASSIVE (N = 90)	SUBMASSIVE (N = 70)
Symptoms			
Dyspnea	81	79	83
Pleuritic pain	72	62	84†
Apprehension	59	61	56
Cough	54	50	60
Hemoptysis	34	27	44
Sweats	26	27	24
Syncope	14	22*	4
Signs			
Rales	53	50	57
Elevated S_2P	53	60*	44
Thrombophlebitis	33	42	21
S_3, S_4 gallop	34	47*	17
Diaphoresis	34	41	24
Edema	23	24	21
Murmur	23	20	7
Cyanosis	18	28*	6

* Significant positive association with massive pulmonary embolism (CR ≅ 3.0).
† Significant positive association with submassive pulmonary embolism (CR ≅ 3.0).
From Sasahara et al. *The Urokinase Pulmonary Embolism Trial: A National Cooperative Study.* New York, Amer. Heart Assoc., also Supplement II to Circulation Vols. 47–48, 1973. By permission of The American Heart Association, Inc.

ment of the pleural surfaces against each other. From these observations, Bray concluded that the pain of pleurisy was not due to rubbing of the pleural surfaces together but rather to tension on the nerve endings in the parietal pleura attached to the intercostal muscles. Pleuritic pain occurred in 72 per cent of all patients in the national cooperative study,[34] the incidence with massive embolism being 62 per cent and with submassive embolism 84 per cent. The higher incidence in patients with submassive emboli is believed to be due to the more frequent involvement of the pleural surfaces with smaller emboli. Dalen[75] also found a high incidence of pleural pain. He reported[58, 60] that dyspnea and pleuritic pain were the two most common symptoms, one or the other occurring in 94 of 100 patients with angiographically proved pulmonary embolism. The discrepancy between clinical and pathologic studies is best explained by differing definitions, as noted earlier. An additional and additive explanation is that autopsy studies indicate that isolated single emboli are rare. Most patients have multiple emboli, so that the patient with the massive embolus may at the same time have many peripheral, smaller emboli, resulting in infarction and pain.

APPREHENSION

It has long been a clinical anecdote that a patient is apt to become apprehensive and to have a recognition of impending danger prior to sustaining a fatal massive pulmonary embolism. This premonition of doom has been encountered by many clinicians; the regularity with which it is fulfilled causes one to wonder if some occult yet definite sign is being overlooked. In the recent national cooperative study,[34] apprehension was present in 59 per cent of patients with proved massive pulmonary embolism (Table 8-4).

OTHER SYMPTOMS

Cough occurred in 54 per cent of the patients; hemoptysis in 34 per cent; sweats in 26 per cent; and syncope in 14 per cent (Table 8-4). The incidence of syncope differs significantly in patients with massive emboli and in those with submassive emboli, which is not unexpected.

Signs

TACHYPNEA

Dalen[75] pointed out that the respiratory rate is the most important single physical finding. In the past the true significance of this was not generally recognized, and little attention was paid to it. Respiratory rates, accurately recorded by nurses and other paramedical personnel, are indeed a useful tool for the early diagnosis of pulmonary embolism.

OTHER SIGNS

No other sign occurrs with sufficient frequency (Table 8-4) to be of great diagnostic importance. But it is to be noted that three signs, viz., elevated S_2P, cyanosis and S_3, S_4 gallop, were present more often in patients with massive embolism than with submassive embolism. The typical picture of a patient gasping for breath and clutching his chest, with shock, central cyanosis, and distended neck veins, is only occasionally seen; however, when seen, it is highly suggestive of massive pulmonary embolism.

WHEEZING

When present on one side of the chest, wheezing is suggestive of pulmonary embolism; its response to heparin[67] is confirmatory evidence of the diagnosis.

Other physical signs include pleural friction rub, fine rales, and splinting of the chest.

LABORATORY TESTS

The most helpful laboratory tests are studies of the blood gases.[34, 45] The arterial oxygen (pO_2) was reduced in the majority of patients; however, it was above 80 mm Hg in 12 per cent of the patients. In massive pulmonary embolism, the pO_2 was less than 70 per cent in 56 patients, between 71 and 80 mm Hg in 11 patients, between 81 and 90 mm Hg in 2 patients, and above 91 mm Hg in 1 patient.

Caution must be taken in interpreting oxygen tension for diagnostic purposes. Arterial samples should be obtained under anerobic conditions and must be tightly capped and analyzed quickly in an electrode that has been just previously calibrated. Unless such precautions are observed, the measurements could be of questionable value.

Fibrinogen Split Products Tests

A high level of fibrinogen split products indicates that fibrin is being lysed somewhere in the body. Its use as a diagnostic test for thrombophlebitis and pulmonary embolism is promising but not yet established.

Serology

In the urokinase pulmonary embolism trial,[34, 45] it was demonstrated that the changes in the serum glutamic oxaloacetic transaminase (SGOT) and serum lactate dehydrogenase (LDH) with or without serum bilirubin were not significant.

ECG

ECG changes in pulmonary embolic disease are the changes produced by pulmonary hypertension. Therefore, unless approximately 65 per cent of the pulmonary vasculature is blocked, no ECG changes are recorded. In massive pulmonary embolism obstructing the pulmonary arteries, typical ECG changes are observed; they may also be seen in microembolism when an elevated pulmonary arterial pressure is present.[76]

It has been estimated that not more than 10 to 20 per cent of patients who subsequently are found to have pulmonary embolism develop ECG changes. This figure is probably high, as it is becoming increasingly evident that the incidence of pulmonary embolism is greater than previously suspected and that the great majority of emboli are small and produce no symptoms or signs. In reality, the percentage of patients with pulmonary emboli is unknown, since at least half of the cases are undiagnosed; also it cannot even be estimated how many small pulmonary emboli occur that are never symptomatic. Some of the changes secondary to lodgment of emboli are so evanescent[76] that clearing occurs before the first ECG can be taken.

Nevertheless, the importance of the ECG must not be understressed. In acute cardiopulmonary emergency, the differential diagnosis is between pulmonary embolism and myocardial infarction, so that while the evidence of embolism is not clear-cut, the ECG is still important in indicating the presence of myocardial infarction.

P WAVES

Fischer[77] has provided a succinct analysis of the ECG changes in pulmonary embolism.

There are no diagnostic characteristics found in the electrocardiogram. The most fortuitous circumstance in which the ECG may be helpful is when there is a pre-embolism ECG with which to compare the current one when embolus is suspected.

The ECG abnormalities that develop are the result of one or a combination of the several pathophysiologic events that may take place in the patient, depending on the percentage of the pulmonary vasular bed that is obstructed.

The most frequent ECG changes are an increase in heart rate and a shift of the electrical axis toward the right and anterior. The mean QRS vector commonly and transiently shifts to point 80° to 110° on the frontal plane (i.e. inferiorly). The QRS complex in the V-leads becomes more diphasic.

If the increased pressure load on the right ventricle is more severe, ST-T changes also occur due to systolic overload. Myocardial ischemia may also be present to account for T-wave abnormalities. The T vector rotatoes progressively more leftward and posterior producing inversions in leads III, AVF, and V_3 through V_3. ST vector changes, if due to sub-endocardial ischemia, point rightward and anteriorly. If the systolic pressure in the right ventricle increases greatly, this vector may rotate with the T vector.

P-wave changes due to right atrial pressure and volume increases are common, causing "P-pulmonale" (tall P-waves in leads II, III, and AVF). Atrial arrhythmias are also common, especially atrial fibrillation and flutter.

Since all of these changes may be subtle as well as temporary, it is to be reemphasized that a **pre-surgical** or pre-embolism ECG for comparison can be most helpful.

The ECGs of patients in the national cooperative study of massive and submassive pulmonary embolism,[34] while frequently abnormal (87 per cent), showed many changes that were nonspecific, the most prominent being T wave inversions in 40 per cent. Of 77 patients with massive emboli whose ECGs were analyzed, 31 per cent showed a change of acute cor pulmonale.[34]

RADIOLOGIC DIAGNOSIS

Chest Film

PULMONARY EMBOLISM

There is no pathognomonic radiologic sign of pulmonary embolism. The following are some suggestive signs.[78]

OLIGEMIA. This is particularly suggestive if one lung appears oligemic and the other shows increased markings (pleonemia). In most instances, the radiologist cannot detect oligemia unless the patient has a prior film for comparison. If different techniques (posteroanterior vs. portable film) are used in the two studies, no comparison can be made.

ENLARGED PULMONARY ARTERY. Obviously, such increase can only be detected from study of successive films.

SMALL PLEURAL EFFUSIONS. While not specific for pulmonary embolism, small pleural effusions with oligemia are suggestive.

PULMONARY INFARCTION

There are no absolute specific roentgen patterns of pulmonary infarction. The following are features that should be looked for.[79]

DISTRIBUTION AND DENSITY OF SHADOWS. Shadows should be segmental in character and homogeneously dense.

SITE OF DENSITY. The base of the right lower lobe, frequently in the costophrenic sinus, is the commonest site of infarction. In the early stages, increasing density is apt to be ill-defined. Like the majority of pneumonias, infarction involves the visceral pleural surface.

INTERVAL BETWEEN LODGMENT OF THE EMBOLUS AND RADIOLOGIC DETECTION. Increase in density may be observed, at the earliest, at 10 to 12 hours or, at the latest, at 1 week after the occlusion.

The so-called classic configuration of an infarction as a truncated cone is uncommon. Most infarctions are completely reversible. The disappearance may take from 5 days to 5 weeks; the average is 1 to 3 weeks. Cavitation seldom occurs. Line shadows probably constitute one of the most frequent manifestations of embolism and infarction. "Plate-like" atelectasis consists of linear areas of increased density, almost always in the lung bases, 1 to 3 cm above the hemidiaphragm. Pleural effusion is common.[79]

COR PULMONALE

Again, there is no pathognomonic sign, but certain signs are suggestive.[78]

OLIGEMIA. The lung may appear to be totally oligemic, i.e., vascular markings have disappeared. A prior film is necessary for comparison.

HILAR ARTERIES. A very marked increase in the size of the hilar arteries may be noted.

RADIOISOTOPE SCANNING

Radioisotope scanning makes possible the measurement of bloodflow to various regions of the lungs.[79, 80] In the absence of right-to-left shunting of blood, regional pulmonary bloodflow measured in this way represents the blood provided by the pulmonary artery, although in certain patients with congenital heart disease the bronchial circulation may be involved as well.

Macroaggregated human serum albumin, labeled earlier with I^{131} and now with technetium-99m, is injected intravenously and assumed to mix uniformly before reaching the pulmonary artery.[80, 81] Because of their size, the macroaggregates become lodged in the pulmonary arterioles and capillaries, where their concentration is determined by radioisotope scanning techniques. The concentration of the radioactivity in various regions of the lungs is directly related to pulmonary bloodflow. The albumin aggregates are metabolized after phagocytosis, and their metabolic products are excreted in the urine.[81]

Lung scanning in the diagnosis of pulmonary embolism is easy, safe, and effective. A positive scan in the presence of a normal chest x ray is highly suggestive of pulmonary embolism, particularly if there is increased radiolucency on chest x ray. Similarly, a negative scan rules out pulmonary embolism. On the other hand, if the avascular areas correspond to opacities on chest x rays, one cannot distinguish between primary vascular disease and secondary involvement of the pulmonary vasculature. Pneumonia, atelectasis, neoplasia, abscesses, sarcoidosis, and, particularly, lung cysts and bullae may appear as areas of increased radiolucency in a manner similar to pulmonary emboli.[81] In the words of a Cincinnati radiologist,[82] "the most classical picture of positive pulmonary embolism by lung scan is produced by bronchial asthma; it looks more like a pulmonary embolism than an embolus does itself."

PULMONARY ANGIOGRAPHY

Pulmonary angiography provides the final confirmation of pulmonary embolism in the living patient, and it should be more widely used.[83] Currently, the preferred method is to inject contrast material directly into the pulmonary artery by a catheter through the antecubital vein. If the examination is performed some days after the incident, some of the contrast medium may slowly pass around the obstruction, and delayed opacification of the vessels occurs beyond the embolus. This delay may be due to clot retraction or to partial lysis of the clot.[83]

With rapid cassette changers, pictures can be taken continuously, and the aorta and its branches can be shown. If carried out immediately, pulmonary angiography is an almost certain method of diagnosing pulmonary embolism. If performed after 48 hours, however, the possibility always exists that the embolus may have dissolved and will not be visualized.[84]

SUMMARY

A history of sudden onset of chest pain, particularly pleuritic pain, with cough and hemoptysis in a patient with a known predisposition to thromboembolic disease should make pulmonary embolism a working diagnosis until proved erroneous. Regrettably, this clear-cut syndrome is not common, and the physician must continually suspect pulmonary embolism and order scans and simultaneous chest x ray as a matter of habit for patients with such a tentative diagnosis. Should any vestige of doubt remain, a pulmonary angiogram should be obtained.

MANAGEMENT OF PATIENTS WITH PULMONARY EMBOLISM

Properly speaking, the only "treatment" of pulmonary embolism is enzymatic therapy,[34] which at present has not attained complete development, and pulmonary embolectomy, which is rarely indicated. All other forms of so-called therapy are in reality (1) prophylaxis directed against lodgment of new emboli, either by anticoagulant agents or by venous interruption, or (2) temporary measures in support of the cardiorespiratory system while waiting for the normal bodily processes to dissolve the clot and restore pulmonary function to normal. It is our belief that one of the functions of the normal lung is to lyse debris and small clots delivered to it by the venous return. Therefore, it is not surprising that many emboli, both small and large, undergo spontaneous resolution. A review of pathologic studies[85] documents the existence of new and old pulmonary emboli in patients in whom this diagnosis had been totally unsuspected. Similarly, in clinical practice patients are encountered who have an almost certain history of pulmonary embolism following an illness, injury, or operation and who have made a complete recovery without treatment and, indeed, without the diagnosis of pulmonary embolism ever having been considered. When managing patients with pulmonary embolism, it is our policy to allay their fears by assuring them that the clot in their lungs will dissolve and their lungs completely restored to normal and that treatment, whether anticoagulants or venous interruption, is entirely prophylactic in nature, i.e., intended to prevent new and possibly larger emboli from lodging in the lungs. The fact that physicians and surgeons speak confidently of directing their "therapy" only to prophylaxis reflects their conviction that the lung will recover spontaneously under ordinary conditions. In follow-up studies of their patients with massive pulmonary embolism, Dalen and associates found only 12 per cent with unresolved embolism when examined at an average of 29 months after the embolic episode.[84]

CLASSIFICATION OF PULMONARY EMBOLI

Rational management of patients with pulmonary embolism is based on categorization of the various degrees of severity of the disease.

Category I

This is the absence of severe dyspnea. The term "minor" is to be abhorred in reference to such a potentially lethal disease. For this reason, the first category simply includes patients with diagnosable pulmonary embolism.

Category II

This is the presence of severe dyspnea: major embolism.

Category III

This is the presence of severe respiratory distress with sustained hypotension or shock: massive embolism. This definition follows the clinical syndrome described by Bryant et al.,[17] which is believed to be most appropriate. "Massive" refers to overwhelming clinical impact rather than to anatomic proportions as demonstrated by pulmonary arteriography. This interpretation is proper since the physiologic effects of pulmonary embolism are the result of many factors, including size and multiplicity of emboli, the state and size of the available pulmonary bed, and the cardiac reserve.

PROPHYLAXIS BY NONOPERATIVE MEASURES

Category I

In addition to general conservative measures (e.g., elevation of the foot of the bed and rubberized bandages to the extremities, as discussed in Chapter 5 under Prophylaxis), anticoagulant therapy is instituted, initially with heparin and subsequently with the prothrombin-depressant agents, which are then continued for approximately 3 months after discharge. (For a discussion of anticoagulation therapy, see Chapter 5.)

Category II

Management is identical to that for patients in Category I, except that it may be necessary to use oxygen therapy and, on occasion, positive-pressure ventilation.

PROPHYLAXIS BY SURGICAL MEASURES

There are two indications for venous interruption or venous blockade for patients in Categories I and II: (1) contraindications of anticoagulant agents and (2) repeated, multiple pulmonary emboli which are not amenable to the above therapy. (For a detailed discussion of surgical prophylaxis, see Chapter 6.)

FAILURES OF TREATMENT WITH ANTICOAGULANT AGENTS

Failures of treatment with heparin may be due to one of the following: (1) it may be contraindicated (see Chapter 5); (2) the prescribed dose may be inadequate; or (3) the heparin may be ineffective. Obviously, inadequate amounts of heparin will not prevent recurrence of pulmonary embolism. "Adequate" dose in our experience is 25,000 to 30,000 USP units a day; this may be revised upward or downward, according to the patient's response to whatever test is being used as a monitor. The patient with a large pulmonary embolism and extensive venous thrombosis may be resistant to heparin for several days; therefore, a large initial dose must be given. After several days of treatment, the dose is tapered off. Heparin therapy should be continued for at least 2 or 3 days after the prothrombin activity is within the therapeutic range. The prothrombin activity is also depressed by heparin therapy, and a slightly larger dose of prothrombin-depressant agent should be administered on the day that heparin is discontinued.

Recurrent and multiple pulmonary emboli occur at times in a patient who is receiving what are believed to be adequate doses of heparin and whose clotting time is significantly prolonged. This is particularly true of a patient with hidden malignancy. The precise incidence is difficult to estimate, since the recurrence of emboli causes one to question whether or not the dose has been adequate.

Nevertheless, particularly in the postoperative patient, heparin may be administered to the point of hemorrhage and yet multiple emboli keep recurring. In such refractory patients, interruption of the interior vena cava is most effective.

Category III

The management of patients with massive pulmonary embolism has been summarized by several authorities.[17, 60, 86] This catastrophe is far from rare: it has been estimated that on hospital wards, of 8 patients stricken with sudden, massive cardiopulmonary collapse, 1 is sustaining a massive pulmonary embolism.[6] A varying number, furthermore, will be dead within a few minutes, before resuscitative efforts can be made. In Gorham's autopsy series,[32] 44 per cent of patients with massive pulmonary embolism died within 15 minutes after onset of symptoms, and an additional 25 per cent survived only 2 hours. This grim percentage cannot be applied universally, as his population was limited to fatal cases. Donaldson et al.,[87] reviewing their experience at the Massachusetts General Hospital from 1943 to 1963, estimated that of 271 patients for whom the time factor could be ascertained, 25 per cent survived at least 1 hour, 22 per cent survived for 2 hours, and 17 per cent lived 6 or more hours. Turnier and associates[88] reported that 36 per cent of the patients died within an hour, 6 per cent lived 1 or 2 hours, and 58 per cent survived longer than 2 hours.

Management: Emergency Resuscitation

The nurse or paramedical aide who observes a patient *in extremis* immediately calls the emergency team by whatever method is used at that institution. At our hospital, an emergency number is dialed that interrupts and supersedes all other calls; the operator immediately turns up the volume of the public address system and announces three times, "Doctor Allcome!," giving the number of the floor where the catastrophe is occurring. All members of the house staff and all physicians within hearing proceed at once to the scene. Members of the anesthesiology and inhalation therapy departments also head that way, while all available nursing and paramedical personnel in the vicinity hurry with the emergency cart to the patient's bedside. After the first few moments, as the nature of the emergency becomes clearer, those whose services are not required leave, getting out of the way of essential personnel. A small group remains to continue resuscitative treatment.

The team captain is the resident who is on call that day; he may defer, however, to a senior resident or staff physician who may wish to assume care of a particular patient. Fortunately, the initial treatment is the same for massive pulmonary embolism and collapse from myocardial disease.

ADEQUATE VENTILATION AND CIRCULATION. An oxygen mask is applied and ventilation begun while a second member of the team listens to the heart. If no sounds are heard, cardiac massage is begun immediately; an attempt is made to maintain the cardiac rate at 50 to 60 beats per minute, allowing approximately 1 second for refilling of the heart after each compressive maneuver. If the patient's color remains good and he seems to be sufficiently aerated, the face mask is kept in place; otherwise, a member of the team who is experienced in inserting an endotracheal tube does so as rapidly as possible.

A member of the team inserts one or two intravenous catheters while someone else threads a central venous pressure line through the brachial-subclavian or jugular veins. Heparin, 15,000 USP units, is administered intravenously.

All customary vasopressors and pharmacologic agents useful in such a crisis are available on the emergency cart and are given on orders from the team captain, e.g., intracardiac epinephrine 0.5 mg; metaraminol; isoproterenol if arrhythmia is not present and the cardiac rate is not excessively rapid; sodium bicarbonate, 1 ampule every 6 to 8 minutes if the patient is in acute cardiac arrest.

While the above steps are being taken, ECG leads are applied. If the tracing indicates arrest or fibrillation, the patient is given electric shock treatment.

Cardiac massage in the event of massive pulmonary embolism serves a twofold purpose: it resuscitates the heart and it empties the right ventricle, which is greatly overdistended. It not only forces blood mechanically into the pulmonary tree around the clot but also may actually force clot out into the peripheral branches of the lung, thus permitting at least some of the proximal portions of the lung to be aerated.

ESTABLISHING THE DIAGNOSIS. While the above resuscitative measures are underway, the patient's chart is reviewed; the history helps clarify the diagnosis of myocardial infarction or pulmonary embolism or of some other condition causing cardiovascular collapse.

Heparin is believed to be of great value in treatment of pulmonary embolism and of no harm to the patient with myocardial infarction. If the patient survives the first crucial moments, heparin is continued at 4-hour intervals or by continuous drip, depending on clotting time response. The patient with massive pulmonary embolism, similar to the patient with massive venous thrombosis (see Chapter 2), frequently appears to be resistant to heparin, so that doses much larger than what is usually given may be required (in some instances, 10,000 to 15,000 USP units every 4 hours during the first 24 hours) in order to attain therapeutic levels. Gurewich et al.[89] surmise that heparin may provide more benefit than is to be expected from its anticoagulant effect by neutralizing serotonin or other similar chemical released from massive platelet accumulation on the fresh thrombus. Although Puckett et al.[68] have produced rather cogent evidence that serotonin is not implicated, we still recommend large doses of heparin. It is our clinical impression that something very beneficial happens in a patient with massive pulmonary embolism when a large dose of heparin is administered. The patient appears to breathe more easily almost at once and sometimes improves dramatically.

If the patient survives the first few moments of resuscitation, a urinary catheter is inserted. An arterial line is inserted, by means of which accurate blood pressure may be recorded and which makes it possible to obtain frequent samples of arterial blood for monitoring blood gases. Methylprednisolone, 30 mg/kg of body weight, may be given as recommended by Bryant et al.,[17] in whose experience it seems to have been of value.

PULMONARY ARTERIOGRAPHY. If the patient still survives, the team captain should pause and take stock of the overall situation. An accurate diagnosis becomes mandatory; for this, only a pulmonary arteriogram can establish the presence of massive pulmonary embolism with the certainty that would encourage the surgeon to schedule a pulmonary embolectomy. If no operation is under consideration, proof of the diagnosis is extremely worthwhile before the patient is submitted to high doses of heparin therapy and prolonged treatment with anticoagulant agents.

Pulmonary angiography is not yet universally accepted[90] as the supreme diagnostic technique. Some physicians prefer to obtain a lung scan and chest film at this time. If the lung scan is negative, it eliminates the possibility of massive pulmonary embolism; if the scan is positive and a chest film is negative, the diagnosis is greatly supported. However, it would not establish the diagnosis with such certainty that the surgeon would plan embolectomy, utterly confident of finding massive clot in the lung. Pulmonary arteriography, over and above its peerless accuracy, allows one to obtain pressures of vital importance: the wedge pressure, the pulmonary arterial pressure, and the pressure in the right ventricle and auricle.[91]

Postresuscitation Management

Once the diagnosis of massive pulmonary embolism has been established, the patient can be moved either to the recovery room or to the intensive care unit, where he is carefully monitored. As Bryant[17] has emphasized, the response to medical treatment after initial resuscitation may be slow. Systolic blood pressure may persist at low levels of 70 to 80 mm Hg for several hours. The *trend of the change* in the patient's condition is what matters.

Fibrinolytic Treatment

If the blood pressure is stable or gradually improving, conservative measures may be continued. At this point in the management of the patient, urokinase, once a readily available supply is assured, is indicated.[34] (See Chapter 5, section on fibrinolytic therapy.)

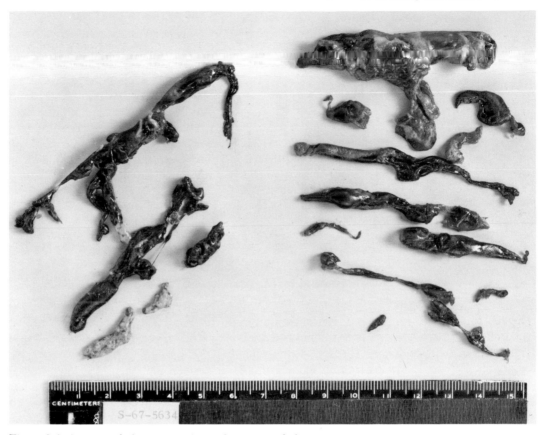

Figure 8-4. Amount of clot extracted at pulmonary embolectomy.

SURGICAL PROPHYLAXIS

If the patient continues to respond and if his blood pressure becomes stable, thought should be given to prophylaxis against recurrent embolization. The inferior vena cava should be ligated or barricaded by placement of an intraluminal filter (see Chapter 6). A subsequent embolus lodging in a lung that is already embarrassed to such a degree would most probably prove fatal.

Surgical Treatment

If the patient's blood pressure gradually falls, particularly if the venous pressure is rising at the same time, preparations should be made for immediate pulmonary embolectomy (Fig. 8-4).

LENGTH OF ANTICOAGULANT THERAPY

The question of how long administration of anti coagulant drugs should be continued remains prob-lematic. It is our policy to continue heparin until the prothrombin time is within therapeutic range for at least 3 days; heparin therapy is never curtailed before 5 to 7 days in any patient.

Long-Term Anticoagulant Therapy as Prophylaxis

Anticoagulant therapy is continued for 3 months in patients who have sustained one episode of pulmonary embolism and for 6 months in those with two bouts. If the patient has had more than two episodes, anticoagulant therapy is continued indefinitely (see Chapter 5).

CONTRAINDICATIONS

The high incidence of bleeding secondary to heparin therapy in patients mentioned in the national cooperative study of massive and submassive pulmonary embolism,[34, 45] viz., 27 per cent, is surprising. For a discussion of patients who should routinely be excluded from anticoagulant therapy, see Chapter 5.

Recurrent Pulmonary Embolism

IN PATIENTS WHILE ON ANTICOAGULANT AGENTS

The recurrence rate of pulmonary embolism was unexpectedly high in 78 patients treated with heparin, viz., 18 (23 per cent).[34,45] In this group, the recurrent embolism was diagnosed by clinical evidence in 6 patients, by pulmonary scan in 5, and by both clinical and radiologic evidence in 7.

IN PATIENTS TREATED WITH UROKINASE

Fourteen (17 per cent) of 82 patients in the national cooperative study of massive and submassive pulmonary embolism[34,45] treated with urokinase were considered to have recurrent pulmonary embolism: 4 by clinical evidence, 5 by scan, and 5 by both scan and clinical findings.

In most clinics, recurrence of pulmonary embolism in a patient who is on adequate anticoagulation therapy constitutes an indication for inferior vena caval interruption.

PULMONARY EMBOLECTOMY
Ernest H. Meese

The first attempt to remove massive emboli from the pulmonary artery was in 1908 by Friedrich Trendelenburg, professor of surgery at the University of Leipzig.[92] He performed embolectomy first in the laboratory on a calf and then clinically on 3 patients. In each case the procedure ended fatally; the patient who lived longest lived 37 hours and died of hemorrhage from an internal mammary artery. However, he did demonstrate the feasibility of the procedure. Kirschner,[93] a pupil of Trendelenburg, in 1924 was the first to perform a successful pulmonary embolectomy; the patient was a long-term survivor following the procedure. However, by the 1930s a review of more than 300 attempted embolectomies showed only 7 successes.[94] The reason that the failures were so numerous can be readily understood from Churchill's[61,62] description of his own attempted pulmonary embolectomies as more of an "immediate postmortem examination than a surgical operation." A patient was observed in the operating room until ready to gasp his last breath; when the heart stopped, operation was performed! The first successful pulmonary embolectomy in the United States was performed by Warren[95] at the Peter Bent Brigham Hospital without the customary observation period and without cardiopulmonary bypass. Vossschulte[96] in 1965 reported a series of 43 Trendelenburg procedures performed at his clinic in Germany between 1957 and 1963. While 13 patients survived the operation, only 7 were long-term survivors, indicating the high mortality associated with this procedure when extracorporeal circulation is not used.

The first successful management of massive pulmonary embolism by open operation with temporary occlusion of the circulation and hypothermia was performed by Allison et al.[97] at Oxford University in 1960.

In 1961 Sharp[98] first used extracorporeal circulation in pulmonary embolectomy. This is considered the ideal method for the performance of pulmonary embolectomy because it allows support of the circulation and permits the operation to be done with deliberation. A large number of patients have undergone this procedure with successful results; when indicated, this technique is the most satisfactory surgical method available for massive pulmonary embolism.[87,99–141]

Some new procedures have recently been reported which seem to have merit. Rothman and Frater[142–144] have described a procedure for removing pulmonary emboli from both lungs through a single incision in the left pulmonary artery without cardiopulmonary bypass. This procedure is designed for use when no extracorporeal circulation was available or when the patient was deteriorating too rapidly for cardiopulmonary bypass to be instituted. It is not meant to supplant embolectomy with extracorporeal circulation.

Another promising development is transvenous pulmonary embolectomy by catheter device. This has been reported with and without cardiopulmonary bypass but does not require thoracotomy in the moribund patient with massive pulmonary embolism.[145-147]

Two forms of massive pulmonary embolism must be considered. Acute embolism has received increasing attention as improved methods of diagnosis have been developed along with improved techniques for accomplishing emergency pulmonary embolectomy or treating the acute condition medically. The diagnosis and treatment of chronic massive pulmonary arterial thromboembolism has aroused less enthusiasm. This disparity in interest is undoubtedly related to the less dramatic clinical picture of chronic thromboembolism, the ease with which it masquerades as or is masked by diverse cardiopulmonary disorders, and the concept that it is not amenable to surgical correction. Chronic pulmonary embolism and hypertension are thought to be more common than is generally recognized, and it is now feasible to establish an accurate preoperative diagnosis and to consider a surgical approach in management.

Carroll in 1950 reported[148] the first patient in whom a diagnosis of chronic occlusion of a pulmonary artery was made before death. In 1956 Hollister and Cull[149] first suggested the operative removal of thromboembolic material from a chronically occluded pulmonary artery. Since then, there have been several direct attempts to restore patency in a pulmonary artery chronically occluded by an embolus, with varying degrees of success in restoring bloodflow to all or part of the involved lung.[150-159]

ACUTE MASSIVE PULMONARY EMBOLISM

Surgical Indications for Embolectomy

Following a flurry of enthusiasm over pulmonary embolectomy in the early and mid 1960s, there has been increasing appreciation of the natural history of pulmonary embolism and its characteristic tendency for spontaneous lysis. This lytic process is augmented by the administration of anticoagulants and thrombolytic agents and has brought about a definite reduction in the number of patients considered as appropriate candidates for embolectomy.[160-166]

How many and what type of patients might be considered candidates for pulmonary embolectomy? Only 25 per cent of patients with massive pulmonary embolism survive for 1 hour, and approximately 22 per cent survive for 2 hours.[87] Of this group, a major proportion have incurable neoplasms or irreversible brain damage or the diagnosis is not suspected. Using these criteria, Gifford and Groves[167] found that only 6 of 101 patients with pulmonary emboli proved at autopsy might have been candidates for pulmonary embolectomy.

At present, the primary indication for pulmonary embolectomy is persistent and refractory hypotension in a patient with massive embolism documented by lung scan or, preferably, by pulmonary angiography. Involvement of the major pulmonary arteries by accessible pulmonary emboli should be greater than 50 per cent. The immediate treatment of such patients is supportive, and many respond to oxygen administration, heparinization, vasopressors, thrombolytic drugs, and ionotropic agents. Every effort should be made to manage the patient by these means as a vigorous regimen of this type has had a favorable clinical response in many patients previously thought to require embolectomy. If after 1 to several hours, administration of the above agents is effective in maintaining a blood pressure of 60 to 80 mm Hg mean arterial pressure by continuous intra-arterial recording, embolectomy may be deferred, particularly if renal and cerebral function is maintained.

Technique

As soon as massive pulmonary embolism is suspected, heparin therapy is instituted, an emergency pulmonary angiogram is obtained, and if shock is not present, a lung scan is also performed. If severe hypotension is present, preliminary support of the patient by partial venoarterial bypass through the femoral vessels with a portable disposable bubble oxygenator (if available) is indicated. This partial bypass alone often corrects the hypotension, and patients who survive with this support for several hours have an excellent chance for recovery without surgical embolectomy.[118, 160, 168]

EMBOLECTOMY WITH CARDIOPULMONARY BYPASS

Primary candidates in refractory shock are usually taken to the operating room immediately after the

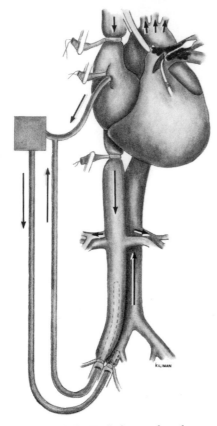

Figure 8-5. Technique of pulmonary embolectomy with cardiopulmonary bypass. Cannulations are completed, and cardiopulmonary bypass is instituted. Main pulmonary artery is opened longitudinally. Emboli are removed from right and left pulmonary arteries and their major tributaries by combination of forceps, suction, and Fogarty catheter.

diagnosis. The pump oxygenator (disposable bubble type) is primed with a mixture of ACD blood and Ringer's lactate solution. If a portable system has not been used previously, the femoral vessels are exposed with the patient under local infiltration anesthesia. The artery is cannulated first and connected to the outflow side of the heart-lung machine. The venous cannula is attached to the coronary suction line of the pump oxygenator and advanced into the inferior vena cava with mild suction in order to retrieve any clots that may have lodged in the iliac vein or vena cava. The blood removed during this maneuver may be returned in-

stantly through the femoral arterial line. The venous line is then transferred to the inflow side of the pump oxygenator, thus completing the peripheral circuit for extracorporeal circulation. Bypass is usually not instituted until hypotension deepens, cardiac arrest occurs, or exposure of the heart for embolectomy is completed. If partial portable bypass has been used, it is continued until it can be converted to total bypass through a second venous cannulation of the right atrium and superior vena cava.

Anesthesia is induced; a median sternotomy provides excellent exposure of the main pulmonary artery. The pericardium is opened, and the right atrium is explored digitally for intracavitary thrombi. After cannulations are completed, cardiopulmonary bypass is instituted. The main pulmonary artery is exposed and incised longitudinally. It is usually free of emboli, although partially obstructing emboli may be present. The emboli are removed from the right and left pulmonary arteries and their major branches by means of curved sponge forceps and suction. A Fogarty catheter is then passed with inflation of the balloon and withdrawal to recover emboli from the smaller pulmonary arterial branches (Fig. 8-5). Finally, the pulmonary arterial tree on both sides is copiously irrigated with saline. During this portion of the procedure, both lungs are massaged with the hands centripetally to dislodge peripheral clots and force them into a location more accessible for aspiration. The right ventricle is explored for residual clots. Following closure of the pulmonary artery, cardiopulmonary bypass is gradually discontinued, and the heart and lungs are allowed to resume their normal function. After closure of the median sternotomy, appropriate venous interruption, usually inferior vena cava ligation, plication, or clipping, is accomplished in order to prevent further embolization.

EMBOLECTOMY WITHOUT CARDIOPULMONARY BYPASS

If extracorporeal circulation is not available, three other methods may be successful, using the same indications as previously described.

UNILATERAL EMBOLECTOMY. In most patients with massive pulmonary embolism, one or the other pulmonary artery is primarily affected. Therefore, the side with the major amount of emboli can be approached without extracorporeal circulation being necessary. An anterior thoracotomy in the third interspace provides good exposure for the pulmonary artery. It is dissected to its origin, clamped, and opened for removal of the emboli while circulation and pulmonary function in the opposite lung are allowed to continue.[169–172]

BILATERAL PULMONARY EMBOLECTOMY THROUGH THE LEFT MAIN PULMONARY ARTERY.

Another procedure has been described for removing emboli from both lungs without cardiopulmonary bypass. Bilateral pulmonary embolectomy[142–144, 173] is performed entirely through the left main pulmonary branch. The left main pulmonary artery is approached through a left posterolateral thoracotomy incision. The pleural space is entered at the fourth intercostal space. The lung is retracted inferiorly and posteriorly. The left main pulmonary artery is gently palpated for thrombus. The pericardium is incised 2 cm anterior and parallel to the phrenic nerve in order to gain access to the main pulmonary and right pulmonary arteries, which are then also palpated for emboli. The left main pulmonary artery is dissected free at its origin, and an umbilical tape with tourniquet is passed about the vessel. A similar tape with tourniquet is passed around the common pulmonary artery.

A small longitudinal incision is made in the left main pulmonary artery after the proximal tourniquet is occluded (Fig. 8-6). The embolus in the left pulmonary vessel is removed with forceps and aspiration. The left lung is compressed to further mobilize distal emboli. A Fogarty catheter is then passed to the more distal branches and withdrawn to remove any residual and long-standing adherent clots. Backflow of blood is usually brisk after these procedures. A clamp or tourniquet placed distally on the left main pulmonary vessel helps control blood loss until the arteriotomy can be closed.

At this point, a sucker or forceps is introduced into the proximal left main pulmonary artery, and the common pulmonary artery tourniquet is temporarily tightened as the tourniquet on the proximal left main pulmonary artery is loosened. The forceps is passed down the right main pulmonary artery,

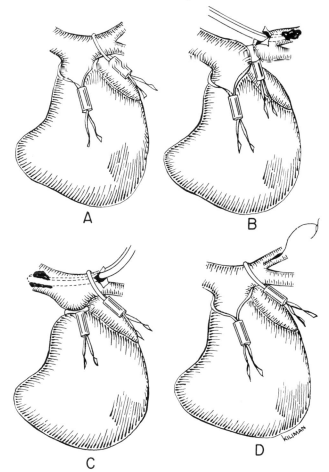

Figure 8-6. Technique of bilateral pulmonary embolectomy through the left main pulmonary artery. **A.** Tourniquets are placed about the common and left main pulmonary arteries. **B.** A small incision is made in the proximal left main pulmonary artery after occluding its proximal tourniquet. Embolus is removed by forceps, aspiration, and Fogarty catheter. **C.** A sucker or forceps is introduced into proximal right pulmonary artery as tourniquet is tightened on common pulmonary artery and left main pulmonary arterial tourniquet is loosened. Emboli are removed during one-minute intervals of occlusion. **D.** After flushing the arteriotomy, left main arterial tourniquet is tightened as common tourniquet is released to allow resuturing of pulmonary arteriotomy.

and emboli are removed. This is usually accomplished in less than 1 minute, without loss of cardiac action. This maneuver must be done in a minimum of time to prevent dilatation of the right heart and brain hypoxia. The procedure may be repeated using a Fogarty catheter, if necessary, to assure removal of all significant right-sided clots. After the arteriotomy is flushed, the left pulmonary artery is re-bound, as the tourniquet on the main pulmonary artery is released to allow suturing of the arteriotomy with continuous 5–0 arterial suture. Administration of anticoagulants is rebegun 48 to 72 hours postoperatively, following removal of chest tubes.

BILATERAL PULMONARY EMBOLECTOMY WITH INFLOW OCCLUSION OF THE VENAE CAVAE.

A third method of pulmonary embolectomy without cardiopulmonary bypass can be performed by a competent surgeon at a smaller hospital.[96, 174–176] The sternum is split longitudinally and the pericardium opened. The cavae are snared and intermittently occluded for 3-minute periods; the pulmonary artery is opened vertically, suctioned clean, and then side-clamped to allow the caval snares to be released (Fig. 8-7). The caval occlusion reduces the blood loss from the pulmonary artery to controllable levels. The patients died in the older Trendelenburg procedure because there was no method for controlling blood loss once the pulmonary embolus was removed. This technique is performed with the patient under normothermia.

TRANSVENOUS PULMONARY EMBOLECTOMY

The relatively high mortality rate associated with the operative procedures for pulmonary embolectomy prompted a search for other methods of management which would obviate the need for general anesthesia, thoracotomy, and cardiopulmonary bypass in a moribund patient. A preliminary report on the successful application of a vacuum-cup catheter device to remove experimental emboli in dogs by Greenfield et al.[177] in 1960 suggested the feasibility of this approach in patients; in 1971 he reported[145, 146] the successful management of 3 patients with acute massive pulmonary embolism using this technique, with immediate hemodynamic improvement and subsequent complete recovery.

In the cardiac catheterization laboratory, after

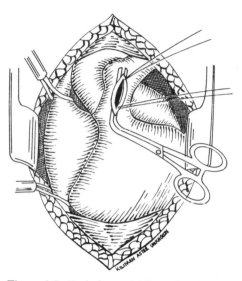

Figure 8-7. Technique of bilateral pulmonary embolectomy with inflow occlusion of the venae cavae. The cavae are snared and intermittently occluded, while the pulmonary artery is opened vertically, suctioned clean, and then side-clamped to allow the caval snares to be released.

pulmonary angiography has demonstrated the presence of massive emboli, usually the left common femoral vein is exposed and a 1-cm longitudinal incision is made. A vacuum-cup device attached to a No. 12 French double-lumen balloon-tipped catheter is introduced under fluoroscopic image intensification and guided through the right heart into the pulmonary artery (Fig. 8-8). Intermittent balloon inflation and injection of contrast medium (50 per cent sodium diatrizoate) in 6-cc increments permits direct visualization of the pulmonary arterial branches. This is performed on both the right and the left side to locate the emboli. Suction is applied to the catheter, and the absence of aspirated blood confirms the capture of the embolus within the cup. The balloon is deflated, and the catheter is withdrawn with the thrombus firmly held in the cup by suction. This maneuver is repeated until all major emboli are removed. There usually is immediate symptomatic improvement. Care must be taken to prevent dislodgment of thrombus from the cup during withdrawal; when this occurs, it is usually in the vicinity of the tricuspid valve or in

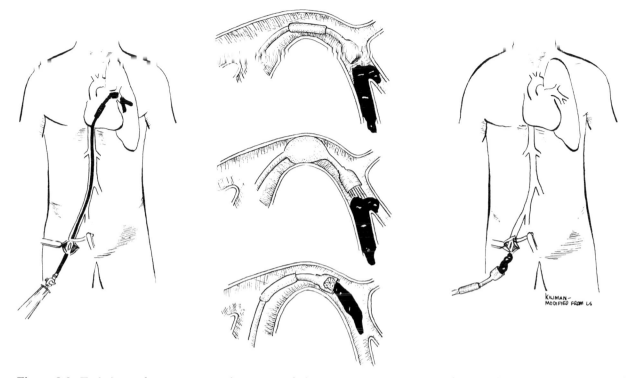

Figure 8-8. Technique of transvenous pulmonary embolectomy. A vacuum-cup device attached to a No. 12 French double-lumen balloon-tipped catheter is introduced through femoral vein into the pulmonary artery under fluoroscopic guidance. Intermittent balloon inflation and injection of contrast medium permits visualization of artery and emboli. Suction is applied to the catheter, and the embolus is captured within the cup and then withdrawn while suction is maintained.

the common femoral vein. Care must also be taken not to damage the endocardium or to stimulate arrhythmias during manipulation with the rigid vacuum cup. Positioning the cup is facilitated by the use of interchangeable catheter tips with different angles to accommodate the various branches. Anticoagulation therapy with heparin and inferior vena caval plication are used to prevent postoperative recurrent embolization.

In the severely ill patient with refractory hypotension, peripheral cannulation of both femoral vessels for partial cardiopulmonary bypass on a portable oxygenator can be utilized to permit definitive pulmonary arteriography.[147, 148] This support while the patient is in the cardiac catheterization laboratory permits safer manipulation of the catheter device and repeated extraction of emboli as necessary. Also, this manipulation can be performed while the operating room is made ready for open pulmonary embolectomy if the catheter procedure is unsuccessful.

This procedure may also be beneficial in patients with nonlethal emboli who have limited cardiopulmonary reserve, so that there is rapid restoration of effective pulmonary bloodflow.

Results

Does an operation with a very high rate of mortality and associated morbidity have any role in the current treatment of pulmonary embolism? In 1967 Cross and Mowlem[168] reported a survey of the results of pulmonary embolectomy in 137 patients. Of these, the diagnosis was incorrect in 9, and all of these patients, who were done on cardiopulmonary bypass, died. The majority of the deaths was considered to be due to myocardial infarction. Of the 128 patients in whose lungs pulmonary emboli were found, 106 were done on cardiopulmonary bypass, and 22 were done without bypass. Of the 128 patients having an embolectomy, 59 (46 per cent) survived the procedure. However, 13 died later, leaving 46 of 128 (36 per cent) survivors. Fifteen of 115 patients done on cardiopulmonary bypass (including those with an error in diagnosis) had central nervous system sequelae. Of the 22 patients operated on without the use of cardiopulmonary bypass, 7 had emboli in one pulmonary artery, permitting a unilateral embolectomy to be performed successfully in all 7 patients. The remaining 15 had bilateral emboli and of these, only 2 (13 per cent) survived operation. Sautter et al.[160] performed 22 pulmonary embolectomies under rigid indications (sustained hypotension unresponsive to vasopressors); mortality was 82 per cent.

Several recent reports reveal a much higher incidence of survival than indicated in previous studies. In 1969 Gentsch et al.[135] reported a series of 10 patients undergoing emergency pulmonary embolectomy with cardiopulmonary bypass, with survival of 7 of the 10 (70 per cent). Twelve patients with massive pulmonary embolism were submitted to pulmonary embolectomy by Stirling and associates,[133] with 9 long-term survivors. In 1973 Berger[141] reported pulmonary embolectomy performed for massive embolism associated with refractory shock in 17 patients, with 13 long-term survivors; three of the four deaths were not related to the operative procedure itself. These encouraging results may be attributed to more rapid and accurate diagnostic measures combined with increased skill in the use of cardiopulmonary bypass.

Refractory systemic hypotension probably is the single most reliable indication for pulmonary embolectomy. However, because clinical experience varies and can be interpreted differently, the indications for pulmonary embolectomy cannot be categoric. The decision must be based on clinical judgment with consideration of the clinical and hemodynamic state of the patient as well as the magnitude of the embolic obstruction. Although pulmonary embolectomy may occasionally be lifesaving, the majority of patients respond to intensive medical management.

CHRONIC MASSIVE PULMONARY EMBOLISM

A nonlethal pulmonary embolus is usually absorbed within 2 or 3 months.[178–181] However, occasionally a patient may present with chronic major obstruction of the pulmonary artery, secondary to thromboembolism. Recently, attention has been directed toward this disorder, which is usually associated with pulmonary hypertension and cor pulmonale. The successful removal of major thrombi many months after the initial embolic episode has been reported.[151–153, 156–159] Chronic massive pulmonary embolism is now an established disorder; however, despite its grave prognosis, little attention has been given to its treatment. The diagnosis has recently been made with increasing frequency, partly as a result of the more widespread use of pulmonary scanning and arteriography.

Indications for Surgical Intervention

Firm indications should be present for surgical intervention. The clinical manifestations of chronic pulmonary embolism are primarily dyspnea with evidence of pulmonary hypertension. The indications were classified by Moser et al.[153] into hemodynamic, respiratory, and pulmonary indications. The hemodynamic indication is significant pulmonary hypertension due to embolic occlusion of a large vessel. The respiratory indication is the presence of a large dead space, as the ventilated nonperfused area impairs ventilation efficiency and imposes an increased workload on the respiratory mechanisms. The patient should have considerable dyspnea and preferably no serious additional cardiac or respiratory problems. The pulmonary indications for surgery are recurrent respiratory infections and repeated hemoptysis.

From data presently available, it appears that patients with persistent occlusion of a main right or left pulmonary artery who show no significant improvement of the pulmonary bloodflow during a 2- to 3-month period after embolization should be considered candidates for pulmonary thromboembolectomy. The patients should be significantly disabled, with gross disturbance of respiratory function but no underlying chronic heart or lung disease.

TECHNIQUE

The advent of bypass techniques has encouraged the surgical approach to this disease by increasing the safety of operative intervention, however, depending on the location of the thrombus, it is sometimes possible to cross-clamp the artery without resorting to bypass. Cardiopulmonary bypass should be available so that if technical difficulties occur, it can be used. The techniques and procedures do not differ from those described previously in this chapter for the treatment of acute embolization. In view of the poor prognosis with conservative management and anticoagulation therapy in chronic massive pulmonary embolism, operation, whenever indicated, seems the better alternative.

Results

The prognosis in most instances of thromboembolic pulmonary hypertension is poor, the patient following an inexorable course with progressive right-sided failure, crippling dyspnea, and ultimate death.

Although the limited experience with thromboendarterectomy for chronic pulmonary embolization is encouraging, it is doubtful whether completely normal bloodflow to an involved lung can be established when there are severe changes due to long-standing obstruction of the pulmonary arterial vasculature. Also, it is not clear to what extent the pulmonary vascular bed remains patent after the chronic obstruction is removed. For these reasons, Symbas et al.[159] have advised strict selection of candidates for surgical treatment and close follow-up studies with serial pulmonary angiography and perfusion lung scans. In general, reported postoperative results have been good as long as surgery is performed before there are irreversible secondary changes in the involved chest and lung, reduction of size of the involved pleural space, and formation of systemic collateral vessels in the affected lung. In such patients, repeated hemoptysis, respiratory infections, and bronchiectasis develop. Unfortunately, lung resection, rather than thromboendarterectomy, then becomes the preferable mode of surgical therapy.

REFERENCES

1. Laënnec, R. T. H. Traité de l'auscultation médiate et des maladies des poumons et du coeur. Paris, 1819.
2. Cruveilhier, J. Anatomie pathologique du corps humain. Paris, Ballière, 1829–1835.
3. Virchow, R. Die Verstopfung der Lungenarterien und ihre Folgen. *Beit exper Path u Physiol 2:*1, 1846.
4. Gray, F. D. *Pulmonary Embolism.* Philadelphia, Lea & Febiger, 1966.
5. Towbin, A. Pulmonary embolism: Incidence and significance. *JAMA 156:*209, 1954.
6. Hume, M., Sevitt, S., and Thomas, D. P. *Venous Thrombosis and Pulmonary Embolism.* Cambridge, MA, Harvard Univ Press, 1970, Chap. 1.
7. Coon, W. W., and Willis, P. W. Deep vein thrombosis and pulmonary embolism. *Am J Cardiol 4:* 611, 1959.
8. Jones, R. H., and Sabiston, D. C. Pulmonary embolism in childhood. In *Monographs in the Surgical Sciences.* Baltimore, Williams & Wilkins, 1966, Vol. 3, No. 1, p 35.
9. DeBakey, M. E. Collective review: Critical evaluation of the problem of thromboembolism. *Surg Gynecol Obstet 98:*1, 1954.
10. Matas, R. Post-operative thrombosis and pulmonary embolism before and after Lister, in retrospect and prospect. *Univ Toronto Med J 10:*1, 1932.
11. Crutcher, R. R., and Daniel, R. A. Pulmonary embolism: A correlation of clinical and autopsy studies. *Surgery 23:*47, 1948.
12. Coon, W. A., and Coller, F. A. Some epidemiologic considerations of thromboembolism. *Surg Gynecol Obstet 109:*487, 1959.
13. Zimmerman, L. M., Miller, D., and Marshall, A. N. Pulmonary embolism: Its incidence, significance, and relation to antecedent vein disease. *Surg Gynecol Obstet 88:*373, 1949.
14. Thomas, W. A., Davies, J. N. P., O'Neal, R. M., and Dimakulangan, A. A. Incidence of myocardial infarction correlated with venous and pulmonary thrombosis and embolism: A geographic study based on autopsies in Uganda, East Africa, and St. Louis, U.S.A. *Am J Cardiol 5:*41, 1960.
15. Rosenthal, S. R. Thromboembolism: Analysis of 1000 autopsies. *J Lab Clin Med 16:*107, 1930.
16. Walsh, P. N., Greenspan, R. H., Simon, M., Simon, A. L., Myers, T. H., Woolsey, P. C., and Cole, C. M. An angiographic severity index for pulmonary embolism. *The Urokinase Pulmonary Embolism Trial:*

A National Cooperative Study. New York, Amer. Heart Assoc., 1973, p 101.

17. Bryant, L. R., Mobin-Uddin, K., Utley, J. R., and Dillon, M. The medical treatment of massive pulmonary embolism. Read in part at Conference on Pulmonary Thromboembolism, Univ of Kentucky Medical Center, Lexington, KY, April 19–21, 1973.

18. Eeles, G. H., and Sevitt, S. Microthrombosis in injured and burned patients. *J Path Bact 93:*275, 1967.

19. Braconier, J. H. Venous thrombi and pulmonary emboli in an autopsy series, 1967, cited by Hume et al. *Venous Thrombosis and Pulmonary Embolism.* Cambridge, MA, Harvard Univ Press, 1970, Chap. 1.

20. Smith, G. T., Dammin, G. J., and Dexter, L. Postmortem arteriographic studies of the human lung in pulmonary embolization. *JAMA 188:*143, 1964.

21. Smith, G. T., Dexter, L., and Dammin, G. J. Postmortem quantitative studies in pulmonary embolism. In Sasahara, A., and Stein, M. (eds.) *Pulmonary Embolic Diseases.* New York, Grune & Stratton, 1965, p 120.

22. Pollack, E. W., Sparks, F. C., and Barker, W. F. Pulmonary embolism: An appraisal of therapy in 516 cases. *Arch Surg 107:*866, 1973.

23. Modan, B., Sharon, E., and Jelin, N. Factors contributing to the incorrect diagnosis of pulmonary embolic disease. *Chest 62:*388, 1972.

24. Carlotti, J., Hardy, I. B., Linton, R. R., and White, P. D. Pulmonary embolism in medical patients. *JAMA 134:*1447, 1947.

25. Allardyce, D. B., Yoshida, S. H., and Ashmore, P. G. The importance of microembolism in the pathogenesis of organ dysfunction caused by prolonged use of the pump oxygenator. *J Thorac Cardiov Surg 52:*706, 1966.

26. Moore, F. D., Lyons, J. H., Pierce, E. C., Morgan, A. P., Drinker, P. A., MacArthur, J. D., and Dammin, D. J. Post-traumatic pulmonary insufficiency. In *Pathophysiology of Respiratory Failure and Principles of Respiratory Care After Surgical Operations, Trauma, Hemorrhage, Burns and Shock.* Philadelphia, Saunders, 1969.

27. Swank, R. L. Alterations of blood on storage: Measurement of adhesiveness of ageing platelets and leucocytes and their removal by filtration. *N Engl J Med 265:*728, 1961.

28. Swank, R. L., and Porter, G. A. Disappearance of microemboli transfused into patients during cardiopulmonary bypass. *Transfusion 3:*192, 1963.

29. Swank, R. L. Platelet aggregation: Its role and cause in surgical shock. *J Trauma 8:*872, 1968.

30. Reuel, G. J., Greenberg, S. D., Lefrak, E. A., McCollum, W. B., Beall, A. C., and Jordan, G. L. Prevention of post-traumatic pulmonary insufficiency. *Arch Surg 106:*386, 1973.

31. Jenevein, E. P., and Weiss, D. L. Platelet microemboli associated with massive blood transfusion. *Am J Path 45:*313, 1964.

32. Gorham, L. W. A study of pulmonary embolism: I. A clinicopathological investigation of 100 cases of massive embolism of the pulmonary artery: Diagnosis by physical signs and differentiation from acute myocardial infarction. *Arch Int Med 108:*76, 1961.

33. Hampton, A. O., and Castleman, B. Correlation of postmortem chest teleroentgenograms with autopsy findings: With special reference to pulmonary embolism and infarction. *Am J Roentg Rad Ther 43:*305, 1940.

34. *The Urokinase Pulmonary Embolism Trial: A National Cooperative Study.* New York, Amer. Heart Assoc, 1973, Chap. 14.

35. Coon, W. W. Personal communication, December 1973.

36. Hardaway, R. M. *Syndrome of Disseminated Intravascular Coagulation With Special Reference to Shock and Hemorrhage.* Springfield, IL, Thomas, 1966.

37. Robb, H. J. The role of microembolism in the production of irreversible shock. *Ann Surg 158:*685, 1963.

38. Robb, H. J. Microembolism in the pathophysiology of shock. *Angiology 16:*405, 1965.

39. Blaisdell, F. W., Lim, R. C., Amberg, J. R., Choy, S. H., Hall, A. D., and Thomas, A. N. Pulmonary microembolism: A cause of morbidity and death after major vascular surgery. *Arch Surg 93:*776, 1966.

40. Lim, R. C., Blaisdell, F. W., Choy, S. H., Hall, A. D., and Thomas, A. N. Massive pulmonary microembolism in regional shock. *Surg Forum 17:*13, 1966.

41. Lim, R. C., Blaisdell, F. W., Goodman, J. R., and Hall, A. D. Electron micrographic study of pulmonary microemboli in regional and systemic shock. *Int Cardiov Surg Soc* Proceedings of VIII Clinical Congress. Vienna, 1967.

42. Blaisdell, F. W., Lim, R. C., Stallone, R. J. The mechanism of pulmonary damage following traumatic shock. *Surg Gynecol Obstet 130:*15, 1970.

43. Blaisdell, F. W. Respiratory insufficiency syndrome: Clinical and pathological definition. *J Trauma 13:*195, 1973.

44. Miller, G. A. H., Gibson, R. V., Honey, M., and Sutton, G. C. Treatment of pulmonary embolism with streptokinase: A preliminary report. *Br Med J 1:*812, 1969.

45. *The Urokinase Pulmonary Embolism Trial: A National Cooperative Study.* New York, Amer. Heart Assoc., 1973, pp II-33; II-51; II-73.

46. von Hayek, H. Ueber einen Kurzschlusskreislauf (Arterio-venose Anastomosen) in der menschlichen Lunge. *Zsch f Anat u Entwklsg 110:*412, 1940.

47. von Hayek, H. *The Human Lung.* New York, Hafner, 1960.

48. Knisely, W. H., and Knisely, N. H. Preliminary observations on the catch-trap architecture of pulmonary artery tips in health and their responses following distant somatic burns. *Anat Rec 118:320* 1954.

49. Krahl, E. V. A method of studying the living lung in the closed thorax and some preliminary observations. *Angiology 14:*149, 1963.

50. Krahl, E. V. In vivo microscopy of the rabbit's lung. *Bibl Anat 4:*400, 1964.

51. Krahl, E. V. The lung as a target organ in thromboemoblism. In Sasahara, A., and Stein, M. (eds.) *Pulmonary Embolic Disease.* New York, Grune & Stratton, 1965, p 13.

52. Burton, A. C. The relation between pressure and flow in the pulmonary bed. In Adams, W., and Veith, I. (eds.) *Pulmonary Circulation.* New York, Grune & Stratton, 1959, p 26.

53. Haggert, G. E., and Walker, A. M. The physiology of pulmonary embolism as disclosed by quantitative occlusion of the pulmonary artery. *Arch Surg* 6:764, 1923.

54. Steinberg, B., and Mundy, C. S. Experimental pulmonary embolism and infarction. *Arch Path 22:*529, 1936.

55. Holden, W. D., Shaw, B. W., Cameron, D. B., Shea, P. J., and Davis, J. H. Experimental pulmonary embolism. *Surg Gynecol Obstet 88:*23, 1949.

56. Dock, D. S., McGuire, L. B., Hyland, J. W., Haynes, F. W., and Dexter, L. The effect of unilateral pulmonary artery occlusion upon calculated pulmonary blood volume. *Fed Proc 19:*97, 1960.

57. Dalen, J. E., Haynes, F. W., Hoppin, F. G., Evans, G. L., Bhardwaj, P., and Dexter, L. Cardiovascular responses to experimental pulmonary embolism. *Am J Cardiol 20:*3, 1967.

58. Dalen, J. C., and Dexter, L. Pulmonary embolism. *JAMA 207:*1505, 1969.

59. Nelson, J. R., and Smith, J. R. The pathologic physiology of pulmonary embolism: A physiologic discussion of the vascular reactions following pulmonary arterial obstruction by emboli of varying size. *Am Heart J 58:*916, 1959.

60. Crane, C., Hartsuck, J., Birtch, A., Couch, N. P., Zollinger, R., Matloff, J. D., Dalen, J., and Dexter, L. The management of major pulmonary embolism. *Surg Gynecol Obstet 128:*27, 1969.

61. Churchill, E. D. The mechanism of death in massive pulmonary embolism. *Surg Gynecol Obstet 59:*513, 1934.

62. Gibbon, J. H., and Churchill, E. D. The physiology of massive pulmonary embolism: An experimental study of the changes produced by obstruction to the flow of blood through the pulmonary artery and its lobar branches. *Ann Surg 104:*811, 1936.

63. Comroe, J. H., Van Lingen, B., Stroud, R. C., and Roncoroni, A. Reflex and direct cardiopulmonary effects of 5-OH tryptamine (serotonin). *Am J Physiol 173:*379, 1953.

64. Thomas, D. P., Tanabe, G., Khan, M., and Stein, M. Humoral factors mediated by platelets in experimental pulmonary embolism. In Sasahara, A., and Stein, M. (eds.) *Pulmonary Embolic Disease.* New York, Grune & Stratton, 1965, p 59.

65. Nemir, P., Hamilton, W. M., and Brody, J. I. Intravenous cyproheptadine hydrochloride in the treatment of pulmonary embolism: An experimental study. *Surgery 72:*920, 1972.

66. Gurewich, V., Thomas, D., Stein, M., and Wessler, S. Bronchoconstriction in the presence of pulmonary embolism. *Circulation 27:*339, 1963.

67. Webster, J. R., Saadeh, G. B., Eggum, P. R., and Suker, J. R. Wheezing due to pulmonary embolism: Treatment with heparin. *N Engl Med 274:*931, 1966.

68. Puckett, C. L., Gervin, A. S., Rhodes, G. R., and Silver, D. Role of platelets and serotonin in acute massive pulmonary embolism. *Surg Gynecol Obstet 137:*931, 1966.

69. Damblé, K. Ueber Thrombose und Embolie. *Z Klin Med 121:*663, 1932.

70. DeBakey, M. E. Editorial. *Ann Surg 132:*158, 1950.

71. Sasahara, A. A., Cannilla, J. E., Morse, R. L., Sidd, J. J., and Tremblay, G. M. Clinical and physiologic studies in pulmonary thromboembolism. *Am J Cardiol 20:*10, 1967.

72. Editorial. Accuracy of death certificates. *Lancet 2:* 1349, 1966.

73. Miller, R., and Berry, J. B. Pulmonary infarction: A frequently missed diagnosis. *Am J Med Sci 24:* 402, 1958.

73a. Sevitt, S. Venous thrombosis and pulmonary embolism: Their prevention by oral anticoagulants. *Am J Med 33:*705, 1962.

74. Bray, H. A. Tension theory of pleuritic pain. *Am Rev Tuberc 13:*14, 1926.

75. Dalen, J. H. Remarks during Conference on Pulmonary Thromboembolism, Univ of Kentucky Medical Center, Lexington, KY, April 19–21, 1973.

76. Littman, D. Observations on the electrocardiographic changes in pulmonary embolism. In Sasahara, A. A., and Stein, M. (eds.), *Pulmonary Embolic Disease.* New York, Grune & Stratton, 1965, pp 186–198.

77. Fischer, D. C. Personal communication, March 1974.

78. Fleischner, F. G. Observations on the radiologic changes in pulmonary embolism. In Sasahara, A. A., and Stein, M. (eds.) *Pulmonary Embolic Disease.* New York, Grune & Stratton, 1965, pp 206–213.

79. Fraser, R. G., and Paré, J. A. P. Diagnosis of diseases of the chest. In *An Integrated Study Based on the Abnormal Roentgenogram.* Philadelphia, Saunders, 1970.

80. Wagner, H. N., Sabiston, D. C., Ilio, M., McAfee, J. G., Meyer, J. K., and Langan, J. K. Regional pulmonary blood flow in man by radioisotope scanning. *JAMA 187:*601, 1964.

81. Wagner, H. N. Radioisotope scanning in pulmonary embolic disease. In Sasahara, A. A., and Stein, M. (eds.) *Pulmonary Embolic Disease*. New York, Grune & Stratton, 1965, pp 225–235.

82. Duffey, W. C. Personal communication, December 1973.

83. Simon, M., and Sasahara, A. Observations on the angiographic changes in pulmonary thromboembolism. In Sasahara, A. A., and Stein M. (eds.) *Pulmonary Embolic Disease*. New York, Grune & Stratton, 1965, pp 214, 224.

84. Paraskos, J. A., Adelstein, S. J., Smith, R. E., Rickman, F. D., Grossman, W., Dexter, L., and Dalen, J. E. Late prognosis of acute pulmonary embolism. *N Engl J Med 289:*55, 1973.

85. Freiman, D. G. Pathologic observations on experimental and human thromboembolism. In Sasahara, A. A., and Stein, M. (eds.) *Pulmonary Thromboembolic Disease*. New York, Grune & Stratton, 1965, p 81.

86. Dalen, J. Natural History of pulmonary embolic disease. Read at Conference on Pulmonary Thromboembolism, Univ of Kentucky Med Center, Lexington, Ky., April 19–21, 1973.

87. Donaldson, G. A., Williams, C., Scannell, G., and Shaw, R. S. A reappraisal of the application of the Trendelenburg operation to massive fatal embolism. *N Engl J Med 268:*171, 1963.

88. Turnier, E., Hill, J. D., Kerth, W. J., and Gerbode, F. Massive pulmonary embolism. *Am J Surg 125:*611, 1973.

89. Gurewich, V., Thomas, D., Stein, M., and Wessler, S. Bronchoconstriction in the presence of pulmonary embolism. *Circulation 27:*339, 1963.

90. Del Guercio, L. R., Cohn, J. D., Feins, N., Coomaraswany, R. P., and Mantle, L. Screening for pulmonary embolism shock. *JAMA 196:*751, 1966.

91. Wechsler, B. M., Karlson, K. E., Krasnow, N., Garzon, A., and Chait, A. Pulmonary embolism: Influence on cardiac hemodynamics and natural history on selection of patients for embolectomy and inferior vena cava ligation. *Surgery 65:*182, 1969.

92. Trendelenburg, F. Ueber die operative Behandlung der Embolie der Lungenarterie. *Arch Klin Chir 86:* 686, 1908.

93. Kirschner, M. Ein durch die Trendelenburgsche Operation geheilter Fall von Embolie der Art. pulmonalis. *Arch Klin Chir 133:*312, 1924.

94. Hume, M., Sevitt, S., and Thomas, D. P. *Venous Thrombosis and Pulmonary Embolism.* Cambridge, MA, Harvard Univ Press, 1970, p 427.

95. Steenburg, R. W., Warren, R., Wilson, R. E., and Rudolph, L. E. A new look at pulmonary embolectomy. *Surg Gynecol Obstet 107:*214, 1958.

96. Vossschulte, K. The surgical treatment of pulmonary embolism. *J Cardiov Surg (Suppl)197,* 1965.

97. Allison, P. R., Dunnill, M. S., and Marshall, R. Pulmonary embolism. *Thorax 15:*273, 1960.

98. Sharp, E. H. Pulmonary embolectomy: Successful removal of a massive pulmonary embolus with the support of cardiopulmonary bypass: A case report. *Ann Surg 156:*1, 1962.

99. Cooley, D. A., and Beall, A. C. A technic of pulmonary embolectomy using temporary cardio-pulmonary bypass. *J Cardiov Surg 2:*469, 1961.

100. Couves, C. M., Sproule, B. J., and Fraser, R. S. Pulmonary embolectomy using heart-lung by-pass. *Canad Med Assoc J 86:*1056, 1962.

101. Rosenberg, D. M., Ekwan, P. J., and Pearce, C. W. Surgical treatment of massive pulmonary embolism with the use of extracorporeal circulation. *J Cardiov Surg 3:*428, 1962.

102. Cooley, D. A., Beall, A. C., and Alexander, J. K. Acute massive pulmonary embolism: Successful surgical treatment using temporary cardiopulmonary bypass. *JAMA 177:*283, 1961.

103. Storey, W. S., Jacobs, J. K., and Collins, H. A. Pulmonary embolism and embolectomy. *Surg Gynecol Obstet 116:*292, 1963.

104. Cross, F. S., and Mowlem, A. Pulmonary embolectomy utilizing cardiopulmonary bypass. *Surg Gynecol Obstet 117:*71, 1963.

105. Baker, R. R. Pulmonary embolism. *Surg 54:*687, 1963.

106. Hume, M. Pulmonary embolism: Historical aspects. *Arch Surg 87:*193, 1963.

107. Haimovici, H. Pulmonary embolectomy with cardiopulmonary bypass. *J. Cardiov Surg 4:*671, 1963.

108. Sautter, R. D., Lawton, B. R., Maguin, G. E., and Emanuel, D. A. Pulmonary embolectomy: Report of a case with preoperative and postoperative angiograms. *N Engl J Med 269:*997, 1963.

109. Cross, F. S., Jones, R. D., and Mowlem, A. Acute pulmonary embolism. *Arch Surg 89:*159, 1964.

110. Rosenberg, D. M. L., Pearce, C., and McNulty, J. Surgical treatment of pulmonary embolism. *J Thorac Cardiov Surg 47:*1, 1964.

111. Paton, B. C., and Marchioro, T. The indications for pulmonary embolectomy. *Ann Surg 160:*325, 1964.

112. Beall, A. C., Al-Attar, A. S., Mani, P., and Tuttle, L. L. D. Resuscitation after acute massive pulmonary embolism. *J Thorac Cardiov Surg 49:*419, 1965.

113. McGuire, L. B., and Smith, G. W. Pulmonary embolectomy: report of a case, with a note on indications and technic. *N Engl J Med 272:*1170, 1965.

114. Sabiston, D. C., and Wagner, H. N. The pathophysiology of pulmonary embolism: Relationship to accurate diagnosis and choice of therapy. *J Thorac Cardiov Surg 50:*339, 1965.

115. Marable, S. A., Winegarner, F. G., Moore, F. T., Olin,, D. B., and Molnar, W. Pulmonary embolism and the indications for embolectomy. *Arch Surg 93:*258, 1966.

116. Gahagan, T., Manzob, A., Mathur, A. N., and

Grodsinsky, C. Removal of impacted pulmonary emboli by retrograde injection of fibrinolysin into the pulmonary veins: Report of three cases and experimental studies. Ann Surg 164:315, 1966.

117. Stansel, H. C., Hume, M., and Glen, W. W. L. Pulmonary embolectomy: Results in ten patients. N Engl J Med 276:717, 1967.

118. Rosenberg, D. M. L., Schmidt, R., Warren, S., Cohen, S., and Stern, F. Partial circulatory support in massive pulmonary embolism. Ann Thorac Surg 2:217, 1966.

119. Baker, R. R., and Wagner, H. N. Pulmonary embolectomy in the treatment of massive pulmonary embolism. Surg Gynecol Obstet 122:513, 1966.

120. Sautter, R. D. The technique of pulmonary embolectomy with the use of cardiopulmonary bypass. J Thorac Cardiov Surg 53:268, 1967.

121. Beall, A. C., and Cooley, D. A. Experience with pulmonary embolectomy using temporary cardiopulmonary bypass. J Cardiov Surg (Suppl)131, 1965.

122. Marchioro, T. L., Hermann, G., Waddell, W. R., and Starzl, T. E. Pulmonary embolectomy in a patient with recent renal homotransplantation. Surgery 55:505, 1964.

123. Timmis, H. H. The diagnosis and management of massive pulmonary embolism. Surgery 59:636, 1966.

124. Beall, A. C., and Cooley, D. A. Use of cardiopulmonary bypass for resuscitation and treatment of acute massive pulmonary embolism. Pac Med Surg 75:67, 1967.

125. Heimbecker, R. O., Keon, W. J., and Elliott, G. Pulmonary embolectomy. Arch Surg 95:576, 1967.

126. Nichols, H. T., Morse, D., Blanco, G., Adam, A., and Gonzalez-Lavin, L. Pulmonary embolectomy: Two successful cases. Vasc Surg 1:87, 1967.

127. Khazei, A. H., Dembo, D. H., and Cowley, R. A. Recognition and management of massive pulmonary embolism: A report of successful embolectomy. Arch Surg 94:884, 1967.

128. De Takats, G. Pulmonary embolism: A second look. J Cardiov Surg Special issue VIII, Confer. of Internat. Cardiovasc Soc, Vienna September 6–9, 197, p. 3.

129. Greenfield, L. J., Pearce, H. J., and Nichols, R. T. Recovery of respiratory function and lung mechanics following experimental pulmonary embolectomy. J Thorac Cardiov Surg 55:160, 1968.

130. Cooley, D. A., and Beall, A. C. Embolectomy for acute massive pulmonary embolism. Surg Gynecol Obstet 126:805, 1968.

131. Juanteguy, J. M., and Wilder, R. J. Experimental pulmonary embolectomy by retrograde flush and balloon catheter. Surg Gynecol Obstet 126:1230, 1968.

132. Stelner, P., Biringer, A., Slamen, J., Kulisek, D., Steinerova, M., and Mazuch, J. Pulmonary embolectomy. J Cardiov Surg 10:67, 1969.

133. Stirling, K. N., Morris, K. H., McLean, K. H., Mirams, J. A., Rubinstein, D., and Wagner, G. R. Surgical aspects of pulmonary embolism. Med J Aust 1:571, 1968.

134. Williams, G. D., Westbrook, K. C., and Campbell, G. S. Two successful pulmonary embolectomies in the same patient: Failure of vena cava plication. J Thorac Cardiov Surg 58:140, 1969.

135. Gentsch, T. O., Larsen, P. B., Daughtry, D. C., Chesney, J. G., and Spear, H. C. Community-wide availability of pulmonary embolectomy with cardiopulmonary bypass. Ann Thorac Surg 7: 97, 1969.

136. Fred, H. L., and Natelson, E. A. Selection of patients for pulmonary embolectomy. Dis Chest 56: 139, 1969.

137. Keon, W. J., and Heimbecker, R. O. Massive pulmonary embolism: Modern surgical management. Canad J Surg 12:1, 1969.

138. Garcia, J. B., Barankay, A., Grimshaw, V. A., Deac, R., Ionescu, M. I., and Wooler, G. H. Pulmonary embolectomy using heart-lung bypass: Report of successful case. J Cardiov Surg 10:165, 1969.

139. Lemole, G. M., Swartz, B. E., and Ingber, C. Bilateral pulmonary embolectomy: Discussion of current concepts and case report. J Cardiov Surg 11: 482, 1970.

140. Heimbecker, R. O. Massive pulmonary embolism: a new look at surgical management. Circulation 2:176, 1971.

141. Berger, R. L. Pulmonary embolectomy with preoperative circulatory support. Ann Thorac Surg 16:217, 1973.

142. Rothman, D., Frater, R. W. M., Amirana, M., Silver, L., and Weber, C. Bilateral pulmonary embolectomy through the left main pulmonary artery: Experimental study in dogs. Arch Surg 96:970, 1968.

143. Rothman, D., and Frater, R. W. M. Removing emboli from both lungs: Without cardiopulmonary bypass. JAMA 201:39, 1967.

144. Frater, R. W. M., Schneider, I. J., and Del Guercio, L. R. M. Unilateral embolectomy. N Engl J Med 272:321, 1965.

145. Greenfield, L. J., Reif, M. E., and Guenter, C. E. Hemodynamic and respiratory responses to transvenous pulmonary embolectomy. J Thorac Cardiov Surg 62:890, 1971.

146. Greenfield, L. J., Bruce, T. A., and Nichols, N. B. Transvenous pulmonary embolectomy by catheter device. Ann Surg 174:881, 1971.

147. Taguchi, K., Okumori, M., and Kay, J. H. Treatment of massive pulmonary embolism with pulmonary artery aspiration employing cardiopulmonary bypass. J Thorac Cardiov Surg 59:645, 1970.

148. Carroll, D. Chronic obstruction of major pulmonary arteries. Am J Med 9:175, 1950.

149. Hollister, L. E., and Cull, V. L. Syndrome of

chronic thrombosis of major pulmonary arteries. *Am J Med 21:*312, 1956.

150. Hurwitt, E. S., Schein, C. J., Rifkin, H., and Lebendiger, A. A surgical approach to the problem of chronic pulmonary artery obstruction due to thrombosis or stenosis. *Ann Surg 147:*157, 1958.

151. Synder, W. A., Kent, D. C., and Baisch, B. F. Successful endarterectomy of chronically occluded pulmonary artery. *J Thorac Cardiov Surg 45:*482, 1963.

152. Houk, V. N., Hufnagel, C. C., McClenathan, J. E., and Moser, K. M. Chronic thrombotic obstruction of major pulmonary arteries. *Am J Med 35:*269, 1963.

153. Moser, K. M., Houk, V. N., Jones, R. C., and Hufnagel, C. C. Chronic massive thrombotic obstruction of the pulmonary arteries. *Circulation 32:*377, 1965.

154. Frater, R. W. M., Beck, W., and Schrire, V. The syndrome of pulmonary artery aneurysms, pulmonary artery thrombi, and peripheral venous thrombi. *J Thorac Cardiov Surg 49:*330, 1965.

155. Castleman, B. (ed.) Case records of the Mass Gen Hos: Case 32–1964. *N Engl J Med 271:*40, 1964.

156. Makey, A. R., and Bliss, B. P. Pulmonary embolectomy: A review of five cases with three survivors. *Lancet 2:*1155, 1966.

157. Nash, E. S., Shapiro, S., Landau, A., and Barnard, C. N. Successful thromboembolectomy in long-standing thrombo-embolic pulmonary hypertension. *Thorax 23:*121, 1968.

158. Moor, G. F., and Sabiston, D.C. Embolectomy for chronic pulmonary embolism and hypertension: Case report and review of the problem. *Circulation 41:*701, 1970.

159. Symbas, P. N., Jacobs, W. F., and Schlant, R. C. Chronic pulmonary arterial embolization or thrombosis. *Am J Cardiol 28:*342, 1971.

160. Sautter, R. D., Meyers, W. O., and Wenzel, F. J. Implications of the urokinase study concerning the surgical treatment of pulmonary embolism. *J Thorac Cardiov Surg 63:*54, 1972.

161. Gracey, D. R., Kwaan, H. C., and Cugell, D. W. The treatment of pulmonary embolism. *Chest 63:*1006, 1973.

162. McIntyre, K. M., Nabi, N., and Sasahara, A. A. Management of pulmonary embolism. *Contemporary Surgery 4:*57, 1974.

163. Coon, W. W. Operative therapy of venous thromboembolism. *Mod Concepts Cardiov Dis 43:*71, 1974.

164. Sasahara, A. A., and Barsamian, E. M. Another look at pulmonary embolectomy. *Ann Thorac Surg 16:*317, 1973.

165. Parmley, L. F., Senior, R. M., McKenna, D. H., and Johnston, G. S. Clinically deceptive massive pulmonary embolism. *Chest 58:*15, 1970.

166. Sasahara, A. A., Wheeler, H. B., McIntyre, K. M., and Criss, A. J. Pulmonary embolectomy (editorial). *Dis Chest 56:*89, 1969.

167. Gifford, R. W., and Groves, L. K. Limitations in the feasibility of pulmonary embolectomy: A clinicopathologic study of 101 cases of massive pulmonary embolism. *Circulation 39:*523, 1969.

168. Cross, F. S. and Mowlem, A. Survey of the current status of pulmonary embolectomy for massive pulmonary embolism. *In* Kittle, C. F. (ed.) *Cardiovascular Surgery,* Amer Heart Assn Monograph 16, 1966. Suppls. to *Circulation 35* and *36* (Suppl I): I-86–I-91, 1967.

169. Bradley, M. N., Bennett, A. L., and Lyons, C. Successful unilateral pulmonary embolectomy without cardiopulmonary bypass. *N Engl J Med 271:*713, 1964.

170. Camishion, R. C., Pierucci, L., Fishman, N. H., Fraimow, W., and Greening, R. Pulmonary embolectomy without cardiopulmonary bypass. *Am J Surg 111:*723, 1966.

171. O'Connell, T. J., and Schreiber, J. T. Selective pulmonary embolectomy without cardiopulmonary bypass. *Ann Surg 165:*466, 1967.

172. Janke, W. H. Pulmonary embolectomy: Retrograde approach without use of a heart-lung bypass. *JAMA 206:*127, 1968.

173. Borja, A. R., and Lansing, A. M. Technique of selective pulmonary embolectomy without bypass. *Surg Gynecol Obstet 130:*1073, 1970.

174. Linder, F., Schmitz, W., Encke, A., Trede, M., and Storch, H. H. A study of 605 fatal pulmonary embolisms and two successful embolectomies. *Surg Gynecol Obstet 125:*82, 1967.

175. Browse, N. L. Current thoughts on venous thromboembolism. *Surg Clin North Am 54:*229, 1974.

176. Clarke, D. B. Pulmonary embolectomy using normothermic venous inflow occlusion. *Thorax 23:*131, 1968.

177. Greenfield, L. G., Kimmell, G. O., and McCurdy, W. C. Transvenous removal of pulmonary emboli by vacuum-cup catheter technic. *J Surg Res 9:*347, 1960.

178. Freiman, D. G., Wessler, S., and Lertzman, M. Experimental pulmonary embolism with serum-induced thrombi aged *in vivo. Am J Path 39:*95, 1961

179. Wessler, S., Frelman, D. G., Ballou, J. D., Katz, J. H., Wolff, R., and Wolf, E. Experimental pulmonary embolism with serum-induced thrombi. *Am J Path 38:*89, 1961.

180. Orell, S. R. The fate and late effects of non-fatal pulmonary emboli. *Acta Med Scand 172:*473, 1962.

181. Poe, N. D., Swanson, L. A., Dore, E. K., and Taplin, G. V. The course of pulmonary embolism. *Am Heart J 73:*582, 1967.

9

Chronic Venous Insufficiency: Varicose Veins. The Postphlebitic Syndrome.

CHRONIC VENOUS INSUFFICIENCY CAUSED BY INCOMPETENT SUPERFICIAL VEINS (VARICOSE VEINS)

Among Western people over the age of 45, it has been conjectured that 1 in 5 women and 1 in 15 men have varicose veins, making this lesion one of the commonest ailments.[1] It has been estimated[2] that 10 times as many people suffer from chronic venous disease of the lower extremity as from arterial disease with leg symptoms. In almost all instances, however, the symptoms of varicose veins can be treated and their complications prevented either by the use of a well-fitted elastic stocking or by surgical excision. Failure is attributable to insufficient recognition of the degree of support that the stocking must afford in order to relieve the symptoms and of the extent of surgical excision necessary to offer hope that the limb will remain symptom-free. With a fuller understanding of the etiology of varicosities may come better methods of preventing their initial formation and of controlling their occasional recurrence despite radical surgical extirpation of all visible varicosities.

HISTORICAL REVIEW

For a complete historical review of venous insufficiency, Anning's survey in Dodd and Cockett's[1] textbook may be consulted; the following is a condensed summary of his survey. The papyrus of Ebers (approximately 1550 B.C.) mentions varicose veins and advises against operation for this condition. Hippocrates (460–377 B.C.) associated ulcers of the leg with varicose veins; he also noted that varices did not occur before puberty. A votive relief from the Asklepieion in Athens (Fig. 9-1) depicts an enormous human leg with varicose veins.[3] In Plutarch's *Lives* there is an early operative note on Caius Marius (a Roman tyrant who died in 86 B.C.), who underwent excisional therapy for varicose veins, naturally without anesthesia. It is reported that he stoically endured the procedure until the surgeon approached the opposite extremity, at which point the patient declined further

253

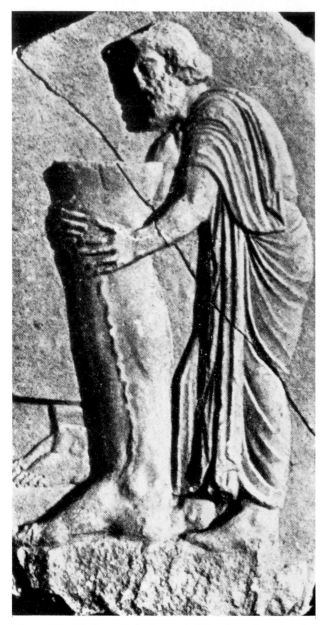

Figure 9-1. Votive relief of man holding huge leg showing varicose veins. (*From Laignel-Levastine,* Histoire de la medicine, I. *Paris, Albin Michel, 1936.*)

treatment, observing, "I see the cure is not worth the pain."

Aurelius Cornelius Celsus (25 B.C.–50 A.D.) advised the use of plasters and linen roller bandages for leg ulcers. Varicose veins were treated by exposure followed by avulsion with a blunt hook or by a touch of the cautery. Claudius Galen (130–

200 A.D.) likewise tore out varicose veins with a blunt hook. He applied wine to leg ulcers and was opposed to frequent changing of the dressing.

The first to ligate varicose veins seems to have been the Byzantine physician Aetius of Amida on the Tigris (502–575 A.D.). Paulus Aegineta (607–690) also performed this operation, but he preferred to carry out ligation of veins on the inner part of the thighs "where they generally arise."

Prior to the discovery of the circulation of the blood by Harvey (1628),[4] there was general acceptance of the concept of to-and-fro movement of the blood, as propounded by Hippocrates and Galen. During this time a number of physicians considered it harmful to heal ulcers of the leg, which were thought to be an outlet for the evil humors of the body. Harvey, however, studied the valves in veins and taught that to-and-fro movement of blood is not possible. In 1676 Wiseman[5] realized that valvular incompetence results from dilatation of the veins; although Hippocrates had noted the association of varicose veins and ulcers, Wiseman seems to have been the first to consider that ulcers might be the direct result of a circulatory defect, and he accordingly used the term *"varicous* ulcer." During the 19th century, ulceration of the leg was mainly attributed to varicose veins, and the term "varicose ulcer" became established. In 1868 Spender[6] and Gay[7] noted that venous thrombosis also could play an important part in ulceration and that severe varicosities might exist without ulceration. They denied the validity of the doctrine of varicose ulcers and agreed with Chapman[8] that the term should be discarded. Gay pointed out that with superficial varicosities there may be other serious lesions affecting both arteries and deep and superficial veins, that were causative factors in ulceration. The wisdom of his ideas has become more and more manifest during the 20th century, when the fact began to be recognized that some ulcers of the leg are secondary to venous thrombosis, others secondary to varicose veins, and still others secondary to arterial thrombosis.

The therapeutic value of firm compression of the leg was appreciated by Celsus and by many ancient writers, including Guy de Chauliac (1363), Ambroise de Paré (1553), and Wiseman (1676). Wiseman introduced a soft leather, laced stocking, the amount of pressure controllable by the lacings.

In the 19th century, Brodie[9] and Spender[6] reported the treatment of ulcers by bandaging. Cooper[10] believed that compression allowed the venous valves to recover their lost action.

Keller in 1905[11] removed the internal saphenous vein by passing a wire loop through the vein, securing it distally, and pulling it out. In 1906 Mayo[12] designed an extraluminal stripper; in 1907 Babcock[13] introduced an intraluminal stripper similar to the type currently in use. The Linton-type intraluminal stripper has the advantage of being semirigid, permitting manipulation of the distal end from the proximal end. Homans[14] emphasized the importance of saphenofemoral ligation in the prevention of recurrent varicosities and advocated radical excision and stripping of varicose veins.

DEFINITION

The word *varix* is derived from an Indo-European root that is represented in Latin by the names for several lesions, including *varus,* a pimple, and *verruca,* a wart, and is represented in Sanskrit by the noun *varṣman,* meaning surface or top. In Latin *varix* means enlarged and tortuous vein, artery, or lymphatic vessel. In common usage, however, *varix* refers only to veins, and a *varicosity* is defined as a "vein that is enlarged in diameter, frequently tortuous, due to enlargement in the longitudinal plane" and one whose valves are incompetent or absent. In general, *varicosity* refers to varicose veins of the lower extremity.

In clinical practice, however, the definition of a varicosity as an abnormally dilated vein does not suffice, because the patient's idea of such a vein may differ markedly from that of the physician. To the female patient, a varicose vein is any visible vein in her lower extremity, even though she may ignore much larger veins on the back of her hand. There are three varieties of visible veins in the lower extremity which the patient may complain of as "varicose veins," viz.:

1. *Minute visible veins that lie within the skin* (see Color Plate II. A). These are frequently called "spider veins" or "spider bursts." Their presence understandably arouses concern in the woman who is appearance conscious. They have no serious clinical significance and, as a rule, are asymptomatic. However, a great number of women insist they have felt a sharp sting just at the time a new spider burst appeared. Occasionally, a patient reports that the spider-type vein causes continual stinging. One wonders, however, whether this is reliable history or merely the patient's effort to exaggerate her discomfort so that the physician will propose some method to rid her of these blemishes. Such veins are too small for surgical excision; the only partially successful treatment is injection with sclerosing solution. Our policy is to inject only a few selected patients, using a 27-gauge needle and a dilute sclerosing solution (0.5 per cent sodium tetradecyl sulfate [Sotradecol]). Occasionally, when the needle enters the vein cleanly, the whole cluster can be eliminated at once; however, if the sclerosing solution is deposited outside the vein, an unsightly brownish pigmentation remains.

2. *Visible subcutaneous veins.* Such veins are tributaries of the long and short saphenous veins.

3. *Dilated main trunks of the long and short saphenous vein, along with some major tributaries.* The vein is enlarged in diameter to the point of valvular incompetence and enlarged longitudinally with resultant tortuosity and irregularly placed areas of local dilatation. When these veins are examined at operation, they are found to be grossly thickened and opaque. The normal vein is so thin that it is translucent, and at times blood can be seen swirling through it. An opaque vein is abnormal despite an absence of dilatation at operation.

ETIOLOGY OF VARICOSE VEINS

Varicose veins may be primary or secondary. Although the true etiology of primary varicosities is unknown, certainly there is an hereditary factor, as noted by all researchers in the field. In order to estimate the extent of such etiologic factors as sex and heredity, a review was undertaken of the charts of 300 of our patients presenting with varicosities who were treated by operation. The study was limited to operative cases in order to exclude patients with only minor varicose veins of little or no clinical significance; this partially removed bias in favor of female patients. Yet, 82 per cent of the 300 patients were women, a ratio of 4 to 1 (Tables 9-1 and 9-2). Furthermore, 61 per cent of these women reported a family history of varicose veins (Tables 9-3 and 9-4), while only 32 per cent of the men reported a positive familial history of chronic venous insufficiency of the lower extremity.

TABLE 9-1. Sex and Age Distribution in 300 Consecutive Patients Treated Surgically for Varicose Veins

	NO.	%	AVERAGE AGE AT OPERATION
Females	247	82	37.7 yr
Males	53	18	44 yr

TABLE 9-2. 300 Consecutive Patients: Ages by Decades at Time of Operation for Varicose Veins

AGE	MALES NO. %	FEMALES NO. %
10–19	3 5.0	0 0.0
20–29	7 12.0	28 12.0
30–39	7 12.0	80 32.0
40–49	15 30.0	90 37.0 } 68.5%
50–59	15 30.0 } 57%	35 14.0
60–69	6 11.0	14 5.5
Total	53 (18)	247 (82)

TABLE 9-3. Heredity Factor in 300 Consecutive Patients With Varicose Veins Treated Surgically

	NO. OPERATED	NO. POSITIVE FAMILIAL HISTORY	%
Males	53	17	32
Females	247	152	61

TABLE 9-4. Familial History of Varicose Veins in 169 Patients Treated Surgically

VARICOSITIES PRESENT IN	152 FEMALES NO. %	17 MALES NO. %
Parents and siblings	29 19.0	2 12
Both parents	11 7.0	1 6
Mother only	76 50.0	10 60
Father only	15 10.0	3 18
Uncles-aunts only	3 2.0	0 0
Grandparents only	2 1.0	0 0
Sisters only	15 10.0	1 6
Brothers only	1 0.6	0 0

Typically the female patient notices the onset of varicose veins in the second decade of life (Table 9-5); the veins become more prominent during pregnancy and increase in size and symptoms with each succeeding child. It is not known if the defect is caused by some inherited weakness in the vein wall, some fault in the valve which permits easier destruction, or by fewer valves. Obese patients seem to have a greater tendency to develop varicose veins.[15] All writers on the subject have suggested the possibility that during pregnancy the enlarged uterus compresses the pelvic veins; in reality, this surmise is an over-simplification, since the patient's veins usually dilate long before the uterus is of sufficient size to obstruct the venous flow in the pelvis. It is not uncommon for a patient to state that one of the first signs of pregnancy is a feeling of discomfort in the legs and enlargement of the veins. For this reason, some writers have considered the possibility of hormonal effects on the veins. Since the estrogenic hormones dilate smooth muscle, it is not unreasonable to assume that smooth muscle of the vein as well as of the uterus is thus affected. The tremendous augmentation of bloodflow during pregnancy is also a possible causative factor. The blood from the extremity, flowing up through the external iliac veins, is probably impeded by the river of blood flowing from the uterus through the internal iliac vein to the common iliac vein.

Varicose veins tend to develop in persons who work in a standing position which permits of little bodily movement and in sedentary persons. Varicosities are less common in those who regularly walk or exercise, e.g., athletes or postmen. This fact suggests that prolonged orthostatic venous hypertension may stretch the veins beyond their elastic limits, resulting in incompetent valves.

It is reasonable to assume (but difficult to prove) that coughing and straining affect the venous valve and the vein wall itself.

TABLE 9-5. Age at Onset of Varicose Veins*

	AVERAGE AGE	YOUNGEST PATIENT	OLDEST PATIENT
Males	31	7	52
Females	27	10	57

* Given as reasonably accurate by 252 of 300 surgically treated patients.

The etiology of secondary varicose veins is clearer. The most common cause is the postphlebitic syndrome, in which varicose veins are a complication of thrombophlebitis. No hereditary factor can be detected in such patients. It is quite common for a person who has varicosities secondary to thrombophlebitis in one extremity to have a completely normal opposite limb. After venous thrombosis subsides, the clot is gradually recanalized. During recanalization, the valves of the veins of the lower extremity are destroyed.[16] Phlebography in the early years after venous thrombosis shows a sponge-like, porous, recanalized clot in which valvular action is impossible. The phlebogram later shows a patent, valveless venous tube in the extremity. Cockett,[1] however, has noted that the veins of the pelvis do not recanalize after thrombophlebitis like those of the leg. In order to detect such chronic pelvic obstruction of the veins, phlebograms of this area should be performed more routinely than is now our practice. In the typical postphlebitic extremity there is daily nocturnal edema of the ankles, followed by the development of pigmentation of the skin due to hemosiderin, induration of the subcutaneous tissue, excoriation of the skin, and, finally, ulceration. Varicose veins in such extremities are caused by transmission of the high pressure in the deep veins of the leg to the superficial veins through communicating veins whose valves have become incompetent.

PATHOLOGY

Clinically, a varicose vein is an abnormally dilated vein. The dilatation in the diameter of the vein causes incompetency of the valve. In addition, most varicosities are elongated and tortuous. Grossly, at operation, the vein walls are thickened and much more opaque than the normal vein. Dilatation occurs most commonly in veins that are subjected to increased hydrostatic pressure but which are poorly supported by surrounding tissue, viz., the superficial veins of the lower leg, the hemorrhoidal veins, the veins of the pampiniform plexus (varicocele), and the veins in the distal portion of the esophagus in patients with portal hypertension. The large veins of the back of the hand might be termed varicose, but they are not usually referred to as such. The pathologic anatomy of the varicose vein has been well described.[17,18]

Ochsner and Mahorner[18] have tabulated the nine features that grossly distinguish full-blown varicose veins.

1. Elongation and tortuosity
2. Loss of elasticity
3. Ectasia or dilatation
4. Increased or decreased thickness of vein wall
5. Thickening of intima
6. Hypertrophy or atrophy of muscularis
7. Disappearance or atrophy of valves
8. Thrombosis—calcification
9. Enlargement of collaterals (easily seen in phlebograms)

Elongation is a characteristic feature of varicosities and may cause the vein to double back on itself (Fig. 9-2). When removed from the body, varicose veins have less elasticity than a normal vein; this finding is due to increased connective tissue and is not related to the amount of elastic tissue, which is likewise increased in varicosities.[18] In ectasia or dilatation the lumen of a vein may become many times its normal diameter; occasionally it may enlarge to such an extent that it is mistaken for a hernia in the groin[18] (Fig. 9-3). The walls of varicose veins may be either thicker or thinner than normal. In the lower leg the superficial veins may be so thin-walled that perforation occurs; however, portions of a varicosity, e.g., a saphenous trunk, may be very much increased in thickness. Thickening of the intima of veins is due to an increase in the subintimal connective tissue. Though this process normally occurs with advancing age, intimal thickening appears to be more marked in certain patients with varicosities than in patients of similar age with normal veins.[18]

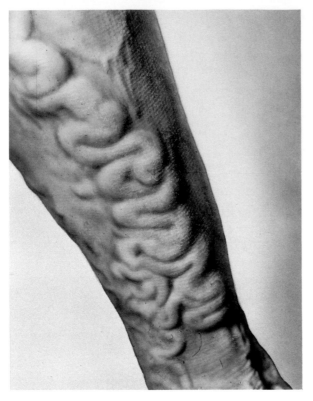

Figure 9-2. Exceptionally large varicosities, demonstrating extreme tortuosity and saccular dilatation.

Microscopically, the most marked change in thick-walled veins is an increase in the thickness of the media. The muscle, which at times becomes tremendously hypertrophied, has relatively little intramuscular connective tissue, and microscopically it resembles the media of arteries. Thin-walled veins show atrophy of the media and replacement by connective tissue.[18] Atrophy may result in the valve entirely disappearing. Thrombosis may occur spontaneously in varicose veins; the processes of repair and eventual recanalization reduce the original lumen. Calcification is an occasional finding in a thrombus.

Increasing venous pressure secondary to propagation of the existing varicosities eventually involves more tributaries in the process of valvular incompetence. Enlarging collaterals frequently usurp the retrograde flow that has been corrected in the main branch by surgical division and ligation and perpetuate the disturbed physiology of the extremity.

Figure 9-3. In dilatation the lumen of a vein may enlarge to such an extent that it is mistaken as a hernia in the groin. (*From Ochsner, A. and Mahorner, H. R. In* Varicose Veins. *St. Louis, Mosby, 1939.*)

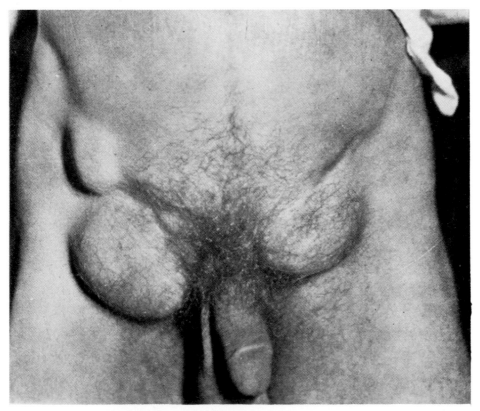

Pathogenesis

The pathogenesis of varicose veins is obscure. In primary varicosities the disease process appears to spread down the saphenous vein in most instances. This makes it probable that the higher pressure above the valve stretches the vein until the valve becomes incompetent. In varicose veins secondary to deep vein insufficiency, the varices appear first in the leg, and the progression is upward. In acquired arteriovenous fistulas, the disease process spreads in both directions, away from the fistulous site of high pressure.

CLINICAL PICTURE

Approximately 30 per cent of the patients who come to us with a chief complaint of "varicose veins" are complaining of veins whose size and number do not warrant surgical treatment, or are too old or disabled to undergo excisional vein therapy. It usually takes the surgeon only momentary inspection to decide whether the patient is a likely candidate for surgical treatment; nevertheless, it is important for him to listen attentively to the history and to examine the patient carefully in order to be certain that the visible veins are causing the symptoms of which the patient complains. Vanity may prompt a young woman to exaggerate her discomfort in the hope of having what she considers blemishes treated surgically. On the other hand, some patients with huge varicosities are surprisingly asymptomatic. Their well-meaning friends or family physician may be alarmed by the size of their varicose veins and insist, even against the patient's will, that consultation be sought. It is our policy not to recommend surgical treatment for varicose veins in an asymptomatic patient, regardless of how large or tortuous the veins are (Fig. 9-4.)

Spider Veins or Spider Bursts

In the majority of patients, spider veins are entirely asymptomatic; however, frequently they are reported to sting, and some observant women have stated that spider veins have appeared immediately after a stinging sensation. This is probably a correct observation.

Tributaries of the Long and Short Saphenous Vein or "Secondary Varicosities"

Secondary varicosities may produce symptoms similar to those caused by large varices of the main trunks, or they may be asymptomatic. The surgeon must determine the true source of the aches and pains in the lower extremity before deciding on operative treatment. Neuralgia is the most commonly reported cause of pain falsely attributed to varicose veins.

SYMPTOMS

The commonest symptoms are those of a tired, heavy feeling in the legs. Other complaints include dull, aching pain in the legs and a feeling of fullness

Figure 9-4. Infrared photo of asymptomatic patient with plainly visible veins. Such veins are not necessarily diseased and should not be removed.

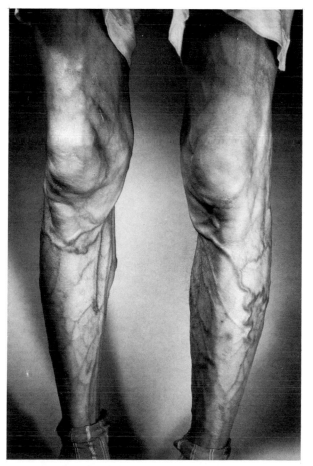

or a "bursting" sensation. None of these symptoms occur when the patient is in bed, nor do they occur immediately upon standing or walking. As the day progresses, the symptoms grow more and more noticeable; they are particularly bothersome toward afternoon or evening, after a long day of the patient being on his feet. The symptoms are aggravated if the patient stands still, e.g., when ironing. Some relief is gained by walking, but all of the symptoms are relieved by elevation of the extremities, especially above heart level, as when lying in bed. Occasionally a patient complains of itching.

MUSCULAR CRAMPS.   Patients with large varicosities may have muscle cramps when at rest. This is an indication to the surgeon that the patient will be relieved of symptoms when the varices are removed.

Many patients without varicosities also have rest cramps. Pregnancy, for example, is one cause of muscle cramps; in such patients, some relief may be obtained from elastic support. Patients who sweat excessively and those on diuretics or salt-free diets may have cramps which are relieved by an increase in salt intake. Many persons have muscle cramps with no obvious cause; such cramps can usually be relieved by the use of quinine sulfate.

SIGNS

The physical appearance of varicose veins is well known by every physician and by most patients (Figs. 9-5 to 9-9). The great majority of patients presenting with varicose veins have no other sign. In a few patients with simple varicose veins, swelling of the ankles is noted as evening approaches. Patients with primary varicosities may expect some relief of mild edema following surgical treatment; however, the physician must not promise relief of swelling by excisional therapy of varicose veins. Swelling usually indicates some incompetence of the deep veins, and in this event, swelling will not be relieved by surgical removal of superficial veins.

The signs of chronic venous insufficiency, such as brownish pigmentation of the skin, induration, and ulceration, may occur in a patient with primary varicosities without deep venous insufficiency. In our experience, ulceration of the leg has been secondary to superficial venous disease or primary varicosities in approximately 30 per cent of pa-

tients treated for ulcer. (See section on chronic venous insufficiency with ulceration.) However, such patients constitute only 10 per cent of the patients seen for varicose veins.

TOURNIQUET TESTS

When we began private practice some 20 years ago, we decided to discard all tourniquet tests; this decision was based on the belief that these tests belonged to a bygone era when surgeons feared that it might be possible to worsen the degree of venous insufficiency by removing the varicose veins. At that time it was thought that in some instances the varicosities might be serving as efficient collaterals in the presence of occluded deep veins. However, it is now believed that only very rarely do varicose veins function as efficient or significant collaterals in a patient with chronic venous insufficiency.[19] Admittedly, occasionally a patient is encountered with acute venous thrombosis and obliteration of the deep veins of the extremity. In such an instance, only the superficial veins are visualized on the phlebogram; however, in such patients the diagnosis is easily made by their greatly swollen limb or by the phlebogram. As a general rule, in the patient with chronic venous insufficiency the incompetent superficial veins do not aid the circulation in any manner but actually impede the normal venous flow of blood. There is no physiologic justification for the surgeon not eradicating the varices, nor is it possible, in our opinion, to remove an excessive number of varicose veins. Testing with the tourniquet thus becomes an unnecessary procedure in office routine. From time to time the Brodie-Trendelenburg test is performed in order to demonstrate to a student or to a patient that the emptied saphenous vein actually fills from above when the tourniquet is released (this does not mean that the blood regularly flows backward in the saphenous vein, however varicosed it may be) (Fig. 9-10). This does demonstrate the competence of the communicating veins, which exists in nearly all patients with primary varicosities. However, the test is frequently equivocal in the patient with combined deep and superficial venous incompetence.

Figure 9-5. A to **D.** Typical varicosities.

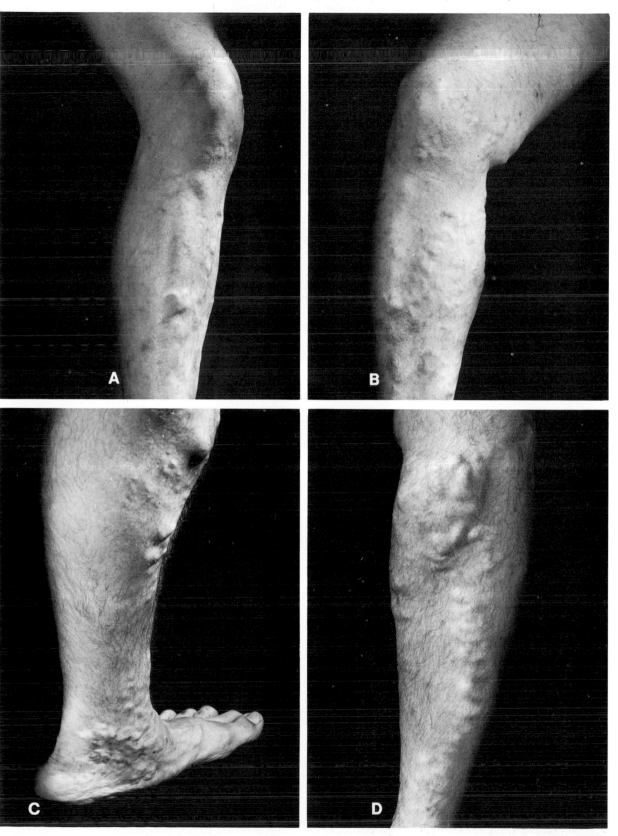

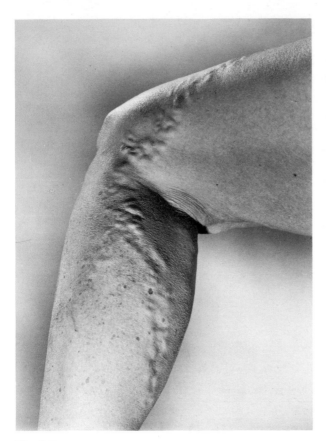

Fig. 9-6.

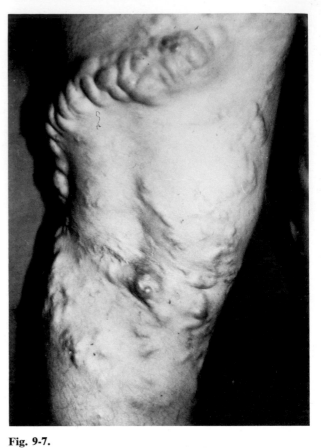

Fig. 9-7.

Fig. 9-8.

Fig. 9-9.

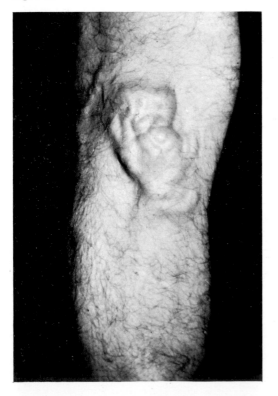

Figure 9-6. Varicose veins of lateral aspect of the thigh. This is a frequently encountered tributary of the long saphenous system, draining the lateral and posterior aspect of the leg, coursing around the lateral aspect of the knee and the anterior aspect of the thigh to join the long saphenous trunk on the medial aspect of the thigh.

Figure 9-7. Unusual course of large varicose vein, a tributary of the long saphenous system coming around from the medial aspect of the leg, directly posteriorly.

Figure 9-8. Isolated cluster of varicose veins in the popliteal space.

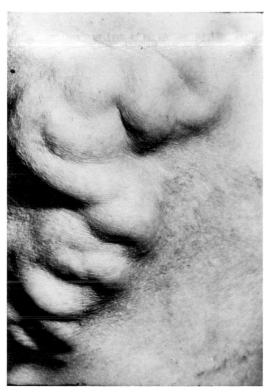

Figure 9-9. Close up of varicosity to show grape-like nature. The vein is enlarged in transverse diameter and is elongated and tortuous.

TREATMENT

Fear impels many patients with varicose veins to seek consultation. They believe or have been told that varicose veins are dangerous for two reasons: the veins may rupture and the patient bleed to death or the varicosities may lead to "fatal blood clots." It is important for the physician to relieve such anxieties and to stress to all patients that the surgical treatment of varicose veins is always elective. Asymptomatic veins need not be treated at all. Symptomatic veins below the knee can easily be managed by well-fitting heavyweight surgical hose. Although it is true that a varicose vein is more likely to become thrombosed than a normal vein (Table 9-6), this type of thrombophlebitis is benign and easily treated. The patient need not assume that excision of the varicosities is necessary in order to prevent "fatal blood clots."

TABLE 9-6. History of Superfical Thrombophlebitis in 300 Consecutive Patients Surgically Treated for Varicose Veins

	NO. PATIENTS	%	2 BOUTS	BILATERAL
247 Females	35*	(14)	2 (4%)	4 (8%)
53 Males	6	(11)	2 (33%)	3 (50%)
Total	41	(13.6)	4 (13%)	7 (2%)

* In 6 (16.7%) patients, the thrombophlebitis was secondary to the postpartum state.

Bleeding Varices

The patient also should not feel undue alarm concerning the possibility of ruptured varices. Such bleeding generally is easily controlled by elevation of the leg and application of pressure by a finger or a handkerchief over the bleeding point.

EXSANGUINATION

Exsanguination has been reported[20] secondary to spontaneous hemorrhage caused by varicose veins in elderly patients who lived alone and who because of physical debility or other reason could not exert pressure over a bleeding varix themselves and were unable to get help. We have not encountered exsanguination in our own practice, nor have we heard of it from our colleagues.

Vulval Varicosities During Pregnancy

Most patients are well controlled by conservative measures, i.e., by wearing a folded towel or napkin inside rubberized leotards (Fig. 9-11). We have operated on no more than 12 patients; in our experience the only indication for operation is the intense pain and discomfort preventing ambulation. The procedure consists of meticulous excision under direct vision with ligation of all veins with absorbable sutures.

SURGICAL TREATMENT

In principle, the elective surgical treatment of varicose veins is exceedingly simple: *remove all the varicose veins and interrupt any detectable com-*

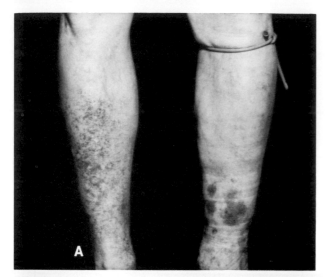

Figure 9-10. The Brodie-Trendelenburg tourniquet test. **A.** The patient's varicosities have emptied by elevation and are compressed by a tourniquet below the knee. He is then asked to stand, and it is noted that the veins do not fill. **B.** Immediately after release of the tourniquet, the large varicosities fill from above. This indicates that the communicating veins are competent and filling is through the valveless saphenous vein itself.

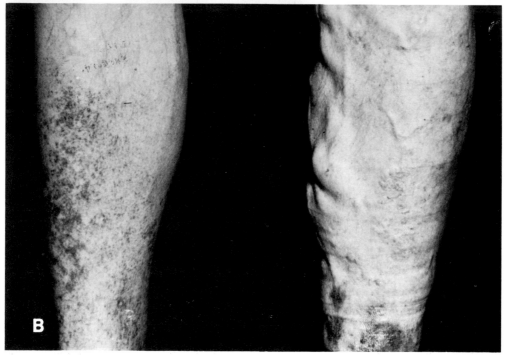

municating veins. The two largest "communicating" veins in the lower extremity are the long saphenous vein itself at its junction with the common femoral vein (Fig. 9-12) and the short saphenous vein at its connection with the popliteal vein. A common cause of "recurrent" varicosities is failure of the surgeon to divide either saphenous vein flush at the junction proximal to all tributaries. When it is divided just a few centimeters below its termination without its tributaries likewise being divided, a direct communication exists through these remaining tributaries between the deep system and the superficial system.

A second source of "recurrent" varices is the surgeon's failure to extirpate all diseased visible veins of the extremity. Total removal of all visible varicose veins requires extensive time and effort in the operating room. It can easily take 4 to 7 hours for a surgeon working alone to remove the long and short saphenous trunks bilaterally and, in addition, all visible incompetent veins. The practical solution for us has been to perform the operation as a team, with two operating surgeons and two assistants suturing the multiple incisions. In this way, operations for varicose veins rarely take more than 1½ hours of operating time (Fig. 9-13).

Operative Preparation

MARKING THE VEINS AND SKIN PREPARATION

It is of utmost importance to mark with ink every vein that is to be removed prior to placing the patient on the operating table. Some surgeons prefer to do this the night before operation; others do the marking in the operating room in order to take advantage of the better lighting. Many types of ink have been recommended: we use an ordinary felt-tipped marker. The ink mark must be placed directly over small veins, so that an incision through the ink mark will expose the vein. If the mark is made parallel to the vein, the vein may easily be missed. Although flecks of ink in the skin have been noted at times, never in our experience has an infection been traceable to the use of ink, nor have we encountered tattooing of the skin by intradermal introduction of ink by the scalpel. If the legs are to be scrubbed after having been marked, some type of indelible ink must be used, e.g., pyrogallic acid, which Myers recommends.[15] Because we use ordinary ink, the legs cannot be scrubbed with soap. Until recently, our preferred preparatory solution was 70 per cent alcohol followed by tincture of benzalkonium chloride (Zephiran Chloride). Presently we prefer to use 1 per cent iodine preparation followed by 70 per cent alcohol.

POSITIONING THE TABLE

Elevation of the lower extremities above heart level is of prime importance, and the steeper the elevation (within reason), the less bleeding there will be. Excessively steep elevation causes undue engorgement of the neck veins and suffusion of the eyes. Elevation of approximately 30 degrees is reasonable. Often the young surgeon forgets to elevate the foot of the operating table, causing much unnecessary bleeding. If the technique herein described is to be utilized (primarily evulsion of most

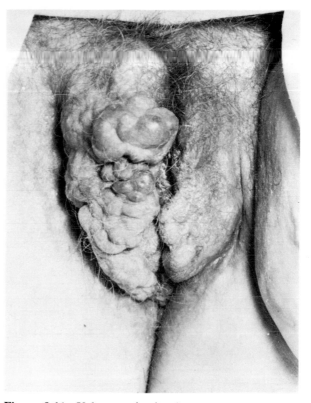

Figure 9-11. Vulvar varicosity in a pregnant woman. Patient was treated conservatively and did not bleed during delivery.

of the varicose veins), then steep elevation of the foot of the table is mandatory.

Operative Technique

The long saphenous trunk is removed in almost all patients; the only exception is in the cosmetic operation on the young female patient who has a few visible varicosities that involve tributaries of the long saphenous vein. The groin incision is placed parallel to and one fingerbreadth below the inguinal crease (somewhat higher in the obese patient), so that it lies approximately one-third lateral and two-thirds medial to the femoral pulse. At his option the surgeon may make a "hockey-stick" incision as recommended by Cockett, letting the medial inferior border curve downward in order to better isolate the large medial accessory trunk. The saphenous vein is seized with a hemostat, divided, and then traced to the saphenofemoral junction. All tributaries are divided and ligated individually; the

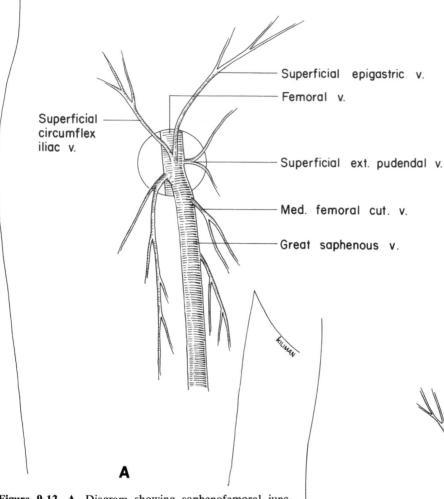

Superficial circumflex iliac v.

Superficial epigastric v.

Femoral v.

Superficial ext. pudendal v.

Med. femoral cut. v.

Great saphenous v.

KILIMAN

A

Figure 9-12. A. Diagram showing saphenofemoral junction. **B.** The saphenous must be divided flush at the junction proximal to all tributaries. **C.** Otherwise, a direct communication exists between the deep and superficial venous systems through these remaining tributaries. Often what appeared to be an enlarged saphenous vein has been encountered in the groin several years after division of the vessel by a competent surgeon. It is believed that one of the tributaries was missed, and it enlarged and migrated to the normal position of the long saphenous vein during the intervening interval.

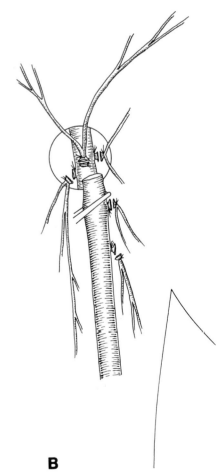

B

C

trunk itself is ligated with a nonabsorbable suture flush with the saphenofemoral junction and a suture ligature placed distal to this. Almost all writers believe that a major cause of recurrent varicosities is failure to divide all tributaries of the long saphenous vein in the groin. On reoperation for recurrent varicosities, at times tributaries of the long saphenous trunk have been encountered in the groin, enlarged to such a degree that they resemble the long saphenous trunk itself. Indeed, such tributaries tend to migrate into the anatomic position of the trunk. Flexion of the patient's knee permits a downward dissection of the long saphenous trunk to permit division and ligation of the large medial tributary.

At the ankle the saphenous vein is exposed through an oblique incision over the vein itself, just above the medial malleolus. An intraluminal stripper is inserted to the groin. If it cannot be passed the entire length of the limb, then it is brought out through a separate incision and a second stripper inserted downward from the groin. Formerly, the saphenous vein was stripped out from the ankle to the foot and brought out near the head of the first metatarsal; this is still our practice in patients with large varicosities of the foot. In patients in whom the saphenous vein does not appear to be prominent in the foot, a different technique has been found to be useful. The vein is seized with a hemostat and slowly drawn downward, with the skin edge being used as a fulcrum until the vein is evulsed. This rarely causes bleeding if the pulling is done *slowly* and gradually, because the lumen is closed by the stretching process. Any remaining visible trunks that can be removed by the stripping procedure are handled similarly. All other varicosities are extirpated by making a small incision, seizing the vein, and avulsing it *slowly*.

After all the veins have been removed from the anterior aspect of the leg, the subcutaneous tissues of the groin are closed with pyrogallic sutures, replacing the 3–0 catgut sutures formerly used. All skin is closed with 4–0 nylon.

To remove the short saphenous vein it is best to turn the patient on his abdomen, because of the need for an unobstructed view in dissecting this vein while simultaneously protecting the sural nerve. The short saphenous vein is exposed by a transverse incision at the ankle and either ligated distally or stripped to the foot. A stripper is then inserted to the knee. The instrument should pass straight up the back of the leg; if it does not, it is lying in an accessory trunk. A transverse incision is made just above or below the crease of the knee in order to pick up the short saphenous vein, which at this point is deep to the fascia. The short saphenous vein is then ligated close to the popliteal vein. The fascia must be opened, and it is closed with two stitches of nonabsorbable suture material.

"MINI"-INCISIONS

When cosmetic results are of minor importance to the patient undergoing operation for symptomatic large varicosities, it is best to use generous incisions, 10 to 15 cm if necessary, in order to visualize and

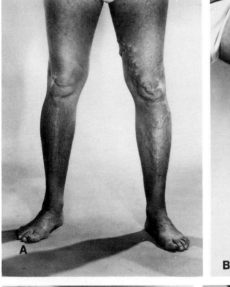
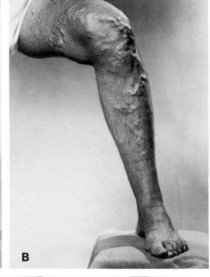
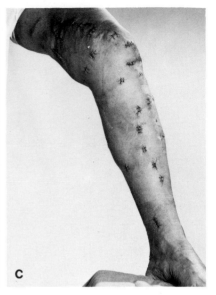

Figure 9-13. A and **B.** Patient with unilateral varicose veins, November 1973. **C.** Early postoperative photo. **D** and **E.** Patient 2 months postoperatively.

eradicate all varicosities that can possibly be extirpated. In patients with bilateral varicosities, it may be necessary to make 40 to 60 incisions; however, this is of little consequence if all varicosities are removed. When the procedure is performed at least partially for cosmetic purposes, it is possible to use very small incisions to remove the tributaries of the long saphenous vein. After the main trunks have been stripped out, one can then use a very sharp pointed knife (No. 11 blade) to make stab wounds 2 or 3 mm in length over the carefully marked veins. These veins can then be seized with a small hemostat (e.g., an especially made small Kocher-type clamp) and teased out quite satisfactorily. The greatest pitfall is missing the veins if they have not been marked with great care. It is not unusual to make more than 100 incisions of this small type that are usually closed with one stitch.

POSTOPERATIVE CARE

The bed is positioned so that the legs are maintained above heart level throughout the hospital stay. On the first day after operation the patient is encouraged to walk as much as desired or to remain in bed, if this is preferred. Sitting in a chair is forbidden. There is no unanimous opinion as to the length of time the bandages should remain in place. Some of our associates change the rubberized bandage on the second day and remove all the padding, replacing the rubberized bandage to the knee only; others replace the bandage all the way to the groin; at times, the entire dressing is left undisturbed for 5 days. The unresolved controversy stems from the question of whether there can be delayed hemorrhage after the second day or whether the ecchymosis that appears and becomes intense on the fourth and fifth days is merely blood that has been present since operation and now becomes obvious.

Complications

The most frequent complication is ecchymosis. Sometimes it is so extreme that it is debatable whether this type of surgery is justifiable. However, in the majority of patients, ecchymosis is moderate. Whether moderate or extreme, it is always gradually resorbed without permanent sequelae. Attempts have been made to find methods of eliminating ecchymosis entirely, but none have been successful.

When larger incisions were being used, we experimented with a long gauze bandage that was tied on the end of a stripper and pulled through the incision; it was permitted to lie in the incision for 10 or 15 minutes to compress small veins and absorb excess blood. This was of minimal value. A second maneuver was to insert perforated tubing (Hemovac suction tubes) the length of the incision and apply suction for two days. This seemed effective for the main trunk area, but it failed to adequately drain the area of tributaries. It did not seem of enough help to justify leaving a drain in place for 2 days and keeping the patient immobilized.

The most effective methods of dealing with ecchymosis are very slow stripping to stretch the veins and thus narrow the lumen and the application of pressure over the area where the trunk has been stripped out. Patience at this time is rewarded by a reduction in postoperative bleeding.

The amount of blood loss is estimated to be 300 to 800 cc. The hemoglobin drops 1 or 2 gm. If the patient enters the hospital with a low hemoglobin level, blood is administered during the operation. It is rarely necessary to give blood to a patient whose hemoglobin level is in the normal range.

INFECTION

By some standards, our operative preparation may seem inadequate, yet surprisingly few incisions become infected. It is our estimate that more than 200 patients are operated on each year for varicose veins and that the number of incisions averages more than 20 per limb, yet infected incisions are rare, several years passing between occurrences. The percentage of infection of incisions or of the patients has not been computed, because when infection does occur, it is localized to 1 incision of possibly 50. One patient, for example, had 7 parallel incisions approximately 1 inch apart on the lateral aspect of the thigh; the middle incision became grossly infected, while all the others healed *per primam*. With such a low incidence of infection, it is difficult to become involved in debates about the superiority of one kind of surgical preparation over another or about the need for prolonged preparation of the skin with antiseptics. We contemplate no change in our program of using ordinary ink for marking and painting rather than scrubbing the skin.

Minor infections are treated with compresses and/or the appropriate antibiotic. On one occasion an infected hematoma developed in the groin that required surgical drainage. This is the most serious infection we have encountered following this operative procedure.

NUMBNESS

Numbness near the incision at the internal malleolus is a frequent complication, due to tearing of small branches of the saphenous nerve as the vein is stripped out. Every attempt is made to separate the vein from the nerve prior to stripping, but the problem persists: approximately 20 to 25 per cent of the patients complain of numbness. Fortunately, the numbness gradually recedes, with return of sensation within a year.

NUMBNESS SECONDARY TO SECTION OF THE SURAL NERVE AT THE ANKLE

Inadvertent severance of the sural nerve results in permanent numbness on the lateral aspect of the foot and should be avoided at all cost. Normally the posterior tibial vein is isolated and a hemostat placed under it; however, this is not clamped until the sural nerve has been positively identified. In the uncomplicated case this is a very simple procedure, and it would be difficult to mistake the sural nerve and vein. However, in a patient with chronic venous insufficiency it is possible for the nerve and vein to be so tightly bound in scar tissue that it is nearly impossible to distinguish them. If such is the case, it is best to cut neither nerve nor vein but to leave the matted mass alone, rather than chance cutting the nerve. A simple expedient at times when it is impossible to differentiate between the two structures is to make a small vertical incision in the structure to determine whether it is a nerve or a vein.

OPERATIVE MORTALITY AND MORBIDITY

There have been no operative deaths in 2838 patients treated operatively for varicose veins; there was 1 patient with a precipitous fall in blood pressure on the operating table which necessitated cancellation of the procedure. Nonfatal small pulmonary embolism occurred in 3 patients (0.01%) postoperatively.

RECURRENT VARICOSITIES

A vein that has been removed cannot recur. However, venous trunks that are normal at the time of operation may dilate to become large varicosities. It is believed that the successful operative treatment of varicose veins is directly proportional to the extensiveness of the surgical excision of the existing varicosities and the division and ligation of all detectable perforating or communicating veins. Varicose veins may "recur," however, despite the most extensive surgical treatment possible. In our experience, the percentage of patients requiring reoperation for recurrent varices is 2 per cent of the females and 0.8 per cent of the males. One male

patient was unique in that he underwent excisional vein therapy twice by other surgeons and three times by our team. At each operation we removed every visible varicosity; nevertheless, within a few years he returned with large varicosities. In the female patient, the extent of recurrence after one or two pregnancies in the interim since initial operation is sometimes astounding. She originally presents with huge varicosities, and the entire long and short saphenous veins bilaterally are stripped out and 50 to 60 other incisions made over visible varicosities. However, 5 years later her extremities look as if they had never been operated on. This is a humbling experience. It is some consolation, however, that the patient is willing to undergo a second and even a third operation. When queried, the patient explains that the operation afforded such relief that she is more than willing to have the varicosities removed surgically a second time, and in some instance a third time.

Case Report 9-1

A 41-year-old male was referred in 1953 for large varicosities secondary to congenital arteriovenous fistula of the lower extremity (Fig. 9-14A) (see Color Plate II. B) He brought along this statement from the referring physician: "I will refer this patient to you if you promise never to discharge him." The patient had been living the life of a semirecluse because many people, including physicians, had told him that if he ever cut his lower extremity, he would bleed to death. He worked part time with his leg wrapped and participated in no other activities outside the home. The veins were so large that no attempt was made to use an intraluminal stripper. The veins were dissected out in three stages on January 18, 21, and 25, 1954.

As the first stage was being completed, he bled excessively. The incisions were reopened, and it appeared that the bleeding was originating from the accidental spearing of one small vein with a suture needle. At operation, the blood in the veins appeared to be under very high pressure. The veins were multiple not only in the horizontal plane, as can be detected from the picture, but also in the vertical plane, one trunk lying directly deep to another. In the first stage the veins of the thigh were excised; in the second stage the veins of the leg were excised; in the third stage the patient was placed in the prone position and the veins were excised posteriorly. A slough developed in a leg incision and had

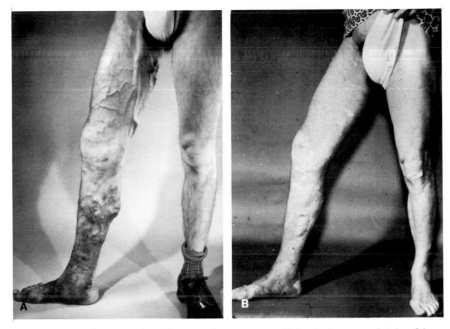

Figure 9-14. A. Large varicosities secondary to congenital arteriovenous fistula of lower extremity. (See Case Report 9-1.) Preoperative photo taken in 1953. **B.** Photo taken in 1969, 16 years after dissection of varicosities.

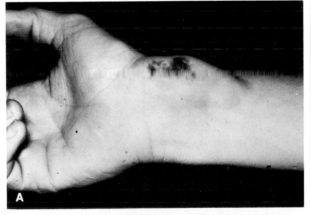

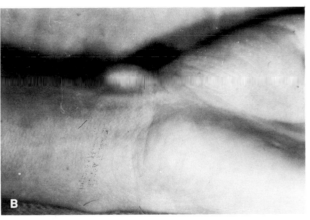

Figure 9-15. A, B, and **C.** Venous aneurysms of hand and arm treated by excision without difficulty.

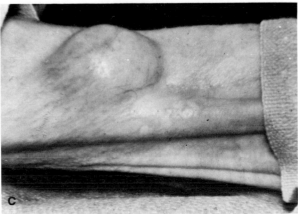

to be excised and grafted on February 2, 1954. After healing was complete, the patient was fitted with a heavyweight elastic stocking. It took a great deal of persuasion to convince him that he could lead a normal life without fear of hemorrhage. It was further explained to him that if bleeding did occur from a varicosity, he (or someone else) needed only elevate the limb and apply pressure with a handkerchief. He began to take up outside activities for the first time, including bowling. He has been our most grateful patient and in 20 years has had no additional treatment other than injection of sclerosing solution into a few small veins in the immediate postoperative period.

Figure 9-14B was taken in 1969. There has been no significant change since then.

VENOUS ANEURYSMS. Most venous aneurysms are found in varicosities of the lower extremity and frequently are mistaken for perforating veins. They are treated by excisional therapy, without difficulty. Venous aneurysms of the hand and arm (Fig. 9-15) are seen less often; however, they also are excised without complication.

COMPRESSIVE SCLEROTHERAPY. The fact that sclerotherapy combined with external compression does at times provide effective therapy for varicose veins encouraged us to search for alternate techniques to traditional excisional therapy that might prove more effective in a higher number of patients. Attempts are being made in our laboratory to do this by mechanical or electric intraluminal intimal destruction which, when combined with external compression, may offer a practical technique for outpatient surgical ablation of varicose veins.

CHRONIC VENOUS INSUFFICIENCY: THE POSTPHLEBITIC SYNDROME

Credit is given to Spender[6] and Gay[7] for first recognizing that all ulcerations of the leg are not caused by varicose veins. In 1868 Gay pointed out that aside from superficial varicosities, there might be other serious lesions affecting the arteries and the superficial and deep venous systems that would bring about ulceration. Homans in 1917[21] clearly distinguished between ulcers secondary to varicosities and those due to incompetent perforating veins. He introduced the term *postphlebitic ulceration* and noted that this variety of ulcers differed very significantly from all others. He was convinced that such ulceration was due to the destruction of the valves of the veins following thrombophlebitis that permitted seepage of blood from the deep veins toward the surface. Furthermore, he believed that the lymphatics, locally at least, were "crippled." In 1948 Linton and Hardy[19] used the term *postthrombotic syndrome* to take cognizance of the fact that many patients with typical symptoms of the postphlebitic syndrome have no clear-cut history of thrombophlebitis. The postphlebitic syndrome, when fully developed, is clearly identifiable clinically, so that a retrospective diagnosis of thrombophlebitis can be made.

CLINICAL SYNDROME

Classically, the patient reports that the limb was normal in all respects until it swelled greatly following a severe injury, an operation, or childbirth. A glimpse of the natural history of the disease without treatment can be obtained from patients who relate an episode of venous thrombosis antedating the advent of heparin and the prothrombin-depressant agents. Some of these elderly patients recall having been kept in bed for 6 to 8 months for treatment of the great swelling of the extremity, which gradually subsided. On questioning, however, they describe daily swelling of the ankle persisting after the swelling of the thigh and leg eventually disappeared. They further recall the onset of symptoms in the affected extremity, as contrasted to the normal limb. During the day the leg became tired and felt heavy or full, and on prolonged standing there was an aching pain in the muscles. Occasionally, as in patients with varicose veins, nocturnal muscular cramps occurred. Over a period of years, a brownish pigmentation discolored the skin of the lower leg, followed by weeping, irritation, "eczema," and, finally, ulceration.

The initial massive swelling of venous thrombosis is attributable to the thrombus completely blocking the main venous channels. In general, the massive swelling to the groin is an indication of occlusion of the superficial, deep, and common femoral, as well as saphenous, veins in the femoral triangle. The gradual disappearance of the swelling is attributable to the development of collaterals and the recanalization of the existing thrombosed veins (Fig. 9-16). The permanent daily swelling of the ankle is secondary to venous hypertension resulting from the now incompetent deep veins. Edwards and Edwards[16] demonstrated that the valves are destroyed in the resolution of the venous thrombus. Thus, daily edema of the ankle is the first permanent, visible consequence of deep venous thrombosis. It is believed that this first swelling consists merely of fluid transudate that is forced out of the circulating blood volume by the higher pressure at the venous end of the capillaries. The daily passage of this fluid through the capillary walls may be compared to a path through the woods. As it is used day by day, the path gradually widens. As the capillaries enlarge, not only fluid but also red cells, white cells, plasma proteins, and other constituents escape into the tissues. Once such elements have left the circulating blood volume, they cannot return, and therefore they accumulate in the tissue spaces instead. The red cells break down, and the hemosiderin thus deposited in the skin causes the typical brownish discoloration by which the venous origin of an ulcer is identified; without this discloration, some other basis must be sought for the ulcerating disease. Gradually the skin atrophies, the hair is lost, the skin becomes scaly, the subcutaneous tissues become indurated, and ultimately the skin ulcerates. The precise mechanism of the destruction of the subcutaneous tissues is not fully understood. However, the fact that the stages of the process are observed regularly

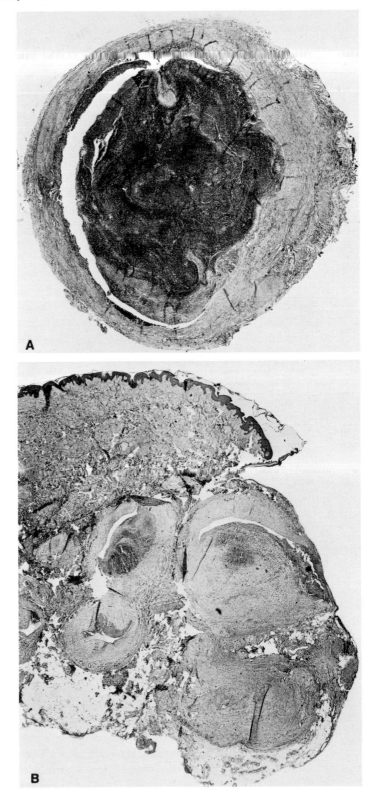

Figure 9-16. A. Vein that had thrombosed, beginning recanalization. **B.** Three veins that are thrombosed and partially recanalized. Any channel, regardless of size, that opens up through a thrombus transmits the full effect of hydrostatic pressure, as the pressure effect is not dependent upon the size of the lumen.

in the postphlebitic syndrome removes all doubt that such degenerative events are related to the basic pathology, i.e., the acquired insufficiency of the venous heart.

The symptoms and swelling are aggravated by sitting or standing still. This observation has partly led to the coinage of the terms "stasis" syndrome and "stasis" ulcer; these terms are not at all appropriate, since they imply that the blood is at a standstill. The total bloodflow out of the limb must at all times equal the volume flowing into the limb; therefore, it is doubtful that the blood is ever completely stagnant in any given portion of the limb. Furthermore, the postphlebitic ulcer is quite vascular; on arteriograms the rate of bloodflow through an ulcerated area appears faster than normal.[1] Blalock[22] showed that the oxygen content of venous blood is not diminished in a patient with varicose veins. Linton et al.[23] confirmed this observation and also demonstrated that this held true even in the presence of chronic postthrombotic ulceration. Finally, the extreme vascularity of an ulcerated area can be observed at operation, even with the limb in the elevated position; the blood frequently appears to be arterial or semiarterial in nature, suggesting that the passage of blood through the area of venous ulceration is swifter than normal if anything and is far from stationary or at a quiet "ebb-tide" level. In view of such experimental and clinical evidence, *postthrombotic syndrome* is probably the most appropriate term for chronic venous insufficiency secondary to incompetent deep veins, but has not become as popular in clinical usage as postphlebitic syndrome.

Patients with various stages of this syndrome are encountered in the vascular clinic or in the practice of vascular surgery. Many patients with pigmented or indurated legs without ulceration show no visible varicosities. In such cases, one may assume that the valves of the deep veins are incompetent but those of the communicating veins are still intact. At a later time, when ulceration occurs, varicose veins are almost invariably present. They may not be visible; however, they can be palpated as soft, lacuna-like areas in otherwise woody, dense tissue. They also can be observed at operation. Such varicosities are considered secondary because they result from an elevated venous pressure transmitted to them through incompetent communicating veins from the deep system.

MANAGEMENT OF THE POSTPHLEBITIC SYNDROME

Control of the postphlebitic syndrome essentially means control of the edema that follows the episode of venous thrombosis (Fig. 9-17). If a patient seeks treatment prior to the actual development of an ulcer, further progression of the disease is almost always prevented if the edema is controlled. In many patients, ulceration has already occurred and healed; by control of the edema, recurrent ulceration is prevented. Control of edema is absolutely essential to the prevention of the postphlebitic syndrome; similarly, sufficient support is the *sine qua non* of any program to combat swelling in the extremity after thrombosis. The *degree* of exogenous support necessary to restore the sufficiency of the damaged venous pump is not widely recognized; therefore, the following is an elaboration of the quality, characteristics, and duration of such support.

Elastic Stockings

Without question, a truly heavyweight two-way stretch elastic stocking is of the greatest value in the treatment of peripheral venous disease. To be effective, support stockings must be heavy enough to control edema and comfortable enough to be worn by patients. However, surprisingly few commercially available elastic stockings are designed to offer an adequate degree of support to control the swelling in the postphlebitic extremity. They are not at all helpful in preventing progress of the disease since edema is not controlled and therefore the symptoms persist. The most that can be hoped for is that the sequelae will advance at a slower pace, delaying the onset of ulceration. On the other hand, the physician need only prescribe (and the patient wear) an elastic stocking heavy enough to control edema for the disease process to be effectively halted (Table 9-7). Hundreds of patients seen in our practice in various stages of the postphlebitic syndrome, including those recently treated for acute deep venous thrombosis, have been successfully managed by elastic support stockings heavy enough to control edema;* nothing else is required.

---

* The elastic stocking regularly prescribed is manufactured by Surgical Appliance Industries, Cincinnati, OH.

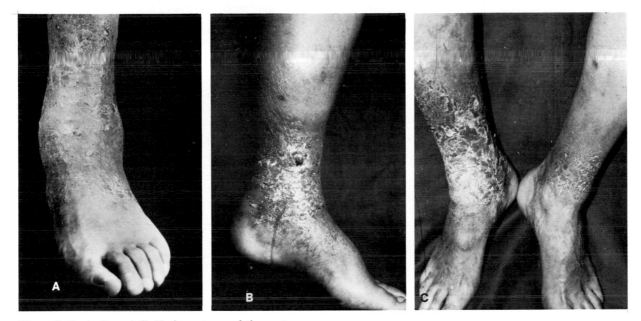

Figure 9-17. A, B, and **C.** Various stages of the postphlebitic syndrome prior to ulceration.

Knee-length elastic stockings are prescribed for the great majority of patients. Occasionally, high-thigh stockings may be worn in the acute postphlebitic period; after a few months, however, these are replaced by below-knee stockings. Stockings that extend above the knee are usually uncomfortable, and patients cannot be expected to continue using them for any length of time. If the swelling of the thigh is of such magnitude as to cause severe discomfort, the patient is advised to continue wearing high-thigh or mid-thigh stockings. However, if the swelling of the thigh, although visible, is

neither disabling nor uncomfortable, he is advised to accept a below-knee stocking for two reasons. First, in our experience, swelling of the thigh is relatively innocuous; only one patient has been encountered with ulceration of the thigh believed to be venous in origin, whereas uncontrolled swelling of the ankle or lower leg frequently results in the typical postphlebitic syndrome and ulceration. Secondly, the knee-length stocking is quite comfortable, unlike the one which extends to the thigh, and is readily accepted for long-term use.

It is most unusual for any stocking but the heavyweight one to be of value in the postphlebitic syndrome. However, very occasionally, a lighter-weight stocking may prove satisfactory. An exceptional patient may be able to discard elastic support with no further progression of the syndrome. These exceptions could be explained by the fact that a rather short segment of the common femoral vein is occluded by thrombus, resulting in great swelling. However, if propagation of the clot is prevented by heparin therapy, the swelling may disappear when this segment of vein recanalizes. Because the main segment of the superficial femoral vein and the veins of the leg were not thrombosed, their valves remain competent. In the few instances in which this has occurred, heparin therapy was begun early.

TABLE 9-7. 869 Extremities With Postphlebitic Syndrome Without Ulceration

	NO. LIMBS	LATER ULCER	%
Conservative treatment			
Swelling with or without pigmentation and induration	832	10	1.2
Dermatitis	37	3	8.0
Total	869	13	1.5

In patients with swelling associated with varicose veins but without the postphlebitic syndrome, stockings of less weight may be beneficial.

All patients with acute deep venous thrombosis and all patients with the postphlebitic syndrome, whether treated surgically or conservatively, are told that their condition is incurable. It is pointed out that they are suffering not from a "disease" but rather from a physical or hydraulic abnormality. Therefore, they must wear elastic support for life, just as a person with poor vision must wear glasses for life. The occasional exception to the rule has been described above, viz., the patient with a circumscribed area of superficial femoral vein thrombosis treated early by heparin, whose lower leg valves remain competent, and who therefore is free of residual swelling. To allow for this exception and to give all patients hope, they are told that daily swelling of the ankle does no great harm unless it occurs for a long period of time. For this reason, they are encouraged to occasionally try going without the stocking, once a year. If there is no swelling, the stocking does not need to be worn. However, when swelling recurs and is detectable at the end of the day, they must resume wearing the stocking. The patient is also advised that if he is able to find a lightweight stocking that controls edema and is comfortable, he is free to use it. In most instances the heavyweight stocking is sufficiently comfortable that the patient willingly wears it for life.

ULCERATIONS SECONDARY TO VENOUS INSUFFICIENCY

INTRODUCTION

Ulcerations of the skin of the leg secondary to venous insufficiency (Table 9-8), whether due to incompetent superficial veins, deep veins, or both superficial and deep veins, differ from one another in two respects: Ulcers due to incompetent superficial veins heal relatively rapidly and are considered curable; radical removal of the varices results in a normal extremity without swelling. Ulcers due to incompetent deep veins, with or without a superficial component (Table 9-9), heal far more slowly and are not curable, even with surgical excision of the incompetent veins. These ulcers are only controllable; unless elastic support is worn for life to control the edema, the ulceration inevitably recurs (Figs. 9-18 and 9-19).

ETIOLOGY AND PATHOLOGY

The causative factors and the basic pathology of venous ulceration do not differ from chronic venous insufficiency without ulceration. (See foregoing sections on etiology and pathology of varicose veins.)

DIAGNOSIS

As a rule, venous ulcers are diagnosable at a glance. One need only observe the brownish pigmentation caused by the deposition of hemosiderin in the

TABLE 9-8. Venous Incompetency With Ulceration

	NO. LIMBS	%
Secondary to varicose veins	392	30
Secondary to deep veins	916	70

TABLE 9-9. 916 Limbs With Ulceration Secondary to Deep Veins

CONTRIBUTING CAUSES	NO. LIMBS	%
History of deep venous thrombosis*	852	93.0
Trauma	230	24.0
Operation	146	16.0
Childbirth	137	15.0
Bed rest	51	5.5
Sclerosing solution	14	1.5
Total	578	63.0
Etiologic factor unknown	274	30.0
Probably silent venous thrombosis	64	7.0
Total	338	37.0

* In these instances the patient was either told he had "thrombophlebitis" or gave a clear-cut history of trauma or illness during which time swelling of the limb occurred and persisted thereafter.

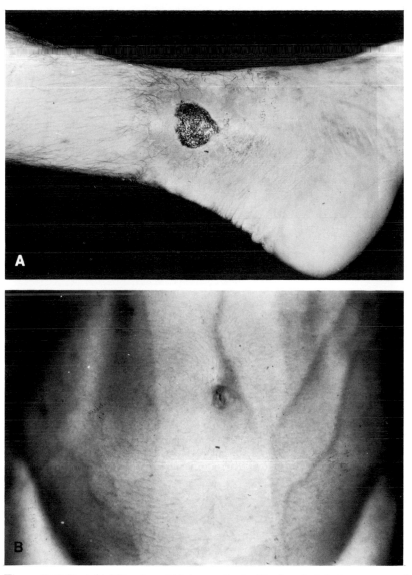

Figure 9-18. Postphlebitic ulcer (**A**) in a patient with chronic inferior vena caval obstruction (**B**).

tissues to be certain of the venous origin of the lesion (See Color Plate, II. C). Indeed, such discoloration is the *sine qua non* of the correct diagnosis; its absence should immediately cast doubt on a venous origin of the ulcer. However, in the non-Caucasian races, the pigmentation may be obscured by the natural dark color of the skin. Also, when acute cellulitis is present in the area of ulceration, the pigmentation may be bright red (see Color Plate II. D and E). Once the infection is

under control, the pigmented area reverts to the typical light tan of hematoid debris (see Color Plate II. F).

The most common site for venous ulceration is the medial surface of the lower third of the leg, just above the ankle; other locations include the lateral aspect above and below the malleolus (see Color Plate II. C). Generally, if an ulcer occurs on the lateral aspect, one will have previously existed on the medial aspect of the limb. The typical ve-

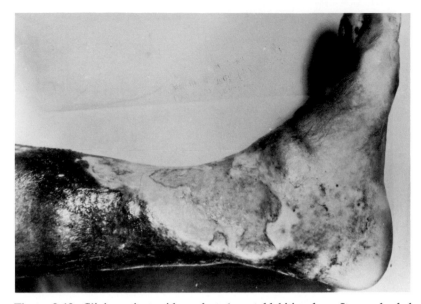

Figure 9-19. Clinic patient with neglected postphlebitic ulcer. It was healed many times in the clinic, but the patient would not wear heavyweight support and would eventually return with recurrent ulceration. Deeply pigmented areas of skin represent previous ulcerations.

nous ulcer is irregular in outline, and it may be large or small. It may be filled with granulation tissue or may be strikingly necrotic. However, the ulceration does not penetrate the deep fascia, as occurs with the arterial ulcer. Penetration of the deep fascia has occasionally been observed in a patient with venous ulceration and associated oblit-erative arterial disease or in a bedridden patient with ulceration complicated by pressure necrosis secondary to resting the ulcerated area on the bed. The presence of deep fascial involvement is of great help in the distinguishing of some arterial ulcers from ulcers of venous origin. Arterial lesions are usually sharply circumscribed and nummular and, as has been said, penetrate the deep fascial layers. An important distinction is the greater amount of pain associated with an arterial ulcer. Patients may be seen with huge venous ulcers that cause them little pain. Large venous ulcers at times are ex-tremely "dirty" (see Color Plate II. G) and appear to be heavily infected, without signs of systemic in-fection. One can frequently observe large varicosi-ties extending directly into the base of the ulcer that is secondary to chronic venous insufficiency of the superficial system (Table 9-8). The pa-tient with an ulcer that is secondary to the post-thrombotic syndrome gives a history of deep venous thrombosis, either overt or related to him by his physician, or recollects an injury to the limb (Table 9-9). In clinical practice the final proof of diagnosis is response to treatment, since it is rare that a venous ulcer cannot be healed.

MANAGEMENT

Initial Healing of the Ulcer

There are two axioms in the management of venous ulcers.

AXIOM 1

Any venous ulcer will heal if the limb can be main-tained above heart level.

There are no exceptions to this rule. Inherent in its application, however, are two limiting provisos: first, the patient must be free of associated oblitera-tive arterial disease with ischemic symptoms, and second, he must not be in cardiac decompensation. Elevation of the limb of a patient with advanced arteriosclerosis obliterans would cause intolerable rest pain; in a patient in congestive heart failure, elevation would add to his difficulty in breathing.

AXIOM 2

All venous ulcers can be healed in the ambulatory patient if the limb can be bandaged tightly enough for a sufficient period of time and if the patient can walk normally. If the patient is crippled or lives a wheelchair existence, this technique will not work. It is also exceedingly difficult to heal an ulcer by this method if the patient is not able to flex his hip, knee, or ankle normally due to crippling arthritis or to surgical fusion. Also exceptions to this axiom are those patients with certain hypersensitivities, such as to the adhesive, the elastic, some element of the bandages, or their own secretions and/or the organisms contained in detritus from the area of ulceration. Under these circumstances, pressure dressings cannot be tolerated.

Elevation

The concept of maintaining the limb above heart level is basically simple, yet many difficulties are encountered in carrying out this directive. Despite daily indoctrination of the nursing personnel in the importance of proper elevation, the physician must look in on his patients personally one or more times a day to assure himself that the limbs are indeed elevated above heart level. Figure 9-20 **A** and **B** shows two methods of achieving elevation. In **A**, 6-inch wooden blocks are placed under the foot of the bed; this is a convenient, practical method of providing an inclined plane which permits the patient to roll and turn and to be quite comfortable. Pillows may be used under his head. In **B**, steep elevation is shown. This method is used for patients with acute thrombophlebitis and lymphedema. It cannot be used for long periods of time because it forces the patient to remain on his back at all times, an uncomfortable position. Figure 9-20 **C** and **D** shows improper elevation, in which elevation of the limbs is lost by greater elevation of the head of the bed. Figure 9-20 **C** depicts elevation of the gatch of the bed while the knee is down, thus forcing the knee to hyperextend; this causes the patient such discomfort that he rebels against maintaining this position. Figure 9-20 **D** shows the futility of attempting elevation by using pillows. By carefully packing under the limb with pillows, good elevation is achieved—for a few minutes. As soon as the patient moves, the effectiveness of this elevation is lost. The pillows tend to migrate

to the ankles, causing painful hyperextension of the knees, or they gravitate up under the knees and cause loss of elevation at the ankles, The physician seems to be waging a losing campaign in his efforts to obtain proper elevation; his only recourse is personal inspection one or more times a day to make certain that the limb is being maintained above heart level and that the ulcer is healing (Fig. 9-21).

LOCAL TREATMENT

With proper elevation, the ulcer will heal; it does not matter what local treatment is used. The ulcer may be left open to the air; this is sometimes very helpful when there is severe skin irritation. However, it may cause some soiling of the bedclothes or prove offensive in some other way. The leg may be wrapped. Any desired local agent may be used, although this is not recommended, primarily because it is counter to the belief that elevation, rather than medication, is curative. The simplest method of local treatment is to apply gauze moistened with saline solution to the ulcerated area. Only *one* piece of gauze is moistened, that which is placed on the ulcer; the rest of the bandage is dry and soft. The purpose is not to saturate the limb with a wet dressing, as this would only increase maceration. It is a deplorable practice to place a dressing on an ulcerated limb and pour saline solution over it every 4 hours to keep it wet; this drenching naturally defeats the very purpose of treatment. Indeed, if the ulcer itself is very moist, dry dressings may be applied. However, whether the ulcer is dry or moist, the dressings should be changed four times daily. It is the change that is important. The exudate and necrotic material absorbed by the dressing are removed; this is the gentlest form of debridement. Gauze moistened with saline solution (which is innocuous and inexpensive) absorbs the detritus rapidly and feels comfortable to the patient's skin.

Pressure Bandaging

In practice, approximately 85 per cent of venous ulcers can be healed by the use of pressure bandages while the patient usually continues his daily activities (see Color Plate III. J). The exact number (Table 9-10) who can be handled in this manner depends on the effort willing to be expended and the comfort and convenience of the patient. Some patients develop sensitivity to various elements of

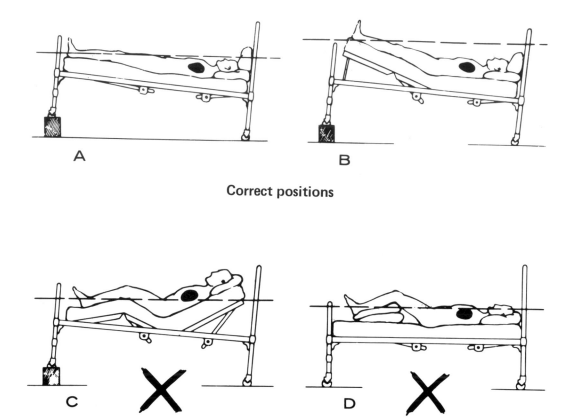

Correct positions

Incorrect positions

Figure 9-20. Correct and incorrect methods of obtaining elevation of the limbs above heart level. **A.** Six-inch wooden blocks placed under foot of bed. **B.** Steep elevation is shown, method used for acute thrombophlebitis and lymphedema. **C** and **D.** Incorrect elevation.

the pressure bandage. In these instances, rather than persist in causing great discomfort and doing more harm than good, the patient is admitted to the hospital for elevation treatment or remains at home in bed with the limbs above heart level.

The basic problem of ulceration is faulty hydrau-

lics. To paraphrase Wright,[24] if one sets the faulty hydraulics straight, the ulcer will heal. Control of leg edema is the crux of the problem; this can be accomplished by applying adequate pressure to the extremity.

The techniques described below (Fig. 9-22) are neither original nor unique. Many methods can be employed to apply pressure; however, the bandage must be smooth and the pressure distributed evenly. Ideally, the bandage extends from the metatarsal heads to the tibial tubercles. An intelligent patient may be taught to bandage his own leg; instructions have been given by telephone and by letter. The one secret to success is the application of sufficient pressure to control the edema. Otherwise, failure results from insufficient pressure to abet the venous

TABLE 9-10. 1308 Limbs With Ulceration: Initial Healing

	NO. LIMBS	%
Healed with pressure	1158	88.5
Healed with bed rest and elevation	103	8.0
Healed with excision and grafting	47	3.5

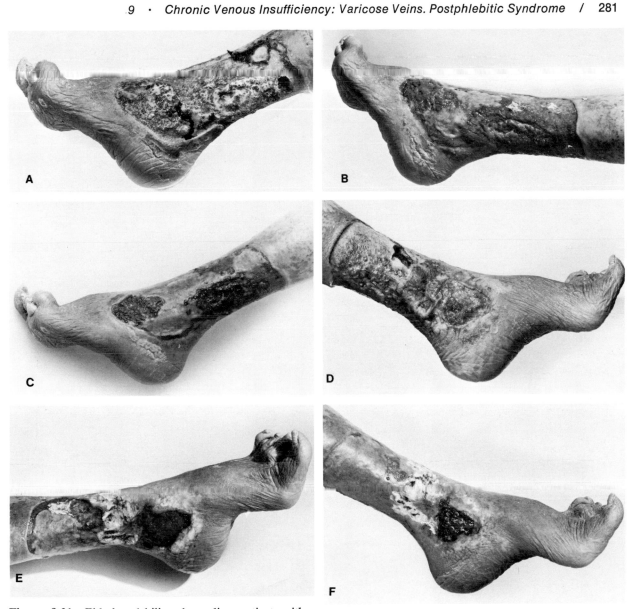

Figure 9-21. Elderly, debilitated cardiac patient with chronic venous ulceration of left lower extremity, aggravated by constant sitting in a chair, due to dyspnea. While her cardiac status was being treated, she was placed in the V position so that her legs and lungs were elevated. **A** (lateral) and **D** (medial). Ulcerated areas as of January 9, 1974; treatment by saline dressings changed four times daily and a minimal amount of debridement begun. **B** (lateral) and **E** (medial). Ulcerations as of January 20, 1974. **C** (lateral) and **F** (medial). Ulcers on January 29, 1974, showing remarkable healing in 20 days; patient had to be transferred to an extended care facility in the care of another physician.

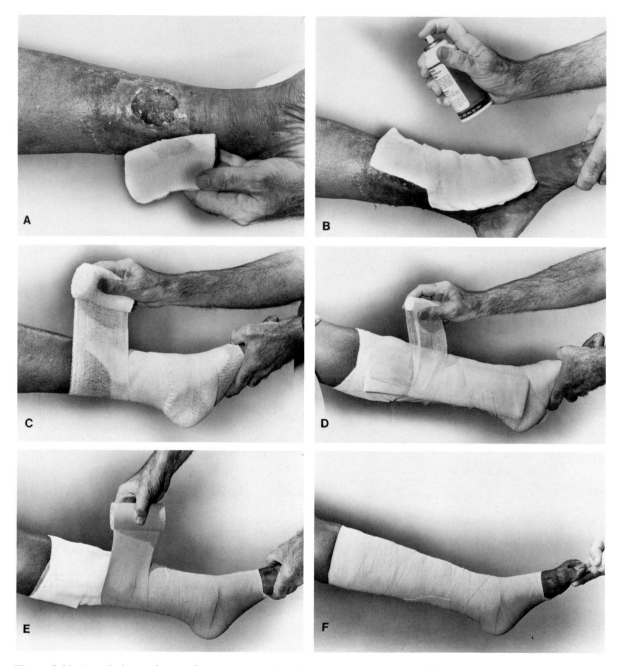

Figure 9-22. A technique of wrapping a venous ulcer. **A.** A 4 × 4 gauze containing a water soluble base (Aquaphor) is applied to ulcer. **B.** Several pieces of gauze are placed on instep to protect against undue pressure at this point. Limb is sprayed with benzoin to help prevent slippage of the bandage. **C.** Soft gauze roll is placed on the limb to protect the skin from adhesive. All bandaging starts at the ankle and is continued down to the metatarsal heads, back up to the tibial tubercle, then down to the ankle again. **D.** A strip of cellucotton is placed over the area of ulceration and along the course of the saphenous vein and held in place by roller gauze. **E.** A 4-inch wide elastic with adhesive is applied tightly; pressure is decreased slightly over instep. It is the compression that does the healing. **F.** Completed bandage. It is worn for 1 week, although it may be left in place for 2 weeks if desired.

return; the limb will not heal, regardless of ancillary measures to combat the infection that is undoubtedly present. Even today many patients are encountered who have been under treatment for months and even years with local antibiotic agents to no avail, only to have the chronic ulcer heal promptly within a few weeks, or months at the most, by the simple application of adequate pressure (Figs. 9-23 and 9-24).

Local Treatment

The ulcerated area is covered with gauze and an innocuous, water-soluble base (Aquaphor), which is used to prevent the bandage from sticking. A small amount of benzoin is sprayed on the rest of the leg to prevent slippage of the bandage. The entire area to which pressure is to be applied is then wrapped using a roll of soft gauze.

Bandaging is started at the point of ulceration and is carried down to the base of the metatarsal heads, back up to the tibial tubercles, and then back down to the area of ulceration. Once the gauze is in place, a padding of cellucotton for extra pressure is applied over the area of ulceration. When the ulcer is on the medial aspect of the leg, the padding extends up the entire length of the leg over the course of the long saphenous vein. The pad is held in place using a roll of gauze. It is believed that the use of cellucotton to apply extra pressure is preferable to sponge rubber.

The heart of the boot is then applied. It consists of elastoplast, 4 inches in width, as recommended by Wright.[24] It is applied as snugly as possible; the greatest pressure is exerted from ankle to knee, and it is somewhat less firm over the instep. It is difficult to apply the boot too tightly; the patient generally feels better when the fit is very snug and will complain on his next visit if the bandaging is applied loosely. The dressing is changed weekly. In patients who have large amounts of exudate, it may be changed twice a week. When healing is progressing satisfactorily without much drainage, the dressing is changed every second week.

After the ulcer begins to turn clean and if the patient is intelligent, rubberized bandages are substituted for the elastoplast dressing. Two 4-inch-wide rubberized bandages are placed tightly over one another in order to apply sufficient pressure to

heal the ulcer. This is advantageous to the patient's comfort and sense of well-being, since it permits him to change the dressing every night. In this way, he can shower comfortably and sleep without a bandage, but with his limbs elevated. This may result in some soiling of the bedclothes, but exposure of the ulcer to the air and removal of the restrictive bandage are very helpful in relieving skin irritation and in accelerating the subsidence of skin reaction.

An alternate method is based on the method advocated by Unna.[25] Occasionally, skin irritation reaches such magnitude that the patient cannot tolerate the elastoplast bandage. In this case, a bandage impregnated with calomine lotion may be superior in aiding healing. Bandages simulating Unna's original paste boot are now available commercially.

DEFINITIVE TREATMENT AFTER HEALING OF THE ULCERATION

After the ulceration has healed, the surgeon reassesses the entire clinical history of the patient in order to arrive at a decision as to the advisability of surgical treatment.

If the ulcer was due to incompetent superficial veins, surgical treatment is recommended unless contraindications are present, e.g., age, debility, or other illnesses. The patient is informed that the operation is elective and need not be performed if he is willing to wear heavyweight surgical hose for life. He can confidently be told, however, that surgical treatment will make his limb more comfortable and that at most he would be obliged to wear a lightweight elastic support. When offered the probability of being free of the need to wear support, most patients choose surgical treatment (Table 9-11).

TABLE 9-11. 392 Limbs With Ulceration Secondary to Superficial Incompetent Veins

TREATMENT AFTER INITIAL HEALING	NO.	%
Conservative	218	56
Surgical		
Division, ligation, and stripping of incompetent veins	174	44

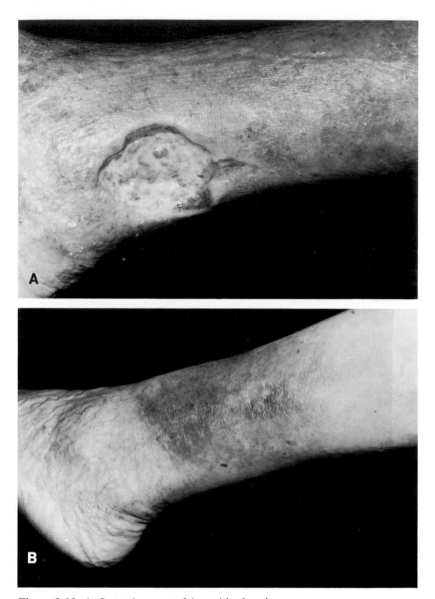

Figure 9-23. A. Lateral aspect of leg with chronic venous disease. **B.** Lateral aspect 11 months later, after treatment by pressure bandages and ambulation.

Surgical Treatment for Chronic Venous Insufficiency Due to Incompetent Superficial Veins

The operation is the same as that carried out for primary varicosities without ulceration, i.e., the most radical removal of all incompetent veins, including those directly under the site of previous ulceration. (See the foregoing section for operative technique under Varicose Veins.)

CHRONIC VENOUS INSUFFICIENCY DUE TO INCOMPETENT DEEP VEINS: THE POSTPHLEBITIC SYNDROME WITH ULCERATION

Conservative Treatment

A different situation prevails when the ulceration was secondary to incompetence of the deep venous system (Table 9-12). The patient is told that a

Figure 9-24. A. Patient with venous ulcer of left leg, lateral aspect. **B.** Close up of ulcer, lateral aspect. **C.** Medial aspect. **D.** Medial aspect 6 months later. **E.** One year later. Lateral aspect took a full year to heal. Patient had an invalid wife and refused hospitalization. Dressings could not be applied for a week at a time due to the tremendous amount of drainage. Therefore, patient was taught to elevate foot of his bed and to wrap his leg tightly each day. He required 9 months for the medial aspect of the leg to heal and a year for the lateral aspect to heal. However, the patient was able to work daily and to care for his wife.

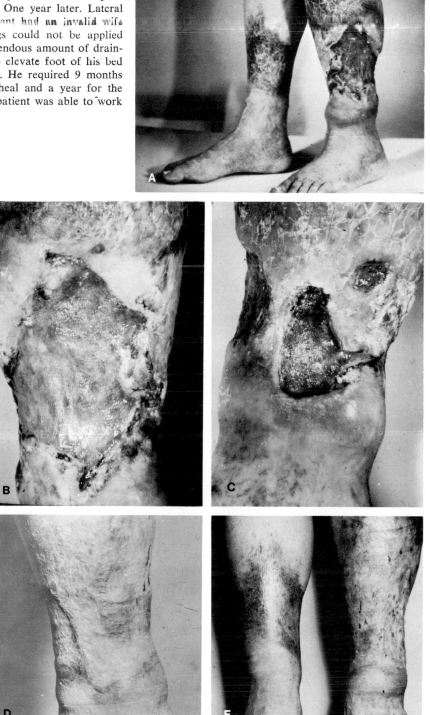

heavyweight surgical stocking will have to be worn for life and that no surgical treatment is available which will eliminate this need. He is advised to leave the foot of his bed elevated and to wear the heavyweight stocking on a trial basis. If he remains healed and is comfortable, surgical treatment is not recommended. If ulceration recurs while the patient is faithfully wearing the heavyweight stocking, then the ulcer is healed as before and surgical treatment is recommended.

If there is recurrent ulceration, every effort is made to elicit a truthful account of whether or not elastic support was continually worn. Many times the patient hesitates to admit having discarded the stocking. If he is told that complete candor on his part allows him to be treated more intelligently, he may acknowledge that he stopped wearing the support because he was getting along so well. He will also acknowledge that he was reminded on every office visit that the stocking must be worn for life. Only recurrence of the ulceration convinced him that he could not discard support except when actually in bed or bathing.

Surgical Treatment

When surgical treatment is elected, the procedure is that described by Linton;[19] however, division and

TABLE 9-12. 916 Limbs With Ulceration Secondary to Incompetent Deep Veins

TREATMENT AFTER INITIAL HEALING	NO. (%)
Conservative	711 (77.6)
Surgical	205 (22.4)
Stripping long and short saphenous veins and ligation of communicating veins	175 (85)
Above plus ligation of femoral vein	30 (15)

ligation of the superficial femoral vein are presently not included.

The essential elements of the Linton procedure (Fig. 9-25) are (1) division and ligation of the communicating veins subfascially on the medial aspect of the leg; (2) fenestration in the fascia of the posterior aspect of the leg to permit radical excision and stripping of the short saphenous vein from the foot to just below the knee; (3) routine careful dissection of the saphenous trunk in the groin and ligation flush with the femoral vein, with division of all tributaries; (4) stripping of the long saphenous trunk from the groin to the ankle or foot; and (5) removal of any visible or palpable varicosities in the leg.

POSTOPERATIVE CARE

The leg is carefully wrapped with soft gauze; pressure padding is placed along the line of the main incision in the leg. A plaster cast may be used, as recommended by Linton. In recent years, however, our preference has been to use rubberized bandages, just as when uncomplicated varicosities have been surgically removed. The patient remains in bed 7 to 10 days with the extremity elevated above heart level.

Complications

Early in our experience, the most frequent complication was sloughing of the skin edge. When this occurs, the best treatment is that recommended by Linton, viz., immediate excision of the slough and application of a split-thickness skin graft. A great amount of healing time is saved in this way. Permitting the slough to separate by itself or excising it and permitting the wound to granulate and heal by secondary intention involves months of treatment. However, when small, the slough may be

TABLE 9-13. Interval to Recurrent Ulceration in 929 Extremities Treated Conservatively

ULCERATION SECONDARY TO	NO. EXTREMITIES	NO. RECURRENCES (%)	< 1 YR NO. (%)	1–5 YR NO. (%)	6–10 YR NO. (%)	> 10 YR NO. (%)
Superficial venous disease	218	10 (4.6)	4 (40)	4 (40)	1 (10)	1 (10)
Deep venous disease	711	108 (15.0)	13 (12)	76 (70)	17 (16)	2 (2)

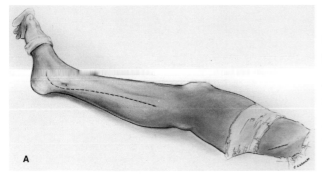

A

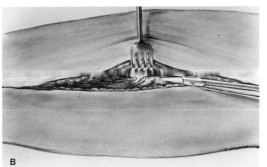

B

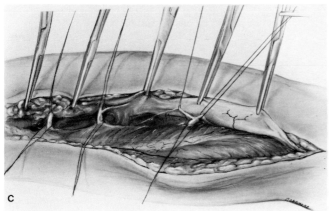

C

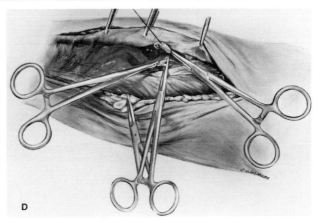

D

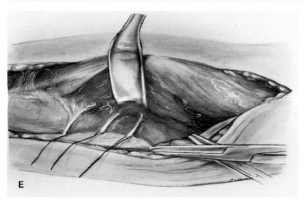

E

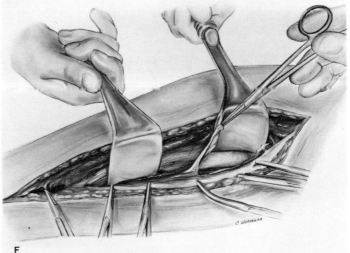

F

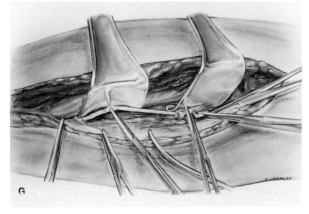

G

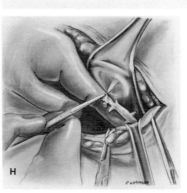

H

Fig. 9-25.
(*Legend for Fig. 9-25 on page 289*)

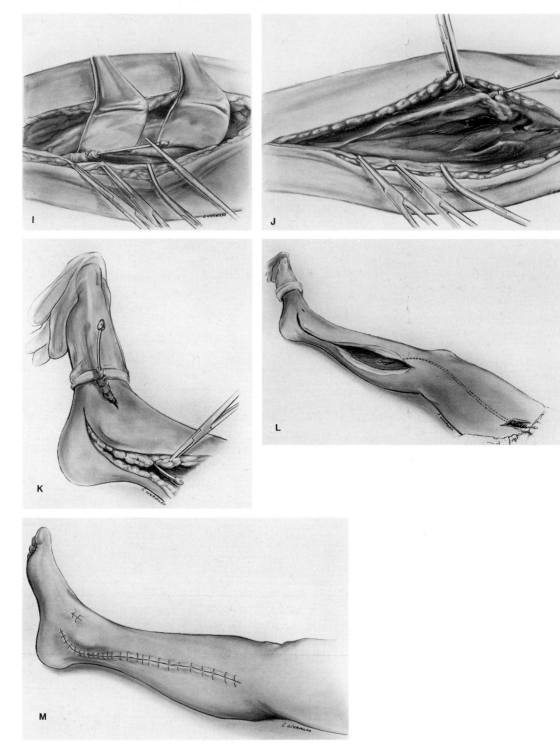

Figure 9-25. Linton procedure: subfascial ligation of communicating veins; stripping and excision of long and short saphenous veins; fasciectomy. **A.** The line of skin incisions. At operation the limbs are elevated 15° to 20°. **B.** Incision is made directly down to the fascia. Any bleeding varices are temporarily ligated. Fascia is cut the length of the incision with a scissors. **C.** After fascia has been cut, it is retracted with a Kocher-type clamp, and the communicating veins can be seen. Their number varies considerably. Normal communicating veins are approximately 1, or possibly 2, mm in diameter. In a patient with chronic venous insufficiency of an advanced nature, they may be 3 to 5 mm in diameter. **D.** Each individual communicating vein is divided and ligated. It is best to ligate them as they are encountered. If they are pulled out of the fascia, it is difficult to control the bleeding. One clamp occludes two divisions of the vein; these are divided and ligated individually. **E.** Posterior fascia is seized with Kocher clamps, and the muscles are separated from the fascia with the fingers and then retracted laterally. This exposes the posterior communicating veins. **F.** A window, approximately 2 × 20 cm, is made in posterior fascia. **G.** The window in the fascia permits visualization of the short saphenous vein and multiple tributaries. The sural nerve is found slightly lateral to the vein and is spared. The sural nerve is not shown in the figure. **H.** Short saphenous vein is traced as far as possible in the wound and is ligated close to popliteal vein with 2–0 silk. **I.** A stripper is inserted into short saphenous vein and pulled through a small incision on lateral aspect of the foot. **J.** Attention is then directed to long saphenous vein, which is dissected free and a stripper inserted, being brought out through a small incision distal to internal malleolus. Any remaining portions of saphenous system that can be seen are dissected out at this time. However, care must be taken not to raise a flap near the ankle, as it is apt to cause a slough. **K.** A small section of long saphenous vein being stripped out without raising a skin flap. **L.** Saphenous vein in groin is treated in usual manner for excising varicose veins, and a stripper is inserted to the main incision below the knee and the trunk pulled through. **M.** Fascia of the leg is closed with heavy absorbable sutures. Nylon skin sutures are used (4–0). In upper portion of the incision or in any portion where skin appears to be normal, mattress sutures are used. However, simple through-and-through sutures are used in areas near the ankle where skin is atrophied.

managed in this way, and the patient may be seen on an out-patient basis after discharge from the hospital while treatment with pressure dressings is continued, just as in the preoperative period. This regimen is less desirable than immediate excision of the slough and application of a split-thickness skin graft.

The cardinal principle in avoiding sloughing is to use meticulous care not to undermine the skin while making the incision and to reduce dissection of the subcutaneous tissue to the absolute minimum while excising the varicosities. The incision should go straight through the skin, subcutaneously down through the fascia. Stripping a vein through subcutaneous tissue, whether it is normal or whether it is grossly indurated as in the postphlebitic syndrome, is less traumatic and causes less total tissue destruction than dissecting a vein out under direct vision by undermining a flap. Analogously, the narrower the path through the woods, the fewer the trees that are destroyed.

Often the varicosities in the postphlebitic limb do not protrude from the skin but are actually lakes or lacunae in dense fibrous tissue. At times they are small, causing the inexperienced surgeon to wonder how they can be so important. The incompetence of the valves, rather than the size of the veins, is significant. Pressure is transmitted through a small tubular incompetent vein just as effectively as through a large vein, as it is not related to the size of the fluid-containing tube.

FOLLOW-UP CARE

As a rule, the patient is discharged from the hospital 10 to 12 days postoperatively, wearing elastic wraps on his limb. The sutures are left in place in the lower part of his leg when he leaves the hospital; these are removed at the office when it seems appropriate, possibly in 2 or 3 weeks. When the limb is fully healed, he is fitted with an elastic stocking. The foot of his bed is usually maintained 6 inches above the floor for at least 6 months postoperatively. These patients are never "discharged" but are advised to return for a check-up once a year or whenever the leg becomes uncomfortable (Figs. 9-26 to 9-28).

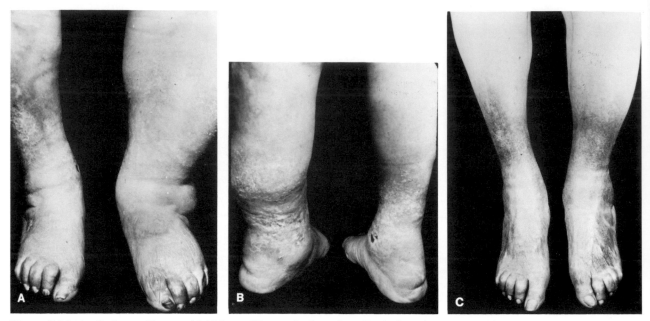

Figure 9-26. A. Patient with postphlebitic swelling and ulceration. Typical neglected postphlebitic syndrome. Frontal view. **B.** Posterior view. **C.** Patient was treated by bed rest, elevation, and saline compresses until ulcerated areas were healed; bilateral Linton operation was then performed. Control of edema is not maintained unless heavyweight elastic stocking is worn, except when patient is in bed.

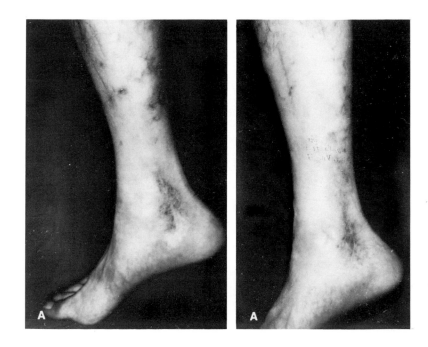

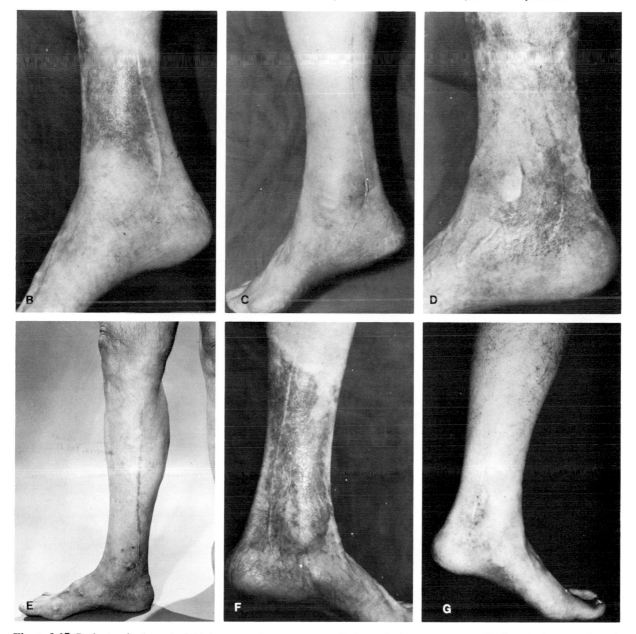

Figure 9-27. Patients who have had Linton procedures are never discharged; they return annually for checkup or when the extremity becomes uncomfortable. **A.** Left and right views of patient with 19-year follow-up. **B.** Patient with 17-year follow-up. **C.** Patient with 14-year follow-up. **D.** Patient with 12-year follow-up. **F.** Patient with 7-year follow-up. **G.** Patient with 9-year follow-up right leg and 4-year left leg.

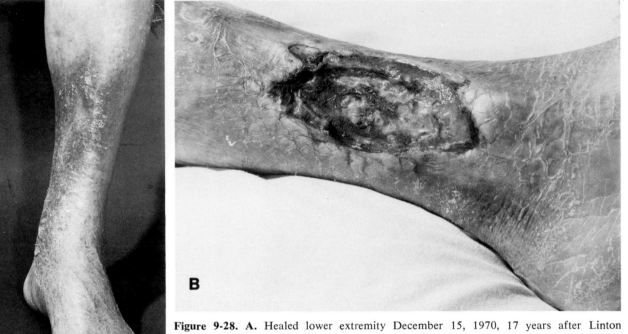

Figure 9-28. A. Healed lower extremity December 15, 1970, 17 years after Linton procedure for recurrent ulceration of leg. The ulceration had recurred innumerable times over a period of 12 years prior to treatment. **B.** Same limb October 21, 1971. Patient had developed severe arterial insufficiency with amputation of his opposite limb. Being old and debilitated, he could no longer use his elastic stocking but sat in a wheelchair most of the day. A new ulcer developed which was both venous and arterial. Note necrosis of fascia. This limb came to amputation.

Skin Grafting

Only rarely is it necessary to employ skin grafts, but grafting has a place in the treatment of some patients (Table 9-14). If for any reason it is not possible to heal an ulcer of the leg on an ambulatory basis, the patient can be hospitalized, the limbs elevated, and the ulcerated areas debrided with saline compresses changed four times daily. When the area is clean, skin grafts are applied (See Color Plate III. K and L). There is nothing basically wrong with this procedure, provided that the surgeon understands that the fundamental problem is not one of grafting but one of incompetent veins in the extremity (Figs. 9-29 to 9-32). As has been said, venous ulcers are healed by elevation of the extremity above heart level. When the ulcerated area is clean, a split-thickness skin graft almost invariably takes well. As long as the patient remains in bed, the limb is in excellent condition; the patient is then discharged from the hospital as healed. Within a few months, his regular physician sees him back in the clinic with a new ulcer. Figure 9-33 shows recurrent ulceration in a patient who had undergone three separate hospitalizations for skin grafting, all of them successful (see Color Plate İI.

TABLE 9-14. 47 Extremities Healed Primarily by Excision and Grafting

ULCERATION SECONDARY TO	NO. EXTREMITIES	NO. RECURRENCES	%
Superficial venous disease	10	0	0
Deep venous disease	37	7	19

H). Her ulcers recurred as soon as she became ambulatory. She had lost all faith in her physicians and refused our recommendation for further hospitalization.

TECHNIQUE

There are two basic approaches for successful skin grafting. Preferably, all the granulation tissue, scar tissue, and fascia are excised down to muscle and tendon. This procedure was included in the basic recommendations of Homans.[14] If all scar and granulation tissue is excised, all incompetent veins in that area are also eliminated automatically. Thus, the skin graft can be nourished normally and not subjected to the pathologic features of venous insufficiency. Swelling of the entire limb is not eliminated; therefore, adequate external support (a heavyweight elastic stocking) is required to control the edema and thus prevent recurrent ulceration.

After the graft has been placed on the muscle and tendons and has taken, surgical removal of the incompetent veins of the thigh and leg above the ulcer is advised (see Color Plate III. K and L).

A primary skin graft was performed in 47 (3.5 per cent) of the ulcerated extremities (Table 9-14 in our series, usually because of age and debility of the patient. Whereas the average age of all patients was 56 years, the age in the group treated with excision and grafting averaged 75 years.

RESULTS OF SURGICAL TREATMENT FOR VENOUS ULCERATION

Ulceration secondary to incompetent superficial veins alone is much more benign than that due to involvement of the deep veins. The recurrence rate after excisional therapy is one-sixth that of ulceration secondary to deep venous incompetence (Table 9-15), which, it may be noted, has doubled since publication of our data in an earlier report.[26] The follow-up period is longer for all operative patients; however, early in our experience an inordinately high proportion of limbs with the most severe form of postphlebitic disease required the most extensive surgical treatment, so that the follow-up period after operation is relatively longer for patients with postphlebitic extremities. (Regarding the Linton procedure in which the femoral vein was ligated, this subclassification has become a fossilized statistic, since the procedure has been performed only once in the last 18 years. As shown in Table 9-15, the recurrence rate for the smaller group is 20 per cent and is 36 per cent for the larger group. In general, reasons for all such recurrences relate first to progression of the disease and secondly to patient neglect, either willful or due to inability because of advancing age and physical debility to pull on the heavyweight stocking or

TABLE 9-16. 9 Extremities With Varicose Ulceration Treated by Division, Ligation, and Stripping of Long and Short Saphenous Veins

CAUSE OF RECURRENT ULCERATION	NO. EXTREMITIES	%
Associated with trauma	5	55
Insect bite	1	11
Patient's height (6' 7")	1	11
Undetermined	2	22

TABLE 9-15. Interval to Recurrent Ulceration in 379 Extremities Treated Operatively

PROCEDURE	NO. OPERA-TIONS	NO. RECUR-RENCES	< 1 YR NO. (%)	1–5 YR NO. (%)	6–10 YR NO. (%)	> 10 YR NO. (%)
Division, ligation, stripping of long and short saphenous veins	174	9 (5.5%)	0	9 (100)	0	0
Division, ligation, stripping of long and short saphenous veins plus ligation of communicating veins	175	63 (36.0%)	9 (14)	38 (60)	11 (17)	5 (8)
Division, ligation, stripping of long and short saphenous veins plus ligation of communicating and superficial femoral veins	30	6 (20.0%)	0	3 (50)	3 (50)	0

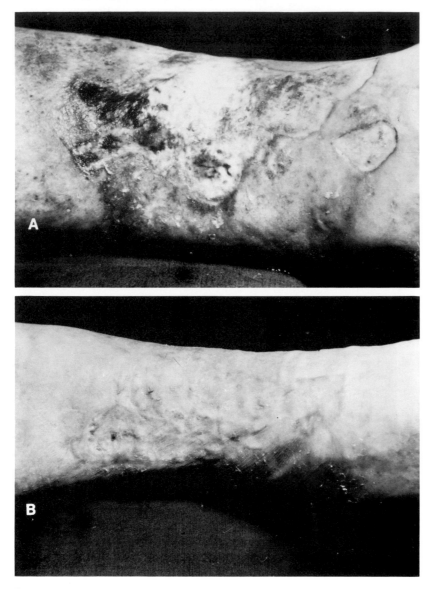

Figure 9-29. A. Dirty venous ulcer in elderly debilitated female patient. **B.** Treated electively by skin grafting.

apply rubberized bandages with sufficient snugness to control the postphlebitic edema. However, failure on our part to remove all the incompetent veins has in some instances contributed to recurrent ulceration, whether secondary to superficial or to deep venous insufficiency.

The value of the Linton procedure cannot be proved statistically from our data; clinically, however, it is believed that operation adds to the patient's comfort and enables many limbs to be maintained in a healed state that could not otherwise be controlled.

Case Report 9-1

The patient's mother told her that when she was an infant she developed great swelling of her left leg and that it remained swollen throughout her childhood. She recalled having the first "sore" on her leg at approximately age 11. When examined in 1953,

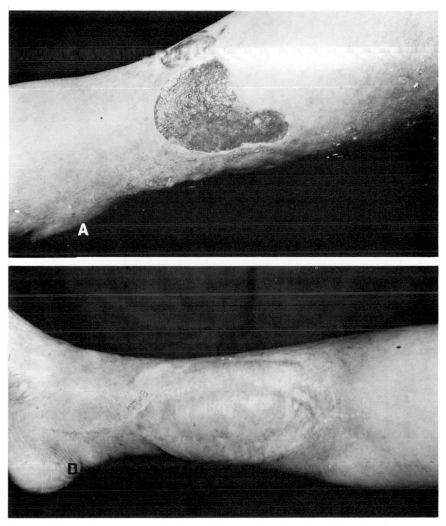

Figure 9-30. A. Venous ulcer. **B.** Treated by combination of excision of subcutaneous tissue and deep fascia with application of skin graft and subcutaneous ligation of communicating veins. (Note fine scar from "Linton-type" operation, difficult to see.)

she was 22 years old; she recalled that the leg had been "open and weeping" almost yearly for the previous 11 years. The leg was healed with pressure bandages, and a Linton operation was performed in April 1953. At operation the superficial femoral vein was found to be completely obliterated and replaced by a fibrous cord. The deep femoral vein was also obliterated at the point of its anastomosis with the superficial femoral vein. The common femoral vein was patent at the point where it drained the saphenous vein. The saphenous vein was enlarged and thickened and was believed to be incompetent. Because in our view an incompetent vein is a detriment to the venous circulation, the Linton-type operation was carried out with subfascial ligation of the communicating veins and complete stripping of the long and short saphenous veins. The superficial femoral vein was divided and sent to the pathologist, who confirmed the obliteration of the lumen and the diagnosis of phlebosclerosis. Although the patient has had many problems during the ensuing period, including alcoholism, morbid obesity, ulceration of the opposite extremity, and recurrent cellulitis of both legs, this limb has nevertheless remained healed, and the swelling is controlled by a heavy-weight elastic stocking (Color Plate III. O and P).

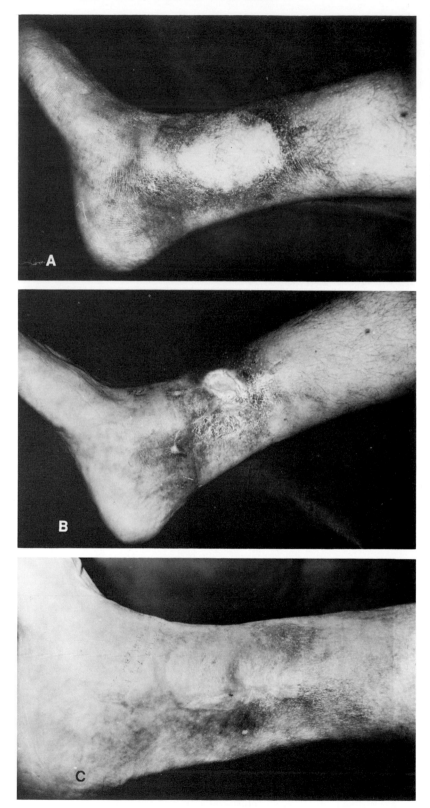

Figure 9-31. A. Photo taken in 1958 of patient with postphlebitic ulcer of leg treated by a plastic surgeon who applied a full-thickness skin graft, using a pedicle from the opposite limb. This graft was flawless and the subcutaneous tissues soft. **B.** Patient did not wear the recommended elastic support; ulceration developed within area of skin graft (1960). He was then treated with compression bandages until healed and instructed to wear heavyweight elastic stocking. **C.** October 1973. Patient has been faithfully wearing heavyweight elastic stocking.

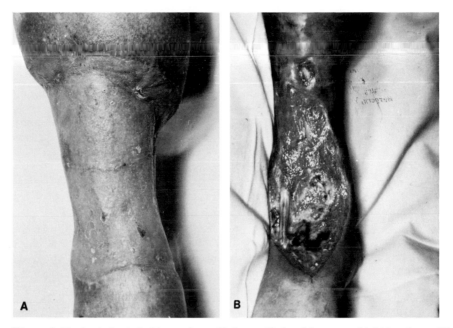

Figure 9-32. A. A healed skin graft applied to a limb with a postphlebitic ulcer. All subcutaneous tissue and deep fascia were excised. **B**. Patient did not wear elastic support of any kind. One year later he returned with ulceration in the skin graft and severe secondary infection, with involvement of tendon and bone. Amputation was necessary.

Case Report 9-2

This patient had six pregnancies and four children. She had experienced swelling during several of her pregnancies and wore an elastic stocking. Her last pregnancy was in 1938, at which time she recalled there was a great deal of swelling of the ankle and leg, with red spots (superficial thrombophlebitis?) on her leg. Following delivery, daily swelling occurred, with the appearance of large varicosities. She had many injection treatments for her varicosities, but over the years they seemed to worsen. During the 1940s she had three hospitalizations for her leg and underwent three operations, consisting of ligation of some varicosities in the leg. At the time of her first visit in late 1952, she had an ulceration of 2 weeks' duration and complained that her leg had been bothering her more and more since her last delivery, 14 years previously. Her leg was swollen, greatly indurated, and ulcerated. The

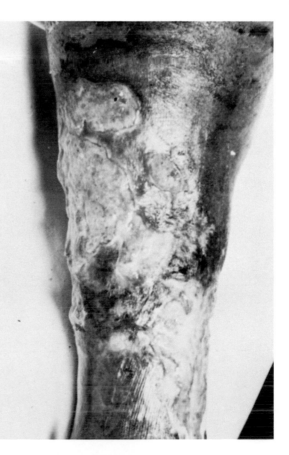

Figure 9-33. Recurrent ulceration in a patient who had undergone three separate hospitalizations for skin grafting, all of them successful. (See also Color Plate II. **H**.) Her ulcers recurred as soon as she became ambulatory.

ulceration was healed with pressure bandages, and operation was performed in March 1953. At that time the femoral vein was explored; it was enlarged but not thickened. The pressure in the vein was normal and did not rise after occlusion of the vein; therefore, it was divided and ligated. The longitudinal incision was then made from just below the knee to the foot on the medial aspect of the leg. The induration of the subcutaneous tissue was so great that a knife blade was broken while attempting to cut it, and it could be cut only using heavy scissors. Because of the heavy induration, the possibility of malignancy arose, and sections were taken for pathologic examination, which proved to be negative.

There was marked necrosis of the fat with a creamy exudate. There was brownish tan speckling around the previously placed black silk sutures, so that one could not be certain whether the dense scarring was due to a reaction to the suture material or to the injectional therapy. Since the veins could not be dissected out through the scar tissue, the scar tissue was excised; this demanded undermining of the skin and resulted in a slough, which had to be treated by a skin graft.

The patient has worn her elastic stocking and remained healed and comfortable for 21 years postoperatively.

REFERENCES

1. Dodd, H., and Cockett, F. B. *The Pathology and Surgery of the Veins of the Lower Limb.* Edinburgh, Livingstone, 1956.
2. Bauer, G. Patho-physiology and treatment of the lower leg stasis syndrome with ulceration of the lower extremity. *Angiology 1:*1, 1950.
3. Laignel-Levastine. *Histoire de la Medicine.* Paris, Albin Michel, 1936.
4. Harvey, W. *Exercitatio Anatomica de Motu Cordis, 1628.* In Keynes, G. (ed.) London, Nonesuch Press, 1928.
5. Wiseman, R. Severall chirurgicall treatises. London, Royston and Took, 1676.
6. Spender, J. K. *A Manual of the Pathology and Treatment of Ulcers and Cutaneous Diseases of the Lower Limbs.* London, Churchill, 1868.
7. Gay, J. On varicose diseases of the lower extremities. The Lettsomian Lectures of 1867. London, Churchill, 1868.
8. Chapman, H. T. *Treatment of Obstinate Ulcers and Cutaneous Eruptions on the Leg Without Confinement,* ed 2. London, Churchill, 1853.
9. Brodie, B. C. Observations on the treatment of varicose veins of the legs. *Med Chir Trans 7:*195, 1816.
10. Cooper, A. *The Lectures of Sir Astley Cooper Bart on the Prinicples and Practice of Surgery.* London, Thomas, 1824.
11. Keller, W. L. A new method of extirpating the internal saphenous and similar veins in varicose conditions: A preliminary report. *NY Med J 82:*385, 1905.
12. Mayo, C. H. Treatment of varicose veins. *Surg Gynecol Obstet 2:*385, 1906.
13. Babcock, W. W. A new operation for the extirpation of the varicose veins of the leg. *N Med J 86:*153, 1907.
14. Homans, J. Operative treatment of varicose veins and ulcers, based upon a classification of these lesions. *Surg Gynecol Obstet 22:*143, 1916.
15. Myers, T. T. Varicose Veins. In Allen, E. V., Barker, N. W., and Hines, E. A. *Peripheral Vascular Diseases.* Philadelphia, Saunders, 1962.
16. Edwards, E. A., and Edwards, J. E. The effect of thrombophlebitis on the venous valve. *Surg Gynecol Obstet 65:*310, 1937.
17. Anderson, W. A. D. *Pathology,* ed 5. St. Louis, Mosby, 1966, Vol. I, pp 596–600.
18. Ochsner, A., and Mahorner, H. R. *Varicose Veins.* St. Louis, Mosby, 1939, Chap. 3.
19. Linton, R. R., and Hardy, I. B. Posthrombotic syndrome of the lower extremity. *Surgery 24:*452, 1948.
20. Evans, G. A., Evans, D. M. D., Seal, R. M. E., and Craven, J. L. Spontaneous fatal haemorrhage caused by varicose veins. *Lancet 2:*1359, 1973.
21. Homans, J. The etiology and treatment of varicose ulcers of the leg. *Surg Gynecol Obstet 24:*300, 1917.
22. Blalock, A. Oxygen content of blood in patients with varicose veins. *Arch Surg 19:*898, 1929.
23. Holling, H. E., Beecher, H. K., and Linton, R. R. Study of the tendency to edema formation associated with incompetence of the valves of the communicating veins of the leg: Oxygen tension of the blood contained in varicose veins. *J Clin Invest 17:*555, 1938.
24. Wright, A. D. Treatment of varicose ulcers. *Br Med J 2:*996, 1930.
25. Unna, P. G. Ueber Paraplasta, eine neue Form medikamentoser Pflaster. *Wien med Wchsch 46:*1854, 1896.
26. Cranley, J. J., Krause, R. J., and Strasser, E. S. Chronic venous insufficiency of the lower extremity. *Surgery 49:*48, 1961.

10

Portal Hypertension

Charles D. Hafner

Portal hypertension means elevation of the portal venous pressure above 25 cm of saline, caused by impedance to portal bloodflow or, less frequently, by an increase in portal bloodflow, as occurs in systemic-portal arteriovenous fistula. This less common type is described as "forward pressure" or "high output" portal hypertension. Classically, however, portal hypertension is often associated with varying degrees of hepatic dysfunction, esophagogastric varices, ascites, and hypersplenism. Rousselot in 1936[1] and Whipple in 1939[2] focused attention on the importance of the portal venous bed in portal venous obstruction; they introduced the term *portal hypertension* into American literature. The pathophysiology and the appropriate treatment of portal hypertension are an enigma for both investigator and clinician.

HISTORICAL REVIEW

Lautenbach's[3] erroneous suggestion that ligation of the portal vein in dogs resulted in death because of hepatic failure provided the necessary stimulus for Eck[4] in 1877 to devise an anastomosis between the portal vein and the inferior vena cava (Fig. 10-1) to demonstrate that ligation of the portal vein did not result in death.

Modifications of the portosystemic fistula have continued to be developed experimentally and clinically.[5-11] An early change was Tansini's[5] forerunner

of the end-to-side portocaval shunt (Fig. 10-2), still used by some surgeons today. In 1912 Franke[6] devised the currently used side-to-side portocaval shunt (Fig. 10-3). These original fistulas were devised primarily for experimental use. It was not until 1945 that Blakemore and Lord[7] introduced into clinical surgery an end-to-end anastomosis between the splenic vein and the left renal vein, utilizing a vitallium tube and removing both the spleen and the kidney. This removal was made unnecessary by Linton *et al.*'s modification,[8] the end-to-side splenorenal venous anastomosis that preserves the left kidney (Fig. 10-4).

The value of portocaval anastomosis in the treatment of ascites was recognized early, and in 1958 McDermott[11] recommended the double-barreled portocaval shunt (Fig. 10-5) for cirrhotic ascites.

To meet the needs of patients with portal vein thrombosis, especially young children, Marion in France[12] and Clatworthy *et al.* in the United States[13] independently demonstrated the usefulness of a side-to-end superior mesenteric-vena caval shunt (Fig. 10-6). Reynolds and Southwick[14] introduced the H graft (Fig. 10-7), employing an autogenous vein as a free graft between the portal vein and the inferior vena cava when a side-to-side anastomosis was difficult or impossible. More recently, Drapanas[15] has reported success using a large-diameter prosthesis as an H graft in porto-

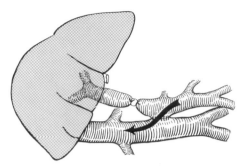

Figure 10-1. Eck's fistula (1877).

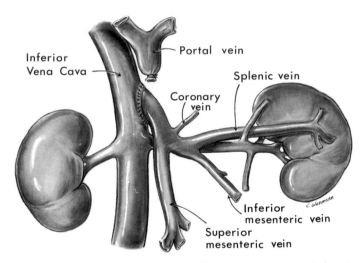

Figure 10-2. Tansini's fistula (end-to-side portocaval shunt) (1902).

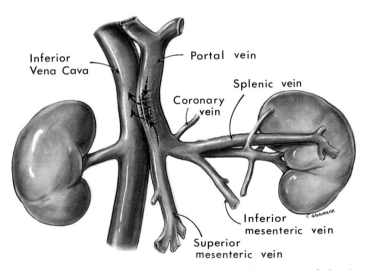

Figure 10-3. Franke's fistula (side-to-side portocaval shunt) (1912).

caval shunts, a technique originally performed experimentally using Teflon by Symbas and associates.[16]

Our preference since 1963 has been a modification of the H type suggested to us by Simeone[17] and reported by Erlik *et al.* in 1964.[18] Here the left renal vein is divided distal to the adrenal, gonadal, and lumbar veins, and the caval end is anastomosed to the side of the portal vein (Fig. 10-8). This requires only one anastomosis and retains continuity of the portal vein. It has the advantages of a double-barreled or a side-to-side portocaval shunt but is technically easier to perform. The left kidney remains viable because of adequate venous drainage through three pathways. When anatomically feasible, when there has been no undue angulation at the renal-caval junction, and when both kidneys have been present, with adequate renal function, this method has been our choice. Warren *et al.*[19] have modified this shunt to facilitate dissection, particularly when surgery in the region of the portal vein is unusually difficult. The left renal vein is divided and anastomosed to the side of the splenic vein (Fig. 10-9). The surgeon is free to perform total decompression or to accomplish a more selective portal decompression by ligation of the splenic vein between the anastomosis and the superior mesenteric vein. Earlier, Warren[20] introduced selective transplenic decompression of gastroesophageal varices by a distal splenorenal shunt (Fig. 10-10) as a possible means of preserving better hepatic function and reducing morbidity from ammonia intoxication encephalopathy. Hemodynamic contrasts between selective and total portosystemic decompression have been demonstrated by Salam *et al.*[21]

For the problem of portal hypertension in children, Martin[22] suggested a retropancreatic portosystemic shunt in which the proximal patent portion of the portal vein is anastomosed to the side of the left renal vein or the vena cava.

Various surgical procedures for the treatment of portal hypertension with ascites and esophageal variceal hemorrhage have been suggested over the past century,[23-26] including omentopexy and Handley's use of silk threads to drain ascitic fluid into the thigh (discussed more fully in the segment on lymphedema). (See Chapter 11.) Around 1926, interest shifted from the treatment of ascites to the management of bleeding esophageal varices.[27-39]

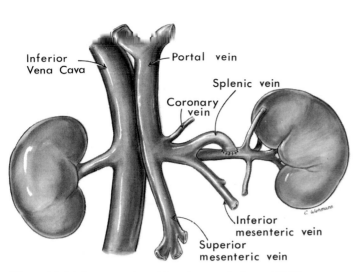

Figure 10-4. Linton's end-to-side splenorenal shunt (1947).

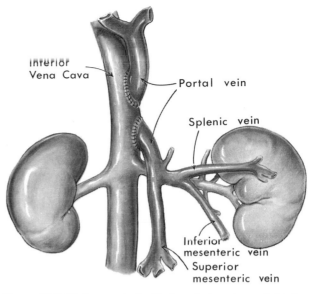

Figure 10-5. McDermott's double-barreled portocaval shunt (1958).

Figure 10-6. Marion-Clatworthy side-to-end mesocaval shunt (1953).

Figure 10-7. Reynolds-Southwick H graft protocaval shunt (1951).

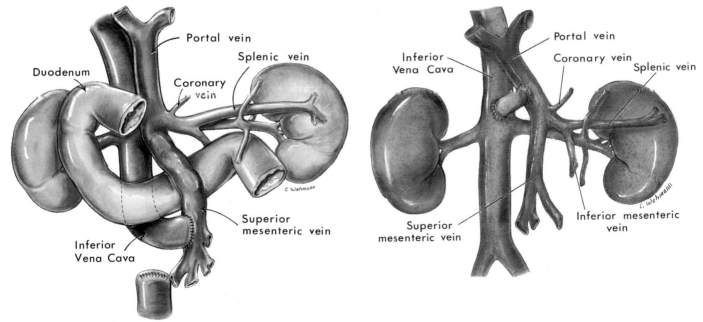

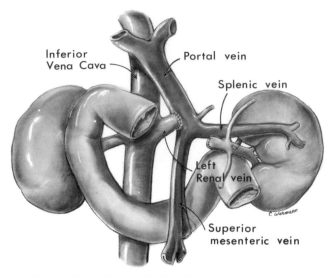

Figure 10-8. Simeone-Erlik side-to-end portorenal shunt (1964).

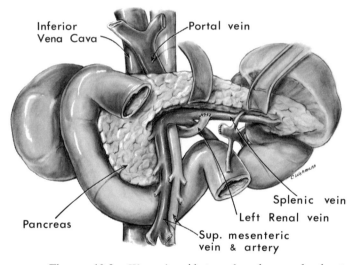

Figure 10-9. Warren's side-to-end splenorenal shunt (1972).

Westphal[29] in 1939 described the first nonsurgical attempt to control bleeding esophageal varices by balloon compression. In 1945 Wangensteen[31] proposed extensive gastric resection for control of massive bleeding. Phemister and Humphreys[32] extended this radical approach to total gastrectomy and resection of the distal esophagus. Linton and Warren[33] and Crile[34] advocated transthoracic suture ligation of bleeding varices of the esophagus and stomach.[35-38] In 1950 Sengstaken and Blakemore[39] proposed an improved balloon tamponade for the temporary control of hemorrhage from esophageal varices.

Nylander and Turunen[40] were the first to transpose the spleen into the left chest to establish collaterals in the treatment of bleeding esophageal varices. In 1963 Berman et al.[41] reported a 5-year experience with omentopexy.

Hepatic artery ligation for portal hypertension was only briefly in vogue following the original, favorable reports of Rienhoff[42] and Berman et al.[43] This operation fell into disrepute following the failure of many surgeons, including Madden[44] and McFadzean and Cook,[45] to demonstrate any merit in the procedure.

Intraoperative portal phlebography[46] and percutaneous splenoportography[47] have been useful diagnostic tools since their introduction in the early 1950s.

The great variety of therapeutic approaches which have evolved over the past century for the diagnosis and treatment of portal hypertension and its sequelae of bleeding esophageal varices, ascites, and hepatic insufficiency, indicates that no unanimity exists as to the optimal methods of therapy. Nevertheless, progress is being made as accumulating experimental and clinical data continue to be evaluated.

CLASSIFICATION OF PORTAL HYPERTENSION

The various conditions which cause portal hypertension may be classified in several ways. The following classification is primarily anatomic, in that it localizes the disease process according to its relationship to the liver.

I. Extrahepatic Portal Hypertension
  A. Suprahepatic (posthepatic) (Budd-Chiari syndrome)
    1. Suprahepatic vena cava and hepatic vein occlusion
      a. Thrombosis
      b. Neoplasm
    2. Heart disease
      a. Chronic constrictive pericarditis
      b. Congenital tricuspid valvular displacement (Ebstein's)
  B. Infrahepatic (prehepatic)
    1. Portal vein occlusion
      a. Congenital
      b. Omphalitis
      c. Exchange transfusions

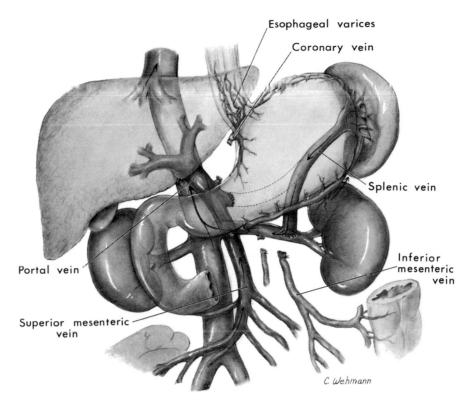

Figure 10-10. Warren's selective distal splenorenal shunt (1967).

d. Peritonitis
e. Trauma
2. Splenic vein occlusion
a. Thrombosis
b. Inflammation
c. Neoplasm
d. Trauma
3. Portosystemic arteriovenous fistulae (high output or forward flow)

II. Intrahepatic
A. Alcoholic-nutritional cirrhosis
B. Posthepatitic cirrhosis
C. Biliary cirrhosis
D. Veno-occlusive disease ("bush-tea" poisoning) (pure postsinusoidal block)
E. Parasitic cirrhosis
1. Schistosomiasis (pure presinusoidal block)
2. Echinococcus
F. Granulomatous lesions
1. Sarcoidosis
2. Histoplasmosis
3. Gummata
4. Amyloidosis
G. Neoplasm
1. Primary
2. Metastatic

3. Hodgkin's disease
4. Leukemia
H. Others
1. Congenital liver fibrosis
2. Wilson's disease
3. Hemochromatosis
4. Lipidosis
5. Polycystic disease

Elevation of Pressure in the Portal System

There are two mechanisms by which pressure in the portal system may become elevated: (1) increased resistance to bloodflow, a concept corroborated by measurements of hepatic bloodflow (which is normal or below normal in portal hypertension) and (2) increased bloodflow, so-called forward pressure or high output, best exemplified by the portosystemic arteriovenous fistula. This second mechanism closely resembles that postulated by Banti[48] whereby profound changes in the portal system were attributed to increased splenic bloodflow. Banti believed that increased flow led to splenomegaly, portal phlebosclerosis, and, eventually, cirrhosis. Later, when it became apparent that

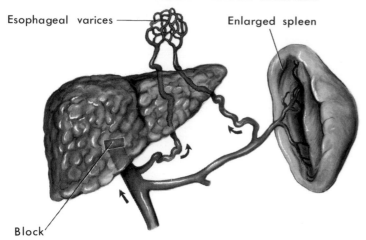

Esophageal varices — Enlarged spleen

Block

Figure 10-11. Obstruction to portal venous flow in intrahepatic portal hypertension.

obstruction to flow rather than its increase was the usual cause of portal hypertension in liver disease, Banti's concept fell into disfavor.

Nonhepatic diseases which produce hypertension by increasing portal flow include myeloproliferative disorders, leukemia, Hodgkin's disease, tropical splenomegaly, portosystemic arteriovenous fistula, and osteopetrosis with splenomegaly.[49]

Whipple's classification[50] of portal hypertension into intrahepatic and extrahepatic blocks according to the site of increased resistance was later amended by Sherlock[51] to also take into account blocks relative to the sinusoids, i.e., prehepatic presinusoidal, intrahepatic presinusoidal, intrahepatic postsinusoidal, and extrahepatic postsinusoidal. This refinement was necessitated by the fact that cirrhosis of the liver at times gives rise to a presinusoidal, as well as a postsinusoidal, block and that other hepatic disease, such as schistosomiasis, congenital liver fibrosis, Hodgkin's disease, and sarcoidosis, appear to cause a presinusoidal block.

PATHOPHYSIOLOGY OF PORTAL HYPERTENSION

Mechanism of Portal Hypertension

Abnormal elevations of pressure in the portal system are caused by obstruction to portal vein flow at various levels or by increased hepatoportal flow, the "high output" portal hypertension observed in ar-

teriovenous fistula. Occlusion of portal vein flow at the posthepatic and the prehepatic level as the cause of portal hypertension is easily understood; increased flow or high output circulation is equally comprehensible. However, the exact mechanism associated with intrahepatic disease such as cirrhosis (Fig. 10-11) is less easily understandable or demonstrable. In 1946 Whipple[52] emphasized that an intrahepatic block characterized portal hypertension associated with cirrhosis of the liver. Later, Kelty et al.[53] observed that the regenerating liver nodule obstructed portal bloodflow. In 1952 Popper et al.[54] demonstrated direct connections occurring between the hepatic arterioles and the portal venules as cirrhosis advances; through these connections a portion of the hepatic arterial pressure is transferred directly to the portal vein, contributing not only to increased portal hypertension but also to the high degree of oxygen saturation often observed in portal blood. The important feature of portal hypertension is the obstruction to bloodflow from the splanchnic system; in cirrhosis of the liver this obstruction is usually postsinusoidal. Compensatory hemodynamic mechanisms develop in an attempt to overcome this obstruction, including dilatation of the portal venous bed, development of extensive collateral veins, elevation in splanchnic vascular resistance, increase in blood volume, and elevation of portal vein pressure.

Hemodynamics of Portal Hypertension

Accurate studies of the hemodynamic pathology in hepatic cirrhosis have been difficult to obtain and to interpret. In recent years, measurements of portal pressure at operation compared with preoperative and postoperative indirect estimations of hepatic bloodflow have provided a more rational basis for the treatment of portal hypertension. Such hemodynamic studies are also useful in selecting an operative procedure for a patient and in gaining a better understanding of the postoperative shunting complications.

In Blakemore's[55] opinion, a side-to-side portocaval shunt had the advantage of permitting some portal blood to continue to flow through the liver, rather than interrupting the flow completely. Linton,[56] however, suggested that all splanchnic portal blood is directed through the side-to-side anastomosis and foresaw that some hepatic arterial inflow may drain through intrahepatic arterioportal shunts retrograde to the anastomosis, with a loss of potentially useful flow. Direct evidence that retrograde hepatic portal flow may occur after a side-to-side shunt has been reported by several investigators using electromagnetic flow probes at operation.[57–59] Retrograde hepatic portal drainage volume has also been measured[60] at operation, and postoperative angiography has been performed by means of a catheter placed through the shunt into the hepatic side of the portal vein.[61] In 1967 Price *et al.*[62] carried out hemodynamic studies at operation in an effort to delineate a more rational approach to the treatment of hepatic cirrhosis with portal hypertension; however, interpretation of the findings and meaningful application of them to the management of the disease have proved difficult because intrahepatic portal hypertension is not a simple, direct hemodynamic phenomenon. On the contrary, a wide variety of forces may be involved in presinusoidal and postsinusoidal blockage, resulting in a multiplicity of intrahepatic shunting and flow patterns. When recognizable, these factors must be considered when planning surgical treatment.

ASCITES

Mechanism of Production

The manner in which ascitic fluid is produced in cirrhosis is not fully understood. It seems to arise from the surface of the liver, the intestine, and the mesentery. Several mechanisms are involved, including lymphorrhea, hypoalbuminemia, retention of sodium and water, alterations in renal functions, and endocrine changes.

LYMPHORRHEA. Lymphorrhea results from interference of venous flow caused by hepatic vein outflow occlusion and from increased lymph production by the liver. The degree of hepatic venous outflow occlusion varies from patient to patient with cirrhosis. The level of occlusion is probably postsinusoidal, with an accompanying decrease in the central hepatic venous bed. This reduction in the hepatic veins of the liver is probably secondary to scarring or to enlargement of new liver lobules

which compress and obstruct the hepatic veins. In addition, obstruction of peritoneal lymphatics results in increased ascitic lymph. High-protein hepatic lymph escaping into the peritoneal cavity results in peritoneal transudation of extracellular fluid to maintain osmotic equilibrium.

HYPOALBUMINEMIA. Hypoalbuminemia occurs as a result of diminished protein production secondary to hepatic impairment and as a result of albumin loss. Hypoalbuminemia accentuates the production of ascites and is apparently one of the main mechanisms in its production.

RENAL AND ENDOCRINE CHANGES. Renal and endocrine homeostatic mechanisms attempt to maintain extracellular fluid by retention of sodium and water; this occurs as a result of impaired glomerular filtration and increased tubular reabsorption. Hyperaldosteronism occurs as a result of increased adrenal production of aldosterone, stimulated by hypovolemia, and due to its accumulation from impaired detoxification by the liver. In turn, increased aldosterone plus increased production of antidiuretic hormone by the pituitary gland causes an increase in water retention. This results in a vicious fluid-endocrine cycle that makes medical management of ascites difficult (Fig. 10-12).

Two or more of the above mechanisms apparently are present in patients who have cirrhosis with ascites. The secondary renal and endocrine homeostatic adjustments probably explain why some patients are resistant to the medical treatment of ascites and fail to mobilize their ascitic fluid in response to reduction of plasma volume by diuretics.

Hepatic vein outflow occlusion seems to play a major role in the production of ascites. In suprahepatic portal hypertension (Budd-Chiari syndrome), ascites is massive and resistant to treatment. Also, since resistant ascites frequently responds to side-to-side or double-barreled portocaval shunt which permits hepatofugal flow and hepatic decompression, it seems certain that outflow block plays an important role in the pathogenesis of ascites. Therefore, McDermott[63] and Welch *et al.*[64] suggested surgical decompression of both the splanchnic and hepatic vascular beds as treatment for intractable ascites.

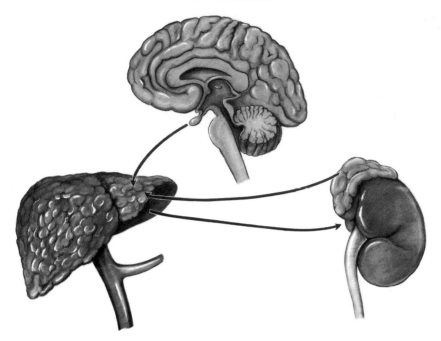

Figure 10-12. Endocrine-renal interrelationship in production of ascites.

Hepatic Metabolic Encephalopathy

Encephalopathy is a relatively common complication of far-advanced cirrhosis of the liver; it is of particular concern in patients who have had portosystemic surgical shunts. This condition is characterized by ataxia, flapping tremors, seizures, confusion, lethargy, coma, and changes in cerebral astrocytes. Emotional disorders and neuropsychiatric symptoms also may occur in postshunt patients who originally had normal livers; Voorhees et al.[65] noted the prevalence of the above symptoms in children and related them directly to the duration of the existence of the shunt. The symptoms are caused by hyperammonemia and other toxic amines. The source of ammonia and toxic amines is bacterial degradation of dietary proteins in the gastrointestinal tract; Nace and Kline,[66] however, produced hepatic encephalopathy of a much milder degree in germ-free dogs with the Eck fistula. The problem was recognized by Hahn et al. in 1893,[67] who described the "meat intoxication" syndrome in dogs following creation of the Eck fistula. In 1954 McDermott and Adams[68] reported neurologic symptoms associated with an Eck fistula in a human as a result of altered ammonia metabolism.

These generally accepted theories regarding the mechanism of ammonia intoxication suggest therapeutic measures for its control, viz., reduction of serum ammonia by protein restriction, mechanical removal of bacteria from the gastrointestinal tract by purgatives and enemas, suppression of bacteria by antibiotics, alteration of environmental pH within the colon, immunization against bacterial enzymes, e.g., urease, and (as a last resort) colectomy to remove the site of bacterial action. More recently, L-dopa has been used to control ammonia intoxication;[69] however, gastrointestinal bleeding is a complication with use of this drug. The type of portosystemic shunt performed to relieve portal hypertension may influence the prevention or limitation of encephalopathy; preserving the continuity of the portal vein may be of some value since there is some evidence to suggest that transient changes of portal pressure associated with normal activities may permit a portion of the portal blood to intermittently pass beyond the shunt into the liver. Selective transsplenic decompression of gastroesophageal varices as suggested by Warren[19, 20] may be effective in minimizing hepatic encephalopathy; however, additional follow-up studies are necessary to determine the usefulness of this procedure.

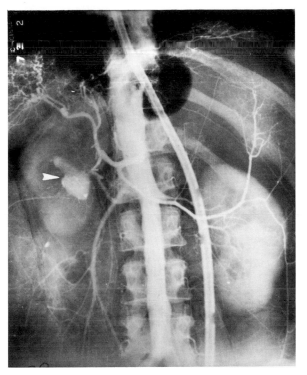

Figure 10-13. Postshunt bleeding duodenal ulcer demonstrated by selective arteriography.

Gastric Hypersecretion Following Portocaval Shunts

Marked hypersecretion has been noted in the Heidenhain pouch (isolated, denervated gastric pouch) in a dog following portocaval transposition[70, 71] and after simple portal diversion.[72] The exact mechanism of this hypersecretion is unknown. In 1969 Newman and associates[73] demonstrated that augmentation of the intestinal phase of gastric secretion seems to be the major reason for the hypersecretion in dogs with portal transposition shunts; they further suggested that gastrin itself may partly contribute to the postshunt hypersecretion. Increased gastric secretion after portocaval shunting is of clinical importance because such patients appear to have an increased peptic ulcer diathesis. Of 42 portosystemic shunts performed, 2 of our patients experienced massive hemorrhage from a duodenal ulcer. One of these actively bleeding ulcers in a postshunt patient is demonstrated by selective arteriography in Figure 10-13.

DIAGNOSIS OF PORTAL HYPERTENSION

The diagnosis of portal hypertension can usually be made without difficulty; at times, however, it may be entirely unsuspected. For instance, a patient may present with cytopenia and secondary hypersplenism; the history, physical findings, and liver function tests may fail to suggest portal hypertension as the causative factor. Similarly, massive upper gastrointestinal hemorrhage may occur without any antecedent signs or symptoms of portal hypertension or liver disease; in such a patient, the immediate diagnosis may not be apparent. In general, however, the patient's history of such things as excessive alcoholic intake, previous hepatitis, jaundice, exposure to parasites, and omphalitis after birth indicates portal hypertension as the underlying disease. Physical examination invariably discloses an enlarged spleen. Indeed, if splenomegaly is not present, the diagnosis of portal hypertension should be doubted. The liver may or may not be palpable. In the early stages of the fatty infiltration that occurs in Laënnec's cirrhosis, the liver may be exceedingly large, rounded, and smooth; in a later stage an enlarged multinodular liver may be palpable; in the advanced stage the liver is nodular but very small, and therefore it is difficult to palpate. Spider angiomas are frequently present on the chest and face. Loss of male hair characteristics, gynecomastia, and gonadal atrophy are frequent findings in Laënnec's cirrhosis. The palms of the hands in patients with advanced liver disease frequently have an erythematous hue. Various degrees of ascites may be found on physical examination. Pendent pitting edema of the legs and ankles may be present secondary to hypoproteinemia. In advanced cases, jaundice may be a sign of severe liver dysfunction.

Diagnostic Procedures

X-ray examination of the esophagus by means of a barium swallow frequently reveals esophageal varices (Fig. 10-14). If the x ray is nondiagnostic and if esophageal varices are still suspected, esophagoscopy may disclose them. Splenoportography (Figs. 10-15 and 10-16) is extremely useful not only in the diagnosis of portal hypertension but also more specifically in the localization of portal occlusion.

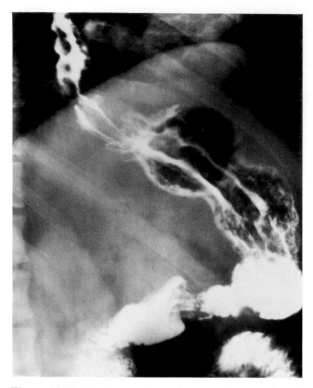

Figure 10-14. Barium swallow demonstrating esophageal varices.

Figure 10-15. Normal splenoportogram.

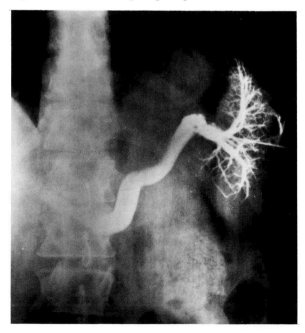

Knowing the site of obstruction is essential in planning an intelligent approach to surgical therapy. At the time of splenoportography, measurements of splenic pulp pressure are helpful in determining the presence of portal hypertension. If the pressure is more than 25 cm of saline, the diagnosis of portal hypertension is established.

To avoid the slight risk of splenic laceration and hemorrhage in percutaneous splenoportography, selective arteriography may be carried out. The portal venous system and varices can be visualized by the injection of radiopaque material selectively into the superior mesenteric artery and celiac axis.

Laboratory Studies

Hepatic function tests not only help to establish the diagnosis of intrahepatic portal hypertension but also provide an estimate of overall prognosis by indicating the degree of hepatic dysfunction. Such information is especially useful in planning operative management. The most useful liver function tests include the retention of bromosulfophthalein (Bromsulphalein BSP) in the absence of jaundice and the measurement of serum albumin, serum bilirubin, prothrombin activity, and serum enzymes. If the prothrombin level is excessively reduced in a patient with chronic liver disease, one should also check for other obscure coagulation defects associated with liver dysfunction which may become manifest during major operative procedures. These include defects in the prothrombin complex (factors II, VII, IX, and X), platelets, factor V, factor XIII, fibrinogen, and fibrinolysin.

TREATMENT OF PORTAL HYPERTENSION AND ITS COMPLICATIONS

Intrahepatic portal hypertension is the most common type of portal hypertension for which patients in the United States seek relief. Treatment is centered around correction of liver dysfunction, improvement of general nutrition, control of ascites, elimination of life-threatening hemorrhage, and relief of hypersplenism. To improve liver function and nutrition, the patient is advised to avoid hepatotoxic agents and drugs (especially alcohol), to eat a well-balanced high-caloric diet, to rest, and to follow prescribed treatment for vitamin deficiency.

Ascites

The treatment of ascites is both medical and surgical. The medical treatment is the **most important** and includes the following measures:

1. Salt restriction (200 mg sodium daily)
2. Diuresis
   a. Thiazides (up to 300 mg daily)
   b. Chlorthalidone (up to 300 mg daily)
   c. Furosemide (Lasix) (up to 120 mg daily)
   d. Spironolactone (Aldactone) (100 mg daily)
3. Potassium supplementation (3 to 6 mg daily)
4. Improvement of serum albumin levels
   a. Through improved liver function
   b. Through serum albumin infusions

PARACENTESIS. The use of paracentesis for the control of ascites is limited, since the ascitic fluid promptly reforms after its removal. However, it may be necessary for the relief of respiratory distress when the abdomen is extremely tight.

SURGICAL PROCEDURES. Unusual surgical procedures for the relief of intractable ascites have been discussed in the section on historical review; they are of minor interest currently. Portocaval shunting has been used successfully for relief of ascites, but in general, intractable ascites is an ominous sign. If portosystemic shunting is contemplated in the presence of ascites, some type of portocaval anastomosis which allows hepatic vascular decompression should be utilized. The end-to-side shunt fails to provide hepatofugal decompression, and the ascites is frequently aggravated. The portorenal shunt is our preference for the relief of ascites; however, the large H shunt, the side-to-side shunt, and the double-barreled shunt have similar hemodynamic results.

Bleeding Gastroesophageal Varices

Although hemorrhage from gastroesophageal varices may be mild, particularly in the initial episode, it usually is massive. The diagnosis should be suspected whenever the vomitus consists of large amounts of bright red blood.

Immediate supportive measures should include restoration of the blood volume. A large nasogastric tube should be inserted for evacuation and lavage of the stomach. Frequent irrigations with iced saline

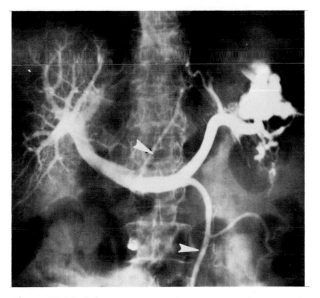

Figure 10-16. Splenoportogram demonstrating intrahepatic portal hypertension with varices and hepatofugal flow with coronary vein and inferior mesentery vein visualized.

solution and neutralization of acid should also be carried out.

BALLOON TAMPONADE. If active bleeding continues despite these initial procedures, balloon tamponade should be instituted by means of the Sengstaken-Blakemore tube (Fig. 10-17) or by means of the Linton balloon.[74] Our experience has chiefly been with the Sengstaken-Blakemore balloon; 40 mm Hg pressure or less should be maintained on the balloon and gastric decompression continued through the triple-lumen tube. These maneuvers gain time for whole blood replacement and for further assessment of the patient's general condition and of the underlying etiologic factors. The balloon should be deflated in 24 to 48 hours; the tube, however, should remain in place. If bleeding recurs, the balloon should be reinflated for an additional 24- to 48-hour period. If there is a third episode of bleeding after the second deflation of the balloon, a surgical approach should be considered; prolonged use of balloon tamponade may cause esophageal erosion. Intravenous Pitressin has appeared to be helpful at times in controlling esophageal variceal bleeding, but the effects are difficult to evaluate; more recently, selective intra-arterial infusion of vasopressin (Pitressin) has been advocated, but this seems to be less effective in the

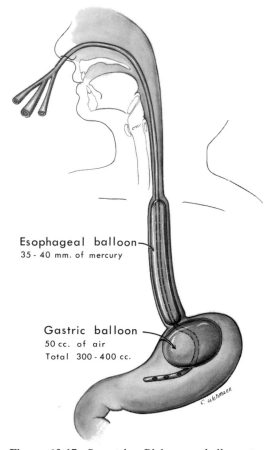

Esophageal balloon
35 - 40 mm. of mercury

Gastric balloon
50 cc. of air
Total 300 - 400 cc.

Figure 10-17. Sengstaken-Blakemore balloon tamponade.

control of bleeding in this condition than it is in other types of gastrointestinal hemorrhage. After it is discontinued, bleeding usually recurs. However, it is frequently useful in temporarily controlling hemorrhage to gain time for better preparation of the patient.

SURGICAL TREATMENT

Several direct surgical procedures have been mentioned in the historical review in this chapter; these are primarily of interest as background. Direct gastroesophageal variceal ligation[33,34] has been beneficial to a limited degree. For the control of continued active bleeding, the most effective surgical procedure is believed to be urgent portal decompression by portosystemic shunting. In this group of patients, operative mortality runs as high as 73 per cent for urgent shunting or direct ligation of varices as reported by McDermott.[35]

Nonbleeding Gastroesophageal Varices

Occasionally, by use of barium swallow, a patient is found to have esophageal varices with no history of gastrointestinal bleeding. Additional studies may disclose further evidence of portal hypertension. The question of portosystemic shunting as prophylaxis of potential variceal hemorrhage[75] is open to debate. Our policy has been not to operate if there is no bleeding. Garceau *et al.*[36] demonstrated no difference in survival rate in patients treated medically and in those treated by prophylactic shunt (Fig. 10-18). However, both medically treated patients and surgically treated patients selected for this randomized study did much better than 288 unselected patients. *Selection for the study itself, rather than subsequent therapy, was associated with a substantial increase in survival.* Jackson[37] reported a lower survival rate in the surgical patients than in the medically treated patients. He therefore advised against prophylactic portocaval shunting, particularly in the nonbleeding patient with established cirrhosis and with recent ascites, jaundice, or encephalopathy. However, others, including Drap-

Figure 10-18. Survival from onset of varices of the study groups compared with survival of 288 unselected patients with varices without hemorrhage. (*Redrawn from Garceau* et al. *Published with permission of New Engl J Med 270: 496, 1964.*)

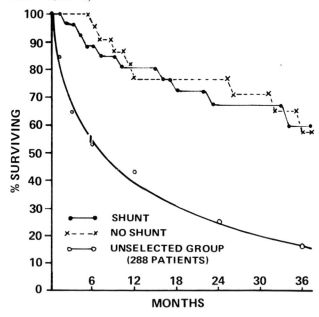

anas,[38] recommend prophylactic shunting in good-risk patients who have no evidence of liver failure.

Portal Hypertension with Hypersplenism

The exact mechanism of the development of hypersplenism is not completely understood; however, the secondary type of hypersplenism associated with portal hypertension and splenomegaly is probably caused by sequestration of one or more of the blood cellular elements, resulting in thrombocytopenia, neutropenia, anemia, or pancytopenia. This complication is one more reason why patients with portal hypertension should be considered for surgical treatment. The choice of shunting procedure depends on the length of time that the hypersplenism has been present. If it is of short duration, then any type of portal decompression should bring about a reversal of the hypersplenism. If it is of longer duration, the hematologic picture may not be reversible by portal decompression alone; therefore, splenectomy plus splenorenal shunting should be the preferred procedure.

ELECTIVE PORTOSYSTEMIC SHUNTING

The preoperative evaluation should define the precise cause of the portal hypertension; the degree of liver dysfunction as determined by the abnormality of the liver function tests; the alteration of coagulation factors, the degree of ascites; the history of bleeding; and the overall nutritional and emotional status of the patient. The response of the patient to intensive preoperative medical therapy must also be assessed: How much have his liver function tests improved? Are his coagulation deficiencies correctable? How well, if at all, does the ascites disappear? To what extent has his general nutrition improved?

These factors are of great significance to the surgeon. After a steady state has been reached, the patient should be classified into one of three groups as described by Child and modified slightly by Turcotte (Table 10-1).

In addition, prothrombin time and BSP retention are very sensitive tests for detecting hepatocellular disease. In the absence of jaundice, the BSP retention below or above 30 per cent at 45 minutes grossly separates patients into good and poor risk groups, respectively.

At present, the type of surgical procedure should be determined by the nature and sensitivity of the patient's disease and the presence of ascites, hemorrhage, and hypersplenism. In the presence of ascites, the shunt selected should provide hepatic decompression by hepatofugal flow; therefore, side-to-side, double-barreled, portorenal, or H type shunts should be made. In the presence of hypersplenism of short duration, any type of portosystemic decompression usually results in a reversal of the hematologic disorder; for hypersplenism of long duration, combined splenectomy and splenorenal shunting may be preferred. However, despite the effectiveness of portosystemic shunting, the prevalence of postoperative progressive liver failure, metabolic encephalopathy, and accelerated mortality is discouraging. In an attempt to circumvent such complications, Warren et al.[19, 20] have been evaluating a new method of decompressing gastroesophageal varices and still preserving hepatic splanchnic bloodflow. They have demonstrated that selective transplenic decompression of varices maintains splanchnic venous perfusion of the liver. Their data thus far indicate that distal selective splenorenal shunting and gastric devascularization prevent variceal hemorrhage and are not accompanied

TABLE 10-1. Laboratory and Clinical Criteria for Estimating Hepatic Reserve

CRITERIA	GOOD RISK (A)	MODERATE RISK (B)	POOR RISK (C)
Serum bilirubin (mg/100 ml)	Below 2.0	2.0–3.0	Over 3.0
Serum albumin (gm/100 ml)	Over 3.5	3.0–3.5	Under 3.0
Ascites	None	Easily controlled	Not easily controlled
Neurologic disorders	None	Minimal	Advanced
Nutrition	Excellent	Good	Poor

From Child, C. G. *Portal Hypertension*. Philadelphia, Saunders, 1974, p. 82.

by encephalopathy and progressive liver failure. A recent communication by Silver[77] lends support to Warren's data.

The Warren shunt, however, is a lengthy, tedious operation that requires disembedding the thin, friable splenic vein and its innumerable tiny tributaries from the pancreas. Therefore, before selecting a patient for this difficult procedure, one should make certain that the goal, viz., preventing further hepatic deterioration by preserving portal venous bloodflow through the liver, is attainable. It cannot be attained if the cirrhosis is so far advanced and the patient has developed such extensive collateral circulation that the portal bloodflow is primarily hepatofugal. If one measures wedged hepatic vein pressure and finds that there is no antegrade portal venous flow to the liver, it seems to be futile to perform the Warren procedure. This operative procedure should not be employed as an emergency shunt.

Nevertheless, in selected patients the procedure appears to be warranted in the hope of preventing some of the postshunt complications, thus improving the long-term survival rate and the quality of survival. However, sufficient data for full evaluation of this procedure are not yet available.

Results

Thirty-two patients in our practice underwent elective portosystemic shunting; all were in Group B. There were 7 (22 per cent) hospital deaths. One patient died with hepatic failure 2 months after discharge. One patient bled to death at home 2 years later from a duodenal ulcer confirmed at autopsy. Another patient died 2 years postoperatively from a bleeding duodenal ulcer after several surgical attempts failed to control bleeding. No patient rebled from varices.

Of the elective cases, there was one mesocaval H prosthetic shunt, one saphenoumbilical shunt, and 3 splenorenal shunts; all the rest were some form of portocaval shunt.

Ten shunts have been performed for the control of massive variceal hemorrhage. Five patients died in the hospital; 5 patients were discharged. One patient died of hepatic failure 6 months later. The 10 patients were in Groups B and C.

Four patients were treated by emergency ligation of bleeding varices. There were two hospital deaths.

One of the survivors was a 2-year-old child with obliteration of the portal vein secondary to omphalitis. Two years later she had an esophagectomy and colon replacement; she is doing well 16 years postoperative.

It is sometimes difficult to evaluate the results of shunt surgery because of the many variable factors involved. Controlled studies have failed to demonstrate an increased 5-year survival rate in patients who underwent therapeutic shunts over those who were treated medically. More recently, however, Jackson et al.[78] in a cooperative study have demonstrated a better survival in those patients treated by therapeutic shunts.

Many studies have been undertaken in an attempt to develop a more scientific approach to the decision for shunting as well as to the type of shunting procedure. One of these was by McDermott, who has analyzed pressure changes in terms of FPP (free portal pressure), HOPP (hepatic occluded portal pressure), and POPP (peripheral occluded portal pressure) in relation to survival and encephalopathy (Fig. 10-19). Eighty-three patients were placed into Groups A, B, and C. They were arbitrarily divided into three groups, depending on the degree of difference between the FPP and HOPP (Table 10-2). If the change was negligible (<5 cm of saline) or if there was an increase in HOPP over FPP, there was a death rate during the first year of 19 per cent and a 19 per cent incidence of shunt encephalopathy. This is in striking contrast to the patients in whom the fall in HOPP was greater than 10 cm of saline. In this group, the mortality during the first year after operation was 30 per cent, and 53 per cent of the patients developed encephalopathy. The intermediate group (a drop of 5 to 10 cm saline) fell between the extremes both of mortality and of incidence of encephalopathy.

Comment

At the present time, the portorenal shunt of Erlik and Simeone is our preference in patients in whom it is technically feasible. This procedure offers excellent decompression of the portal system and maintains continuity of the portal vein. No patient has rebled from esophageal varices following this procedure, and encephalopathy has not been a consistent major problem.

Shunting procedures in young children remain a problem because of the size of the splenic vein and the location of the portal venous occlusion. After the child reaches a suitable size, the splenic vein may be large enough for adequate decompression by splenorenal shunting. In the very young age group, this is virtually impossible. The jejunal interposition procedure has not been totally satisfactory because of recurrent episodes of bleeding. The Marion-Clatworthy[12,13] procedure of side-to-end mesocaval shunt or the large H venous shunt between the superior mesenteric vein and vena cava can be considered. The retropancreatic shunt suggested by Martin[22] can also be considered; in this procedure, the patent portion of the portal vein is anastomosed to the side of the left renal vein or vena cava.

No single surgical procedure is presently (or is likely to become) the complete answer to all problems of portal hypertension. The procedure should be undertaken for a specific need and should be based on the total symptom complex of the individual. As more knowledge of the pathophysiology and hemodynamics is accumulated and as additional data from shunt procedures are assessed, a more rational approach to the surgical and medical management of patients with portal hypertension will become available.

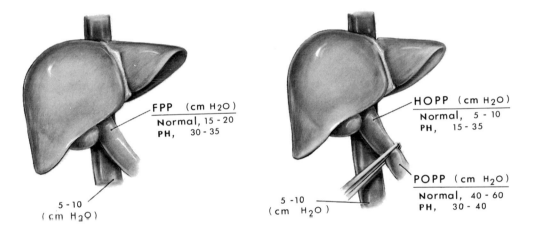

Figure 10-19. Hepatic pressure recordings. (*From McDermott, W. V. Surgery of the Liver and Portal Hypertension. Philadelphia, Lea & Febiger, 1974. Modified from Warren, Fomon, and Zepp. Ann Surg, 169:653, 1969.*)

TABLE 10-2. Relationship of Portal Pressure Changes Measured at Operation to Development of Encephalopathy and Late Survival

DIFFERENCE BETWEEN FPP AND HOPP IN CM SALINE	TOTAL CASES	POSTSHUNT ENCEPHALOPATHY GRADE 1 2 3 4	TOTAL	CATEGORY OF RISK (CHILD'S CLASSIFICATION) A	B	C	DEATHS 3 MO	3–6 MO	6–12 MO	TOTAL (1 YR)
> 10	17	1 1 4 3	9 (53%)	6 (35%)	11 (64%)	0	4	0	1	5 (30%)
5–10	25	2 4 2 2	10 (40%)	7 (28%)	15 (60%)	3 (12%)	4	1	2	7 (28%)
< 5	41	4 1 2 1	8 (19%)	5 (12%)	26 (63%)	10 (24%)	4	1	3	8 (19%)

From McDermott, W. V. *Surgery of the Liver and Portal Hypertension.* Philadelphia, Lea & Febiger, 1974.

REFERENCES

1. Rousselot, L. M. The role of congestion (portal hypertension) in so-called Banti's syndrome. *JAMA 107:*1799, 1936.

2. Whipple, A. O. The medical-surgical splenopathies. *Bull NY Acad Med 15:*174, 1939.

3. Lautenbach, B. F. On a new function of the liver. *Phil Med Times 7:*387, 1877.

4. Eck, N. V. Concerning ligation of the vena porta. *Milit Med J 1,2:*130, 1877.

5. Tansini, I. Diversion of the portal blood by direct anastomosis of the portal vein with the vena cava. *Centrbl f Chir 29:*937, 1902.

6. Franke, The side-to-side anastomosis of the portal vein in the inferior vena cava as a substitute for the Eck fistula. *Ztschr f biol Technik u Methodik 2:*262, 1912.

7. Blakemore, A. H., and Lord, J. W. The technique of using vitallium tubes in establishing portocaval shunts for portal hypertension. *Ann Surg 122:*476, 1945.

8. Linton, R. R., Jones, C. M., and Wolwiler, W. Portal hypertension: The treatment by splenectomy and splenorenal anastomosis with preservation of the kidney. *Surg Clin North Am 27:*1162, 1947.

9. Vidal, E. Discussion of the Eck operation. *Rev Chir Paris 42:*1181, 1910.

10. Satinsky, V. P. Thoraco-abdominal approach for a portocaval anastomosis. *Ann Surg 128:*938, 1948.

11. McDermott, W. V. The treatment of cirrhotic ascites by combined hepatic and portal decompression. *N Engl J Med 259:*897, 1958.

12. Marion, P. Les obstructions portales. *Semaine hôp Paris 29:*2781, 1953.

13. Clatworthy, H. W., Wall, T., and Watman, R. N. A new type of portal to systemic venous shunt for portal hypertension. *Arch Surg 71:*588, 1955.

14. Reynolds, J. T., and Southwick, H. W. Portal hypertension: Use of venous grafts when side-to-side anastomosis is impossible. *Arch Surg 62:*79, 1951.

15. Drapanas, T. Interposition mesocaval shunt for treatment of portal hypertension. *Ann Surg 176:*435, 1972.

16. Symbas, P. N., Foster, J. H., and Scott, H. W. Experimental vein grafting in the portal venous system. *Surgery 50:*97, 1961.

17. Simeone, F. A. Personal communication, 1963.

18. Erlik, D., Barzilai, A., and Shramak, A. Porto-renal shunt. *Ann Surg 159:*72, 1964.

19. Warren, W. D., Salam, A. A., Faraldo, A., Hutson, D., and Smith, R. B. End renal vein-to-splenic vein shunts for total or selective portal decompression. *Surgery 72:*995, 1972.

20. Warren, W. D., Zeppa, R., and Fomon, J. J. Selective trans-splenic decompression of gastroesophageal varices by distal splenorenal shunt. *Ann Surg 166:*437, 1967.

21. Salam, A. A., Warren, W. D., LePage, J. R., Viamonte, M. R., Hutson, D., and Zeppa, R. Hemodynamic contrast between selective and total portal systemic shunting. *Ann Surg 173:*827, 1971.

22. Martin, L. W. A retro-pancreatic portal systemic shunt for portal hypertension in children. *Arch Surg 95:*332, 1967.

23. Drummod, D., and Morrison, R. A case of ascites due to cirrhosis of the liver cured by operation. *Br Med J 2:*728, 1896.

24. Talma, S. Chirurgische Oeffnung neuer Seitenbahnen für das Blut der Vena Porta. *Klin Wsch 35:*833, 1898.

25. Bograz, N. A. La transplantation de la veine mesentère supérieure dans la veine cave inférieure. *Med Russe 2:*63, 1913.

26. Ruote, M. Abouchement de la veine saphène externe au peritoine pour resorber les épanchements ascitiques. *Lyon Med 109:*574, 1907.

27. Flerow, quoted in Spivack, J. L. *The Surgical Technique of Abdominal Operations.* Chicago, DeVour, 1941.

28. Walters, W., Rowntree, L. G., and McIndoe, A. H. Ligation of the coronary veins from bleeding esophageal varices. *Proc Mayo Clin 4:*146, 1929.

29. Westphal, K. Ueber eine Kompressions-Behandlung der Blutungen aus Oesophagus Varizen. *Deutsch Med Wsch 2:*1135, 1930.

30. Crafoord, C., and Fenckner, P. New surgical treatment of varicose veins of the esophagus. *Acta Otolaryngol 27:*422, 1939.

31. Wangensteen, O. H. The ulcer problem (Listerian Oration). *Canad Med Assoc J 53:*309, 1945.

32. Phemister, D. G., and Humphreys, E. M. Gastroesophageal resection and total gastrectomy in the treatment of bleeding varicose veins in Banti's syndrome. *Ann Surg 126:*397, 1947.

33. Linton, R. R., and Warren, R. The emergency treatment of massive bleeding from esophageal varices by transesophageal suture of these vessels at the time of acute hemorrhage. *Surgery 33:*243, 1953.

34. Crile, G. Transesophageal ligation of bleeding esophageal varices. *Arch Surg 61:*654, 1950.

35. McDermott, W. V. *Surgery of the Liver and Portal Hypertension.* Philadelphia, Lea & Febiger, 1974, p 90.

36. Garceau, A. J., Donaldson, R. M., O'Hara, E. T., Callow, A. D., Muench, H., Chalmers, T. C., and the Boston Inter-Hospital Liver group. A controlled trial of prophylactic portocaval-shunt surgery. *N Engl J Med 270:*496, 1964.

37. Jackson, F. C., Perrin, E. B., Smith, A. G., Dagradi, A. E., and Nadal, H. M. A clinical investigation of the portacaval shunt: II. Survival analysis of the prophylactic operation. *Am J Surg 115:*22, 1968.

38. Drapanas, T. Discussion of Jackson *et al. Am J Surg 115:*22, 1968.

39. Sengstaken, R. W., and Blakemore, A. H. Balloon

tamponage for the control of hemorrhage from esophageal varices. *Ann Surg 131:*781, 1950.

40. Nylander, P. E. A., and Turunen, M. Transposition of the spleen into the thoracic cavity in the case of portal hypertension. *Ann Surg 142:*954, 1955.

41. Berman, E. J., Waite, P., Gerig, E. L., and Bakemier, R. E. Omentocopexy. *Arch Surg 86:*1008, 1963.

42. Rienhoff, W. F. Ligation of hepatic and splenic arteries in treatment of portal hypertension with report of six cases: Preliminary report. *Bull Johns Hopkins Hosp 88:*368, 1951.

43. Berman, J. K., Koenig, H., and Muller, L. P. Ligation of hepatic and splenic arteries in treatment of portal hypertension: Ligation in atrophic cirrhosis of liver. *Arch Surg 63:*379, 1951.

44. Madden, J. L. Clinical evaluation of ligation of hepatic and splenic arteries in the treatment of cirrhosis of the liver. *Rev Gastroent 20:*300, 1953.

45. McFadzean, A. J. S., and Cook, J. Ligation of the splenic and hepatic arteries in portal hypertension. *Lancet 1:*615, 1953.

46. Moore, G. E., and Bridenbaugh, R. B. Portal venography. *Surgery 28:*827, 1950.

47. Vahnson, H. T., Sloan, R. D., and Ballock, A. Splenic-portal venography: A technique utilizing percutaneous injection of radiopaque material into the spleen. *Bull Johns Hopkins Hosp 92:*331, 1953.

48. Banti, G. Splenomegalie mit Lebercirrhose. *Beitr Path Anat 24:*21, 1898.

49. Denison, E. K., Peters, R. L., and Reynolds, T. B. Portal hypertension in a patient with osteopetrosis: A case report with discussion of a mechanism of portal hypertension. *Arch Int Med 128:*279, 1971.

50. Whipple, A. O. The problem of portal hypertension in relation to the hepatosplenopathies. *Ann Surg 122:*449, 1945.

51. Sherlock, S. The investigation and classification of portal hypertension. *Min Cardioangiol 9:*303, 1961.

52. Whipple, A. O. The rationale of portocaval anastomosis. *Bull NY Acad Med 22:*251, 1946.

53. Kelty, R. H., Baggenstoss, A. H., and Butt, H. R. Relation of regenerated liver nodule to vascular bed and cirrhosis. *Gastroent 15:*285, 1950.

54. Popper, H., Elias, H., and Petty, D. E. Vascular pattern of the cirrhotic liver. *Am J Clin Path 22:*717, 1952.

55. Blakemore, A. H. The portacaval shunt in the surgical treatment of portal hypertension. *Ann Surg 128:*825, 1948.

56. Linton, R. R. Bleeding esophageal varices and their treatment. *Maryland Med J 2:*400, 1953.

57. Ferguson, D. J. Hemodynamics in surgery for portal hypertension. *Ann Surg 158:*383, 1963.

58. Rousselot, L. M. Discussion of Ferguson, Ref 53.

59. Schenk, W. G., McDonald, J. C., McDonald, K., and Drapanas, T. Direct measurements of hepatic blood in surgical patients: With related observations on hepatic flow dynamics in experimental animals. *Ann Surg 156:*463, 1962.

60. Reynolds, H. D., Mikkelsen, W. P., Redeker, A. G., and Yamahiro, H. S. The effect of a side-to-side portacaval shunt in hepatic hemodynamics in cirrhosis. *J Clin Invest 41:*1242, 1962.

61. Mulder, D. G., Plested, W. G., Hanafee, W. N., and Murray, J. F. Hepatic circulatory and functional alterations following side-to-side portacaval shunt. *Surgery 59:*923, 1966.

62. Price, J. B., Voorhees, A. B., and Britton, R. C. Operative hemodynamic studies in portal hypertension. *Arch Surg 95:*843, 1967.

63. McDermott, W. V. The treatment of cirrhotic ascites by combined hepatic and portal decompression. *N Engl J Med 259:*897, 1958.

64. Welch, C. S., Attariean, E., and Welch, H. F. Treatment of ascites by side-to-side portacaval shunt. *Bull NY Acad Med 34:*249, 1958.

65. Voorhees, A. B., Chaitman, E., Schneider, S., Nicholson, J. F., Kornfeld, D. S., and Price, J. B. Portal-systemic encephalopathy in the noncirrhotic patient. *Arch Surg 107:*659, 1973.

66. Nace, F. C., and Kline, D. G. Eck's fistula encephalopathy in germ-free dogs. *Ann Surg 174:*856, 1970.

67. Hahn, M., Massen, O., Nencki, M., and Pawlow, J. Hohlvene und der Pfortader und ihre Folgen für den Organismus. *Arch Exptl Pathol Pharmakol 32:*161, 1893.

68. McDermott, W. V., and Adams, R. D. Episodic stupor associated with an Eck fistula in the human with particular reference to the metabolism of ammonia. *J Clin Invest 33:*1, 1954.

69. Abramsky, O., and Goldschmidt, Z. Treatment and prevention of acute hepatic encephalopathy by intravenous levodopa. *Surgery 75:*188, 1974.

70. Clarke, J. S., Hart, J. C., and Ozeran, R. S. Increase in Heidenhain pouch secretion after a portacaval transposition in the dog. *Proc Soc Exp Biol Med 97:*118, 1958.

71. Clarke, J. S., Ozeran, R. S., Hart, J. C., Cruze, K., and Crevling, V. Peptic ulcer following portacaval shunt. *Ann Surg 148:*551, 1958.

72. Dubutue, T. J., Mulligan, L. B., and Neville, E. C. Gastric secretion and peptic ulceration in the dog with portal obstruction and portacaval anastomosis. *Surg Forum 8:*208, 1958.

73. Newman, P. H., Reeder, D. D., Davidson, W. D., Schneider, E., Miller, J. H., and Thompson, J. C. Acid secretion following porta-caval shunting. *Arch Surg 99:*369, 1969.

74. Linton, R. R. Emergency and definitive treatment of bleeding esophageal varices. *Gastroenterology 24:*1, 1953.

75. Callow, A. D., Lloyd, J. B., Ishihara, A., Ponsdomenech, E., O'Hara, E. T., Chalmers, T. C., and Garceau, A. J. Interim experience with a controlled study of prophylactic portacaval shunt. *Surgery 57:*123, 1965.

76. Child, C. G. *Portal Hypertension.* Philadelphia, Saunders, 1974, p 82.

77. Silver, D. Personal communication, 1973.
78. Jackson, F. C., Perrin, E. B., Felix, W. R., and Smith, A. G. A clinical investigation of the portacaval shunt: V. Survival analysis of the therapeutic operation. *Ann Surg* 174:672, 1971.

11

Differential Diagnoses of Peripheral Vascular Diseases

DIFFERENTIAL DIAGNOSIS OF SWELLING OF THE LOWER EXTREMITY

One of the commonest problems facing the physician interested in peripheral vascular diseases is the differential diagnosis of swelling of the lower extremity. Lower-limb swelling may be due to cardiac, renal, or hepatic disease; to heat or vasodilatation; to venous obstruction or incompetence of the venous valves; to excessive accumulation of fat; to obstruction to lymphatics; or to purely gravitational forces. As a beginning point in understanding the mechanisms by which the normal physiologic balance is disturbed, it is useful to reconsider the hypothesis of filtration, first propounded by Starling in 1896.[1] This theory describes

> a hydrodynamic process in which physical forces determine the movement of fluid across the capillary wall which is regarded as a semi-permeable membrane in which secretion plays no part. The movement of fluid back and forth across it is governed by the balance between the blood pressure in the capillary which tends to force fluid outwards and the osmotic pressure of the plasma proteins which tend to suck it back. At the arteriolar end of the capillary, blood pressure is high and there is a

tendency for filtration to occur outwards into the tissues. At the venous end the blood pressure is lower and the osmotic pressure of the plasma proteins tends to absorb fluid back into the capillary. The tension of the tissues is an additional factor tending to oppose entry of fluid into the tissues or to return it to the capillary but under normal circumstances it is small compared to the other factors. The small excess of fluids filtered out over that absorbed provides the small volume of fluid which is removed from the tissues by the lymphatics.[2]

A second fundamental hypothesis is Pappenheimer's[3] deduction that in addition to the above-described filtration mechanism, some other principle is involved by which water and dissolved materials pass back and forth through the capillary walls, viz., by a process of diffusion, at a rate many times greater than that which can be achieved by the pure filtration mechanism. According to Pappenheimer, the rates of diffusion of water, salt (NaCl), urea, and glucose in both directions through the capillary wall are estimated to be respectively 80, 40, 30, and 10 times the rates at which these substances are brought to the tissues by the incoming blood. Enlarging on the concept of restricted diffusion, that suggests that small molecules might diffuse through the capillary much more rapidly than larger molecules, Pappenheimer suggested that most, if not all, of the capillary endothelial surface is available for the passage of oxygen, carbon dioxide, and other molecules which are soluble in lipids as well as in water. The rates of transcapillary diffusion of these molecules are correlated with their oil-water partition coefficients, and these rates are many times greater per unit concentration difference than the transcapillary diffusion rates of lipid-insoluble molecules of comparable size.

Utilization of the two hypotheses of filtration and diffusion provides a plausible explanation of at least some of the factors involved in the many types of edema encountered by the clinician. These processes are discussed in the following categories: changes in the arterial filtration pressure; changes in the venous-capillary pressure; changes in the osmotic pressure within the capillary; changes in capillary permeability; changes in tissue pressure; and changes in the osmotic pressure within the tissue spaces.

CHANGES IN THE FILTRATION PRESSURE AT THE ARTERIAL END OF THE CAPILLARY

The arteriole forms an excellent buffer between systemic arterial blood pressure and the capillaries. Thus, under normal circumstances, fluctuations in arterial pressure have a minimal effect on the filtration pressure at the arteriolar end of the capillary. However, during vasodilatation, with relaxation of the arterioles, the filtration pressure at the arteriolar end of the capillary increases markedly and is immediately detectable by measurement of the venous pressure.[4] This probably explains the increased tendency for swelling in hot weather; it is also one of the mechanisms for increased swelling in obese patients, whose hands and feet are almost continuously vasodilated in order to dissipate the heat from the increased metabolic load. Swelling due to salt retention is best explained by an increase in the total circulating blood volume with a consequent increase in capillary filtration pressure.

CHANGES IN THE VENOUS-CAPILLARY PRESSURE

There is no buffer like the arterioles to separate the capillary pressure from the venous pressure; capillary and venous pressure are the same.[5] Wood[4] demonstrated that in a normal subject the venous pressure at the ankle rises to approximately 90 mm Hg on assumption of an upright position; the length of time necessary for this elevation of pressure to occur is markedly shortened by administration of a vasodilating agent, such as tetraethylammonium chloride. This pressure is normally reduced by muscular movements of the venous heart, as has been discussed in previous chapters. Thus, it is readily seen that standing erect while motionless is conducive to pendent edema, even in a normal subject. It is difficult to stand erect without some movement of the lower extremities, and thus the venous heart comes into action. However, the motionless pendency of sitting at rest or the absence of motion due to pain accompanied by a dependent position of the limb or by paralysis is highly conducive to formation of edema. Any obstruction of the venous tree, whether it be intraluminal due to clot or extraluminal due to compression, or an obstruction to the outflow of venous blood, as in right-sided cardiac failure, immediately raises the pressure at the venous end of the capillary, thus not only impeding transference of fluid from the tissues to the capillaries but also actually augmenting passage of fluid from the capillaries to the tissues. Finally, venous valvular incompetence or any interference with the muscular venous heart of the lower extremity is conducive to formation of edema in the extremity.

CHANGES IN CAPILLARY PERMEABILITY

Landis et al.[5] have postulated that increased venous pressure leads to gradual increase in the size of the capillary pores and an increase in capillary permeability. This supposition is employed to hypothesize the natural history of the postphlebitic syndrome, with the extravasation of red blood cells, white blood cells, and proteins into the subcutaneous tissues, resulting in the typical hemosiderin pigmentation and induration. Increased capillary permeability also probably accounts for a significant portion of the swelling secondary to trauma.

CHANGES IN THE OSMOTIC PRESSURE WITHIN THE CAPILLARY

Edema formation is a common finding in hypoproteinemic states from any cause. The hypoproteinemia of nephrosis and cirrhosis are typical examples, although interference with the aldosterone, angiotensin, and renin mechanisms is also involved. Typically, the edema fluid of the hypoproteinemic state has a very low concentration of proteins.

CHANGES IN TISSUE PRESSURE

The subcutaneous tissues and skin offer resistance to the flow of fluid from the capillaries. This is obvious on observing the weeping of any wound, particularly in a dependent portion of the body when the skin is denuded. The patient with lipedema or fatty legs (Fig. 11-1) is susceptible to swelling, probably due to the decreased resistance offered by excessive amounts of fat. The use of external elastic support for the lower extremities increases tissue pressure, thus forcing fluid back into the capillaries or into the lymphatics.

CHANGES IN THE OSMOTIC PRESSURE WITHIN THE TISSUE SPACES

In any form of lymphatic obstruction, whether due to aplasia of the lymphatics, to obstruction secondary to infection, to neoplasm, or to surgical excision, there is a gradual accumulation of protein-rich fluid in the tissues. This in turn has a strong osmotic effect, the less concentrated fluids being drawn from the capillaries to the tissues.

All the above changes fit well into the hypothesis of Starling,[1] and they do not, in our opinion, contradict the hypothesis of Pappenheimer.[3] The latter pointed out that "at high magnification blood appears to flow rapidly through individual capillaries, thus forming a striking contrast to the relatively stagnant extravascular fluid and accentuating the role of the capillary member in providing a phase boundary separating the blood from the tissues." However, he believed that there was good reason to suppose that the capillary blood is in intimate con-

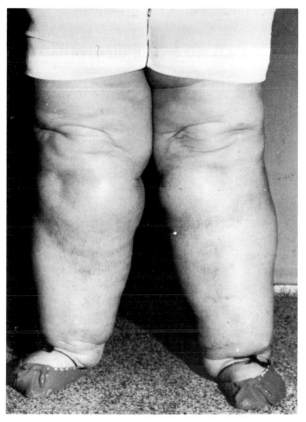

Figure 11-1. "Fatty" legs (lipedema).

tact with extravascular fluid and that the visible flow of blood through the capillaries is in fact very small in comparison with the invisible flow of water and dissolved materials back and forth through the capillary walls. As noted by Kinmonth,[2] this hypothesis would partially explain the differences in degree or rate of occurrence of tissue necrosis in arterial, venous, or lymphatic insufficiency. In arterial insufficiency, the total cessation of blood-flow through the capillaries brings everything to a stop; the filtration of fluid ceases, as does the diffusion of oxygen, carbon dioxide, electrolytes, carbohydrates, and other constituents, and tissue death ensues. In lymphatic edema, except in the most extreme cases, the tissues are well nourished; for while the amount of fluid in the tissues is increased, capillary flow is normal, and nutritive products are brought to the area and diffused in a continuum of fluid from the capillaries to the cells. The necrosis of venous disease has still not been adequately explained. Our supposition is that the capillaries become so dilated that a functional arteriovenous shunt is simulated with rapid passage of blood but with inadequate filtration and diffusion of nutrients to the tissues.

Crockett[6] studied the protein levels of 400 samples of edema fluid collected from more than 200 patients and demonstrated a very clear separation into two major classes of edema: one is caused by cardiac, venous, and hypoproteinemic edema, which are characterized by low protein levels of less than 1 gm/100 cc, the value being independent of the duration; the other class of edema is due to malignancy, surgical excision, idiopathic lymphedema, or paralytic edema, the protein levels of which are always higher (1 to 5 gm/100 cc) and rise progressively with the duration of the edema. Figure 11-2 shows Crockett's diagrammatic representation of edema due to various levels of protein in the edema fluid.

CLINICAL TYPES OF EDEMA OF THE LOWER EXTREMITY

Clinically, five different types of swelling are encountered, and frequently a reasonable judgment of the cause of the swelling can be made by history and physical examination alone.

The Swelling of Trauma

Swelling following injury is localized to the site of injury. The skin color is normal unless ecchymosis is present. The area is painful, and attempts to detect pitting elicit exquisite tenderness. The swollen ankle secondary to sprain or strain is typical.

The Swelling of Venous Insufficiency

Swelling may be due to long-standing varicose veins or may be secondary to deep venous thrombosis.

SWELLING SECONDARY TO VARICOSE VEINS

The patient with long-standing large varicosities may have edema. The swelling is unilateral if the varicosities are unilateral. It subsides overnight. Swelling is usually at the ankle, and it is more pronounced on the medial aspect of the leg than on the lateral aspect. The foot usually is not involved in the swelling. The skin color may be normal, or there may be brownish pigmentation. The edema is pitting and usually painless.

Figure 11-2. Representation of edema due to various levels of protein in the edema fluid. (*From Crockett, D. J. Lancet 2:1179, 1956.*)

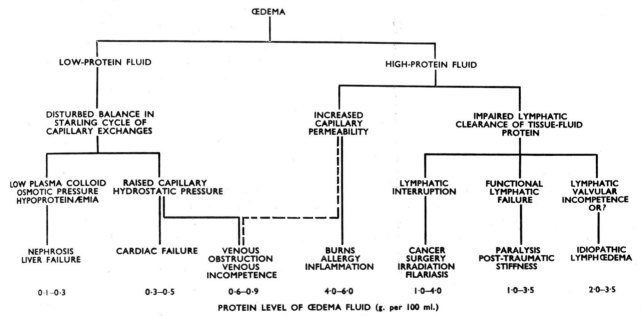

SWELLING SECONDARY TO THE POSTPHLEBITIC SYNDROME

The patient gives a history which suggests deep venous thrombosis or trauma as the original cause of trouble. Swelling is unilateral, centers around the ankle on the medial or lateral aspect, and rarely involves the foot. There is brownish pigmentation of the skin, and in more advanced stages there may be atrophy, dermatitis, or ulceration. Digital compression of the edema may cause slight pain.

The Swelling of Lymphedema of the Extremities

This type of swelling fills the limb as water fills a sack. The limb is uniformly swollen. The most distal dependent parts, such as the ankle, foot, or toes, are involved. The edema is usually unilateral. It is firm and pits with difficulty and is painless. It does not completely subside overnight. The skin color is normal. Lymphedema is not associated with atrophy or ulceration, except in the most advanced stages. The primary type of lymphedema is most common in teen-age females or in patients who have blockage of lymphatics due either to malignancy or to an operative procedure.

The Swelling of Heart Disease

This cause of swelling is suggested by the known presence of cardiac disease. The swelling is painless. It is usually bilateral, symmetric, and centers around the ankle if the patient is ambulatory and wearing shoes. If the patient is sedentary or bedridden or is not wearing shoes, the swelling involves the entire foot. The edema is much softer than the edema of venous or lymphatic swelling. The skin color is normal.

Low-Protein Edema

This swelling may be recognizable by the fact that the patient is known to be ill and has hypoproteinemia. The swelling is painless. It is bilateral, symmetric, and involves the feet. There is pitting, and the edema is so soft that the fluid when palpated may emit a sucking, gurgling noise. This is the softest type of edema, readily classified by palpation. The skin color is normal.

LYMPHEDEMA OF THE EXTREMITIES

Anatomy of the Lymphatics of the Extremity

A lucid review of the anatomy of the lymphatic system is presented by Thompson:[7]

> The lymphatic system is developed embryologically in community with the veins, and it is therefore to be expected that the skin epidermis having no vascular circulation should also be devoid of lymphatics. In the dermis is a closed plexus of unvalved lymphatics draining into a valved plexus in the deepest dermis and subdermal tissues, which in turn drains through valved collecting vessels into the superficial lymph trunks which lie in the subcutaneous fat superficial to the deep fascia. The midposterior axis of the limb is a zone of negative lymph drainage from which the superficial lymph trunks sweep forwards around both borders to converge on the anteromedial aspect of the limb where they accompany the main superficial veins to the regional lymph nodes at the root of the limb.
>
> Knowledge of the lymph trunk anatomy in the upper and lower extremities has been extended in recent years by the use of lymphangiography in living human beings. The superficial lymph trunks drain discrete peripheral areas, with limited means of compensatory lymph communication between them; Ngu by lymphangiography has recently confirmed that lower leg and thigh have quite separate and distinct channels of lymph drainage, so that pathological processes affecting one do not usually affect the other.
>
> In the lower limb two distinct systems of superficial lymph trunks are developed in relation to the two main superficial veins—the greater and lesser saphenous systems. The greater saphenous lymphatics are cannulated most readily on the dorsum of the foot and ascend the medial aspect of the limb to end in the superficial inguinal lymph nodes. They preserve an even calibre and bifurcate as they ascend and show the beaded appearance due to valves every centimeter or so. It occasionally happens that some of the thigh lymphatics bypass the inguinal nodes to end in the lowest lateral iliac nodes. The lesser saphenous lymphatics, if cannulated on the posterior calf, flow laterally round the knee and lower thigh to drain into the superficial inguinal lymph nodes, but if cannulated behind the lateral malleolus ascend the posterolateral aspect of the calf to end in the superficial popliteal lymph node from which efferent flow is via the deep popliteal lymph nodes up the deep

lymphatics of the thigh accompanying the femoral vein.

In the upper limb, cannulation of the superficial lymphatics at the wrist discloses three groups of superficial lymph trunks in the forearm: radial, median, and ulnar which accompany the homonymous veins. The epitrochlear gland lies in the pathway of the ulnar group only and its efferent vessels may be superficial or deep to deep fascia during the ascent to the axillary nodes. Radial lymphatics cross anteriorly from lateral to medial side in the lower two-thirds of the upper arm to reach the axilla, but they may accompany the cephalic vein into a deltopectoral lymph node and thence to the supraclavicular nodes thus by-passing the axilla. Median lymphatics drain direct to the axillary lymph nodes.

In the deep (subfascial) compartment of the limb no lymphatics have been found in muscles, bones, or tendons, but they are present in the intermuscular fascial planes and deep lymph trunks ascend as two to four channels alongside the main veins of the limb to end in the regional (axillary and inguinal) lymph nodes. All lymph trunks, whether superficial or deep, are valved. The flow of lymph is determined in its direction by these valves, but propulsion against the force of gravity is from the intermittent compression of muscular activity, and in the case of the deep lymphatics from the pulsation of adjacent blood vessels. Smooth muscle is present in the walls of lymph trunks but in the limbs is not known to assist lymph flow, and may only be concerned with the regulation of calibre.

Normally, the superficial and deep lymphatic channels are separate, joining only at the inguinal ligament in the inguinal node and at the popliteal node in the leg. In the upper extremity, the junction is at the supratrochlear lymph node. Under normal circumstances, especially when proximal lymphatic obstruction is present, some communication between deep and superficial lymphatics may occur.[8] The infrequency with which such communications are demonstrated indicates that they are not a common occurrence and that when present, they probably function only under abnormal conditions.

LYMPHATICOVENOUS COMMUNICATIONS

Summarizing the available literature, Thompson[7] believes there is sufficient evidence to conclude that lymphaticovenous communications may well exist in all mammals, but only function in the presence of increased lymphatic pressure or volume resulting from lymphatic obstruction, or increased accumulation of fluid and protein in tissues and organs.

PROTEIN CONTENT OF EDEMA FLUID

Crockett in 1956[6] and Taylor et al. in 1958[9] found that the protein content of edema other than lymphedema, i.e., swelling due to venous stasis, cardiac failure, or hypoproteinemia, ranged from 0.1 to 0.9 gm/100 cc. In lymphedema, however, the protein content ranges from 1.0 to 5.5 gm/100 cc.

PRESENCE OF FAT IN EDEMA FLUID

Fat in the edema fluid of the lower extremity[2] means that there is reflux of intestinal chyle downward from the abdomen through incompetent lymph vessels.

LYMPHANGIOGRAPHY

Hudack and McMaster were the first to observe the superficial intradermal lymphatic network by means of lymphangiography.[10] In the following 30 years, Kinmonth[2, 11–15] developed the technique until it is a specialty in its own right.

Physiology of the Lymph Circulation

Kinmonth et al.[2] have presented an admirable explanation of the physiology of the lymphatic circulation:

> The purpose of the lymph vessels is to carry away from the tissues molecules such as those of protein and also larger things such as particulate matter or the various cells which may occur there in health or disease; in short protein molecules or anything larger. A small amount of water also passes through the lymph vessels from the tissues but this is no more than a vehicle or solvent for the substances already mentioned. Removal of water in bulk from the tissues is a function of the blood capillaries and not of the lymphatics.
>
> The physiology of the lymphatics must be considered with the exchanges that take place between the blood capillaries and the tissues. Two main processes are concerned in the exchange of substances between the blood and the tissues.

These two main processes are filtration (Starling's hypothesis) and diffusion (Pappenheimer's deduction). In this concept, molecules may pass backward or forward across the membrane, independent of fluid movement. This diffusion is restricted, because the membrane is only semipermeable. Larger molecules, such as those of proteins, have more difficulty and pass more slowly across the membrane than smaller ones. There is no difficulty, however, in molecules entering the highly permeable lymphatics, which can then remove from the tissue the small amounts of protein which reach them. If there is any obstruction to the lymphatic drainage, the concentration of protein in the tissue rises. This provides a colloid osmotic pressure outside the capillary which counteracts the effect of pressure due to plasma proteins inside. Therefore, filtration tends to be increased and reabsorption hindered. Fluid collects in the tissues, and edema becomes evident. This process continues until the tension of the fluid collecting in the tissues becomes high enough to counteract the filtering effect of the blood pressure in the capillaries.[2]

CLASSIFICATION OF LYMPHEDEMA

In 1934 Allen[16] presented a classification of lymphedema that has stood the test of time; with only minor modifications, it appears in the 1972 edition of Allen *et al.'s Peripheral Vascular Diseases.*[17] Kinmonth[15] added a subdivision under the primary type of noninflammatory lymphedema, viz., *tarda,* to indicate persons developing the disease after the age of 35. He also contributed a classification according to radiologic appearance: aplasia indicates the lack of formed lymph pathways; hypoplasia indicates fewer and smaller lymph channels than usually observed; and hyperplasia indicates larger and more numerous pathways than are normal.[15]

THE "YELLOW NAIL SYNDROME"

A subclass of patients with yellow nails, clinical lymphedema, and pleural effusions has recently been discovered. In 1964 Samman and White encountered 13 patients with yellow nails, 10 of whom also had primary lymphedema.[18] Two years later, Emerson[19] confirmed this association and added pleural effusions as a third finding. Dilley

et al.[20] in 1968 reported 5 additional cases of various combinations of primary lymphedema, yellow nails and pleural effusions, suggesting that some common etiologic relationship might be likely. They did not attempt a search of the literature for cases of idiopathic pleural disease not associated with clinical lymphedema, but they could find no cases of yellow nails and pleural effusions without clinical lymphedema. They added from their own files 6 cases of primary lymphedema and idiopathic pleural effusion without nail changes.

Milroy's Disease

Among the lymphedemas, Milroy's disease is one of the most fascinating. In his original publication,[21] Milroy spoke of an "undescribed" variety of hereditary edema; in his later report he mentioned that Sir William Osler in his *Practice of Medicine*[22] had bestowed the eponym *Milroy's disease* on this congenital and hereditary type of lymphedema. Six years after Milroy's first study, Meige in France published an account of similar cases.[23] Accordingly, in some European countries the condition is called *Meige's disease.* In his original paper, Milroy gave a definitive account of 22 occurrences of this edema in six generations of a family including 97 persons. Thirty-six years later, in 1928, he tried to find out what had happened to them in the interim[24]:

> After a rather prolonged effort of followup investigations, I found it impossible to secure complete and dependable data. However, I located 30 additional descendants of the family in the fifth, sixth, and seventh generations, and of these only 2 exhibited the family edema. They were both children of my original patient. It is obvious that this disease is disappearing from this family quite possibly from attenuation of the taint through marriage.

Milroy described "his" disease as a chronic, hereditary edema consisting of firm swelling.[24]

> It is limited in extent to the toes and to a part or the whole of both feet. It never extends above Poupart's ligament. It is not painful or tender. It is without constitutional symptoms. There is no apparent cause. Hereditary transmission is conspicuous. Edema is permanent. It subsides to some extent with rest in

bed. It occurs in both sexes. It is not inimical to long life, as shown by the family I observed. At the time of my report, four of those in the third generation subject to edema were in good health, their ages being 82, 75, 73 and 66 (Fig. 11-3).

DIAGNOSIS

The diagnosis of lymphedema may be made by inspection alone since the findings are so typical (Fig. 11-4): Swelling fills the entire limb, including the toes. In advanced stages there is the tell-tale *peau d'orange* appearance of the skin with or without associated ulceration of the skin secondary to chronic infection. The arterial circulation is normal. There is no evidence of venous insufficiency, varicose veins, or pigmentation of the skin characteristic of deep venous incompetence. If the clinician is in doubt, a phleborheogram, phlebogram, lymphangiogram, or measurement of the protein con-

Figure 11-3. Patient with congenital lymphedema (Milroy's disease).

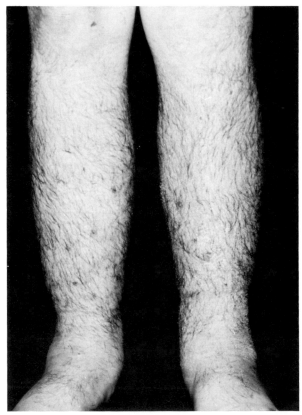

tent of the fluid may be obtained; however, in our experience, difficulties in diagnosis are rarely encountered.

THERAPY

Conservative Treatment

Whereas the diagnosis of lymphedema of the lower extremities requires only a moment's inspection, a full hour may be consumed in efforts to convince the patient that a lifetime of scrupulous attention to the edematous extremity lies ahead. This concept of the problem often is so shocking to the patient that the course of management must be repeated on several return visits before he is completely convinced that there is no method of treatment other than controlling the edema and before he accepts the finality of the situation. The steps for achieving control of edema and for halting infection are relatively minor inconveniences: elastic support to the limb, elevation of the foot of the bed, and scrupulous cleanliness of the feet. By following these rules, the patient can carry on a normal life without incapacitation.

ELASTIC SUPPORT

The elastic support for the swelling of lymphedema of the extremities is the same as that prescribed for chronic venous insufficiency. In most instances, a below-the-knee stocking controls the edema; occasionally, a mid-thigh or high-thigh stocking is necessary. The physical forces exerted on the arterial and venous limbs of the capillaries by osmotic and/or tissue pressure are vital in forcing the fluid back into the circuit of the vascular tree. Thus, a heavyweight supportive stocking should be expected to control edema in most patients. It is rarely necessary to use a rubberized bandage on top of the heavyweight stocking to get increased pressure. The patient is advised to avoid prolonged sitting and to be as active as is reasonably possible. In the vast majority of patients the swelling can be controlled by this regimen (Figs. 11-5 to 11-7; see also Color Plate IV.)

ELEVATION

The patient is advised to elevate the foot of the bed 6 to 8 inches and to keep it in this position permanently. If there is no evidence of pitting of

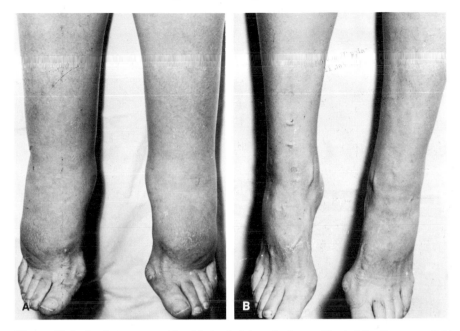

Figure 11-4. A. A teen-age girl with typical lymphedema. She habitually wore tight sandals, which controlled the swelling of her toes. **B.** Complete control of swelling of legs and feet with elastic stockings and elevation of the foot of the bed.

Figure 11-5. Patient had several hospital admissions for acute cellulitis, excoriation of skin, and lymphedema **A.** After approximately 10 days of elevation and antibiotic therapy the cellulitis and swelling were well controlled, and the patient could maintain good control for several months by wearing elastic stockings **B.** Then he would discard the stocking, and the cycle would be repeated.

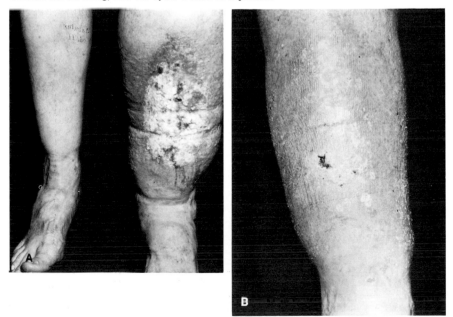

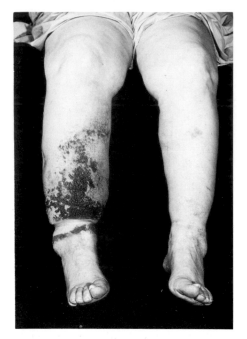

Figure 11-6. Patient with chronic lymphedema and excoriation of skin partially controlled by conservative measures. Surgical excision of three elliptic masses of skin and subcutaneous tissue failed to make his problem manageable.

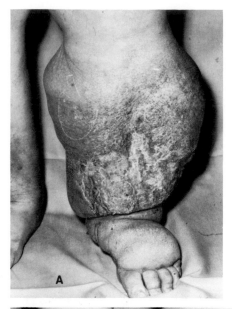

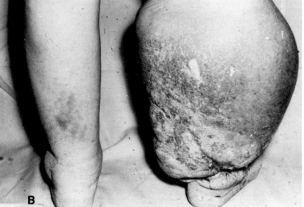

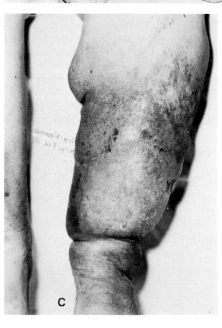

Figure 11-7. Patient with elephantiasis aggravated by years of sitting in a chair most of day and night. **A.** and **B.** Frontal and posterior views. **C.** Degree of improvement obtained preoperatively by conservative measures. Patient died of myocardial infarction between stages of a planned three-stage operative procedure.

the limb at the end of the day, indicating full control of edema, then, and only then, may the foot of the bed be lowered.

DIURETICS

The use of diuretics may be helpful in reducing the edema during the initial phase of treatment. We prescribe them only rarely during this time and never prescribe them for long-term use.

LOCAL TREATMENT

CLEANLINESS. The interdigital spaces of the toes must be cleansed as thoroughly and as frequently as are the hands.

FUNGICIDES. Fungicides are prescribed to prevent trichophytosis of the lower extremity. Since excessive sweating of the feet is conducive to fungus infection of the toes and nails, the patient is advised to avoid strenuous sports. Sunburn may also prove harmful to the edematous extremity. In the younger patient, compliance with these rules means eliminating tennis, baseball, and football.

LYMPHEDEMA OF THE UPPER EXTREMITY

Lymphedemas of the upper extremity usually are comprised in three groups: (1) the postmastectomy edemas, following surgical or radiation treatment for malignant disease; (2) primary edemas, either congenital or delayed; and (3) tumors, such as diffuse lymphangiomas.[15] To control edema of the arm is far more difficult than to control edema of the lower extremity; patients are reluctant to wear a rubber compressing sleeve because of its discomfort. In such patients the application of intermittent pressure with a pneumatic sleeve may be beneficial.

Surgical Treatment of Lymphedema of the Lower Extremity

Kinmonth[15] divided the surgical treatment of lymphedema into two categories, physiologic and excisional (Table 11-1). Physiologic operations are designed to remedy the fault in the lymph drainage of the limb or to improve the drainage in some way. Excisional operations are designed to improve the situation by eradication of swollen disease tissue, and they are not an attempt to change the drainage for the better.

PHYSIOLOGIC OPERATIONS

Handley[25] in 1908 inserted silk threads as subcutaneous wicks in an attempt to carry lymph past obstructions; this proved unsuccessful, as the silk threads became enclosed in scar tissue and ceased to function.[15] Operations similar to Handley's have been described using materials such as silastic rubber, nylon, and polyethylene, without any proved long-term success. In 1935 Gillies and Fraser,[26] believing that lower limb edema was due to a localized block in the pelvis or groin, constructed a bridge of healthy flesh obtained from the arm to lead the lymph to the axillary drainage area.

Thompson's operation[27-31] may be considered

TABLE 11-1. Classification of Operations for Lymphedema

Physiologic		
Handley	1908	Insertion of silk threads
Kondoleon	1912	Window in deep fascia
Gillies and Fraser	1935	Bridge of skin
Thompson	1963	Buried dermis flap
Nielubowicz and Olszewski	1966	Lymphovenous shunt
Excisional		
Charles	1912	Cover with free skin grafts
Sistrunk	1918	Cover with local flap grafts
Thompson	1963	Cover with local flap graft

From Kinmonth, J. B. *The Lymphatics: Diseases, Lymphography, and Surgery.* Baltimore, Williams & Wilkins, 1972, p. 172. (Reprinted with permission of Edward Arnold, Publishers, Ltd., London, England).

both a physiologic and an excisional procedure (Fig. 11-8). His technique of using a buried dermis flap has replaced most other operations for lymphedema in the practice of Kinmonth and associates.[15] Kinmonth has tried to discover the reasons for the success of Thompson's operation but has been unable to uncover evidence by postoperative lymphangiography of lymphatic to lymph anastomoses from the buried flap to the deep lymphatics in the intermuscular compartments. Also, he has not been able to demonstrate lymphaticovenous shunts or drainage of the lymph into the intramuscular tissue planes. However, by using cinelymphangiography he has demonstrated the massaging effect of muscles on the buried flap during exercise, which actually compresses and moves the iodized oil (Lipiodol) in the distended lymphatics not only in the flap but also in the surrounding skin which is pulled and moved by the traction on the flap. Kinmonth also believes that Thompson's operation produces an increase in tissue tension which favors the flow of lymph and the elimination of stagnant pools of tissue fluid.

In 1966 Nielubowicz and Olszewski[32] described an operation in which a lymph node is transected and anastomosed into the lumen of a vein so that the lymph may enter the bloodstream below the level of obstruction. However, Calnan et al.[33,34] carried out this procedure in dogs and found that the lymphaticovenous connections were demonstrably patent for 2 weeks but in 2 or 3 months were universally absent. Kinmonth carried out lymphaticovenous anastomosis in 2 patients and could find no improvement on lymphography.

In 1967 Goldsmith et al.[35,36] suggested omental transposition for primary lymphedema; a year later, Lanzara[37] reported on omental transplantation. Kinmonth carried out this procedure on 2 patients and could find no lymphangiographic evidence, early or late, of a link-up of lymph and omental channels.

EXCISIONAL OPERATIONS

In 1912 Charles[38] described an excisional operation designed for the treatment of tropical filarial elephantiasis. In this procedure, all of the skin, subcutaneous tissue, and deep fascia are excised, and the muscle is covered by a split-thickness skin graft. This remains the preferred surgical procedure for elephantiasis, and in the opinion of many surgeons, it is the most successful operation, although today a full-thickness skin graft would be placed whenever possible. This procedure has completely supplanted Kondoleon's[39] window in the deep fascia, originally designed as a "physiologic" technique but which at best removed quantities of edematous tissue, with some benefit in some patients. To identify the operation, Kondoleon's name is joined with that of Sistrunk,[40] who modified the maneuver in 1918; Auchincloss[41] then modified Sistrunk's

Figure 11-8. Thompson's operation of using a buried dermis flap may be considered both a physiologic and an excisional procedure. (*From Thompson, N.* Surg Clin North Am 47:445, 1967.)

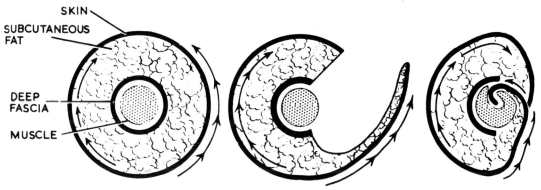

Arrows indicate direction of lymph flow in the limb

method. It is now a purely excisional procedure in which long elliptic incisions are made with little undermining. Homans[42] in 1936 described a method of excising all tissue from skin to the muscle and then suturing the skin. Sloughing of the skin edges presents a problem.

Miller *et al.*[43] have reverted to complete excisional therapy by a staged procedure. Follow-up studies of 2½ to 3½ years have shown this procedure to be satisfactory, as demonstrated by improved postoperative radioiodinated human serum albumin clearance studies. These authors raise the point that Thompson's operation is both "physio-

logic" and "excisional." It is therefore possible that the improvement noted following his procedure is due to the excisional portion of his method rather than to the physiologic portion. They also point out that by reducing the tremendous subcutaneous fat depot, the majority of the tissue mass involved in lymph production as well as lymph accumulation is also removed.

Our own experience is shown in Tables 11-2 to 11-5. Surgical treatment has been necessary in only 2 of our patients; the others were all adequately controlled by the conservative measures mentioned in the foregoing sections.

TABLE 11-2. 201 Patients With Lymphedema

	TOTAL PATIENTS	MALE (%)	FEMALE (%)
Upper extremity	10	1 (10)	9 (90)
Lower extremity	191	29 (15)	162 (85)
Total		30 (15)	171 (85)

TABLE 11-3. Lymphedema of the Upper Extremity in 10 Patients

Noninflammatory	9 (90%)
Primary	7 (70%)
Praecox	5
Tarda	2
Secondary	2 (20%)
Malignant occlusion	2
Postmastectomy	1
Cancer of breast	1
Inflammatory	1 (10%)
Primary (acute, chronic)	0 (0%)
Secondary (acute, chronic)	1 (10%)
Local tissue injury or inflammation, recurrent erysipeloid cellulitis	1

TABLE 11-4. Classification of Lymphedema of the Lower Extremity in 191 Patients

Noninflammatory	135 (70%)
Primary	123 (64%)
Praecox	49 (25.6%)
Tarda	62 (32.5%)
Congenital	12 (6.3%)
Simple	10
Milroy's	2
	(6.3%)
Secondary	12 (6.3%)
Malignant occlusion	10 (6%)
Prostate	3
Pelvis	3
Bowel	1
Cervix	1
Unknown	2
Surgical removal of lymph nodes	0
Pressure	0
Radiation treatment	2
Inflammatory	56 (30%)
Primary (acute, chronic)	5 (2.6%)
Secondary (acute, chronic)	51 (26.7%)
Venous stasis	12
Trichophytosis	7
Systemic disease (OAD)	14
Local injury or inflammation	18
Trauma	1
Recurrent erysipeloid cellulitis	17

TABLE 11-5. Treatment of 201 Patients With Lymphedema

Upper extremity	10 Patients	
Jobst sleeve	1	
Lower extremity	191 Patients	
Operative		2 Charles' excisional procedure
Conservative	189	

RECURRENT ERYSIPELOID CELLULITIS

The association of recurrent erysipeloid cellulitis with chronic lymphedema has long been recognized.[44, 45] Usually it is considered to be due to streptococcal infection.[46] The association of erysipelas with dermatophytosis was noted by McGlasson in 1926.[47] In our experience, recurrent erysipeloid cellulitis may be seen in patients with chronic lymphedema, in those with the postphlebitic syndrome, and in some with neither of these conditions but with fungus infection or some other lesion of the skin epithelium including arterial ulceration.

Typically, the patient states that he was well until he experienced a rather sudden onset of a systemic reaction characterized by fever, malaise, chills, nausea, and vomiting. He went to bed and on awakening in the morning found that one leg was fiery red, swollen, and painful. On examination, the leg is swollen, erythema is present, streaks may be visible along the lymphatics, and tender lymph nodes may usually be palpable in the groin. Examination of the feet frequently shows fungus infection (Fig. 11-9). In our experience with 642 patients treated for cellulitis, 82 (12.6 per cent) had the acute erysipeloid type.

TREATMENT

Immediate treatment consists of bed rest, elevation of the limb, and antibiotic therapy. Almost all of the antibiotic agents have been tried, and all of these have been effective. Fungicides are also prescribed if indicated.

The causative organism is usually considered to be streptococcus, although since there is no drainage, culture usually is not obtainable unless one wishes to scarify the skin or take a biopsy; this we have not done.

Response to treatment is very rapid; within a few days the patient is comfortable, and the swelling and erythema have subsided (Figs. 11-10 and 11-11). If swelling persists, a heavyweight stocking is prescribed. The patient is advised to regularly use fungicide and to wear the prescribed stocking to control the edema.

SIGNIFICANCE

Many patients with cellulitis are erroneously considered to have thrombophlebitis. When a patient gives a history of having had "thrombophlebitis" numerous times, the physician should suspect that the disease was actually cellulitis, perhaps of the erysipeloid type. Specific questioning of such a patient with alleged thrombophlebitis usually elicits the typical history of erysipeloid cellulitis. It is extremely rare for a patient to contract thrombophlebitis 10 or more times; however, the same number of bouts of recurrent erysipeloid cellulitis is not rare at all.

Figure 11-9. Recurrent erysipeloid cellulitis. **A.** Feet of patient presenting with acute cellulitis of leg. **B.** Severe fungus infection, making a portal of entry for bacteria. In many patients, the break in the skin may be very small and overlooked as the site of bacterial invasion.

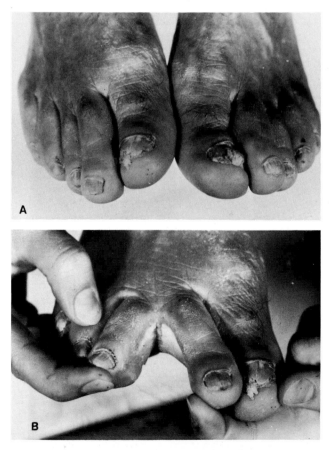

MUSCLE HEMORRHAGE

Muscle hemorrhage is frequently encountered in clinical practice. It produces a distinctive syndrome, easily recognizable by the history and physical examination, that has been known in the literature under other names, e.g., ruptured plantaris tendon, tennis leg, "coup de fouet" "syndrome of the whip blow," or simply muscular tears or rupture. When confined to the calf muscles, as it was in 93 per cent of our patients in whom the lower extremity was involved, it may be mistaken for acute deep thrombophlebitis; in this instance, treatment with anticoagulant agents may have disastrous consequences. Also, if the hemorrhage is confined within the fascial compartment, it may be extensive enough to cause muscle necrosis; to prevent this, prompt fasciotomy must be performed. Prompt recognition of this entity, which is most often benign, saves unnecessary hospitalization and

Figure 11-10. A. Initially area of cellulitis is bright reddish pink. **B.** As it responds to treatment, it becomes a dull purplish color.

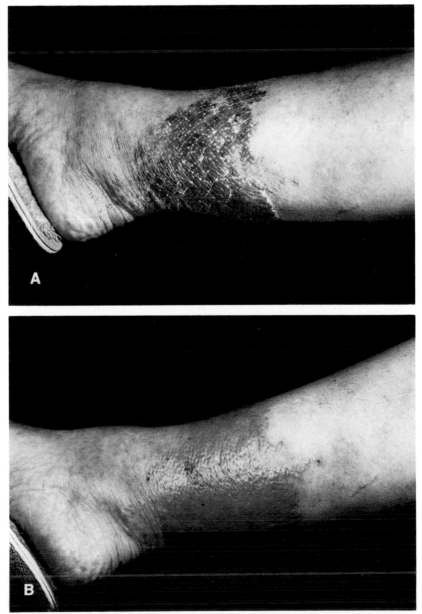

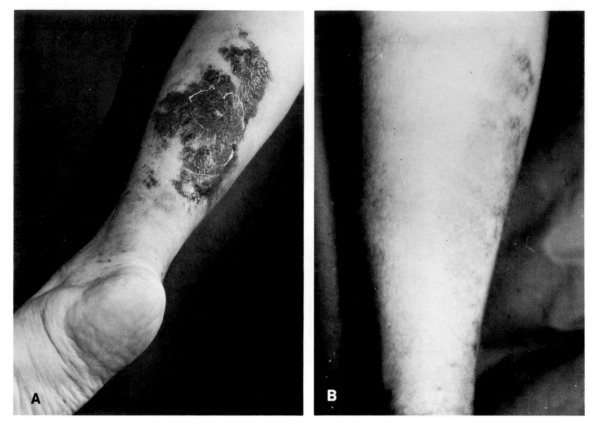

Figure 11-11. A. Patient with acute cellulitis beginning to improve. Color was a deep bluish purple, and it appeared to be turning necrotic. **B.** However, it gradually resolved in approximately 6 weeks with slight permanent discoloration of the skin.

spares the patient and the physician considerable worry.

HISTORICAL REVIEW

Goldberg[48] recently reviewed the literature on this subject after he recognized that the "syndrome of whip blow" as reported by Martorell in 1955[49] was identical to the syndrome previously known as "tennis leg" or "ruptured plantaris." He was able to find 22 reports touching on this subject. The most striking thing he found was the similarity of the clinical picture, which removed all doubt that the different authors were describing the same syndrome. In our earliest experience we characterized these patients as having a ruptured plantaris tendon; however, when it became obvious that various portions of the calf muscle might be involved, as well as muscles of the thigh and even of the upper ex-

tremity, it was recognized that a new category of diagnosis had to be established. On an *a priori* basis it seems that the hemorrhage must come from spontaneous or traumatic rupture of an artery or vein, tear of a muscle fascicle, or rupture of a tendon. Furthermore, it was noted to occur spontaneously in patients on anticoagulant therapy; thus, it seemed that venous hypertension in a patient on anticoagulants might be a predisposing factor.

In only one instance in our experience was it possible to pinpoint the bleeding vessel, viz., a small artery in the forearm. Because it is usually impossible to find a specific source of the hemorrhage and because it is of small consequence as far as diagnosis and treatment are concerned, it seemed best to consider this entity simply as "muscle hemorrhage." Excluded were patients with analogous syndromes, such as abdominal wall hematoma,[50] hemorrhage into a digit or joint, or subcutaneous ecchymosis.

DIAGNOSIS

The history provides the most important clue for the diagnosis. An otherwise normal person has a sudden seizure of pain in a muscle group. At times this follows an abrupt muscle contraction, as when stepping down off a ladder, truck, or curbstone or when catching oneself after slipping on a pebble, follows a sudden minor effort, such as jumping up from a sitting position, or follows the strain of sudden exertion, such as occurs in bowling. However, at other times it may occur without warning as the patient is walking, sitting, or lying down. It is of particular interest and has been reported by many authors that the patient may describe a sensation of being struck in the calf by a stone thrown by an unknown person. Indeed, Martorell[48] stated

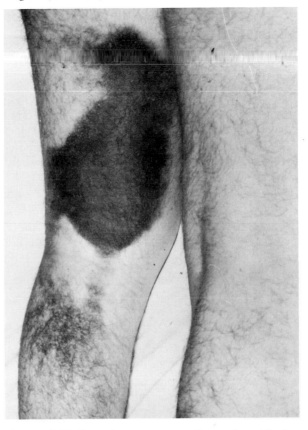

Figure 11-13. Extensive spontaneous hemorrhage. Ecchymosis did not appear for several days following onset of symptoms.

Figure 11-12. Exceptionally large muscle hemorrhage. Initially, when swelling was less marked, patient was referred with diagnosis of thrombophlebitis. Ecchymosis appeared at the ankle a few days after this photo was taken.

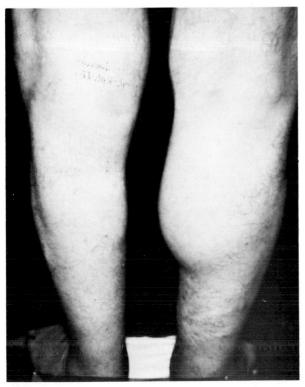

that most of his 21 patients gave such a history. Gilcreest[51] stated that when the calf muscle ruptures, the patient often hears a snap; this is a finding concurred in by others and one which coincides with the concept of Martorell[48] and of Costeas and his associates[52] which led them to the term "whip blow" to the leg.

The history of such an abrupt onset is not obtained in patients with thrombophlebitis. Although the immediate pain subsides somewhat, some discomfort persists and is followed by swelling of the limb. As it swells, the leg becomes more and more painful, again to a degree not usually encountered in deep thrombophlebitis. At this stage it may be difficult to distingiush hemorrhage from deep venous thrombosis. The patient has pain, swelling, and tenderness. Movement of the calf muscle, e.g., by dorsiflexion of the foot, aggravates the pain. Initially, no discoloration of the skin is observed.

However, ecchymosis appears a few days later, frequently around the distal portion of the leg or the foot. This ecchymosis establishes the diagnosis (Figs. 11-12 and 11-13).

By far the greater number of our patients experienced muscle hemorrhage of the lower extremity, the great majority in the calf area (Table 11-6). The source of the hemorrhage in these 193 patients could not be determined specifically; however, it was our clinical impression that the patient actually had rupture of the plantaris muscle in 14 instances (7 per cent); rupture of a portion of the gastrocnemius muscle in 9 (5 per cent) rupture of a vein or venous bleeding without trauma in 13 (7 per cent). In the remaining 157 patients (81 per cent), no reasonably precise judgment could be made as to the exact cause of the hemorrhage.

TREATMENT

If the history is clear-cut or if ecchymosis is noted on first examination, the patient is treated by elastic support and reassurance. If the diagnosis is in doubt, a phleborheogram is obtained. A negative tracing rules out venous thrombosis of the extent that would cause this type of swelling. Before the availability of phleborheography for use in diagnosis, the patient was hospitalized and treated with bed rest and elevation until thrombophlebitis could be excluded.

COMPLICATIONS

If the pathologic process is not recognized and especially if anticoagulant agents are given, the patient may develop hemorrhage into the subfascial compartment of a muscle sufficient to cause muscle necrosis. Two patients in our experience illustrate this complication:

TABLE 11-6. Site of Hemorrhage in 214 Patients

EXTREMITY		NO. PATIENTS
Upper		7 (3%)
Arm	6	
Forearm	1	
Lower		207 (97%)
Calf	193	
Thigh	11	
Anterior tibial	3	

Case Report 11-1

In March 1960 a 63-year-old Caucasian female was hospitalized and under treatment for thrombophlebitis with heparin and a prothrombin-depressant agent. Her prothrombin time was 43 seconds and less than 10 per cent of normal when she developed spontaneous swelling and pain in her left calf. Three weeks prior to this episode, the patient had had a sudden onset of severe pain in the leg, diagnosed as thrombophlebitis; it is possible that the diagnosis was in error. Also, the prothrombin time was at this level for less than 24 hours when she bled. Therefore, it is impossible to establish exactly how great a role the anticoagulant therapy played.

When seen in consultation, the patient had marked swelling of the calf associated with ecchymosis about the ankle. She was taken to the operating room immediately. The leg was opened through a longitudinal incision over the medial head of the gastrocnemius muscle. When the fascia was opened, approximately 300 cc of blood was removed. Almost the entire medial head of the gastrocnemius muscle appeared to be necrotic. It was infiltrated with blood and was a dull, grayish red color and therefore was removed. The fascia was closed without drainage. The incision healed *per primam*. The patient has had a very good result, with residual swelling of the leg controlled by a heavyweight elastic stocking.

Case Report 11-2

In October 1959 a 44-year-old Caucasian male was admitted with a history of having had pain of one week's duration in his left calf. He also had had a temperature of 99 to 100 F and hemoptysis; he described the hemoptysis as having occurred before he developed the calf pain. On admission to the hospital, he had pain, swelling, and tenderness in the left calf and x-ray evidence of a pulmonary infiltrate, which was interpreted as a pulmonary infarct. He was placed on anticoagulant therapy, and the swelling in his leg became much greater and the pain became more severe.

He was seen in consultation; a diagnosis was made of hemorrhage into the leg as a complication of an increase in venous pressure secondary to thrombophlebitis plus anticoagulant therapy. He was taken to the operating room; because his thigh was swollen and there was tenderness over the iliac vein, his inferior vena cava was explored first and found to be almost completely thrombosed up to the renal veins. Thrombectomy and inferior vena cava ligation were performed. The leg was then opened through a longitudinal incision over the medial aspect; when the fascia was opened, a large amount of blood gushed out. The muscle was infiltrated with blood and was necrotic. The entire medial head of the gastrocnemius muscle was excised. A full-thickness skin graft was applied to the denuded area. This graft did not survive because all of the necrotic muscle had not been removed. Subsequently, this dead muscle was excised, and the area was grafted again, this time successfully. In all, the patient lost approximately one-third of the gastrocnemius muscle and one-third of the soleus muscle. He has been followed for 14 years; his leg has been well controlled.

Cases of Special Interest

Case Report 11-3

A 65-year-old Caucasian male was eating lunch after finishing a round of golf. During the luncheon, he noticed gradually increasing discomfort and pain in his right forearm. The pain soon became excruciating. He saw a physician, who referred him for consultation. On physical examination the patient was obviously in great pain. His forearm was tight and painful to touch. There was no visible ecchymosis. His hand was beginning to get numb. The radial pulse was barely palpable; the ulnar pulse was not palpable. A diagnosis of subfascial hemorrhage into the muscles of the right forearm was made.

The forearm was explored through a 6-inch incision on the anteromedial aspect. There was no obvious bleeding in the subcutaneous tissue. The superficial muscles were tense but showed no hemorrhage. When the fascia over the pronator teres was opened, blood gushed out; an estimated 100 to 200 cc of fresh and clotted blood was removed. After evacuation of the blood, one small arterial bleeder was identified and ligated. The postoperative course was completely uneventful. Both the radial and ulnar pulsations were strong immediately after operation.

Case Report 11-4

While bowling, a 57-year-old Caucasian male stopped quickly and turned suddenly. He experienced severe pain in the medial aspect of his right thigh but continued to play. Two days later, discoloration appeared in the skin of the right thigh. He denied the presence of swelling. On physical examination, his arterial circulation was normal. The right thigh measured 56.0 cm, as compared with 51.0 cm on the left side. There was no ankle edema. A large area of ecchymosis with some induration was present on the anteromedial aspect of the right thigh.

Case Report 11-5

A 37-year-old Caucasian female was sled riding; while standing at the top of the hill waiting for her family to catch up with her, she experienced a sudden onset of severe pain in her left leg. The pain increased in intensity so that she was unable to walk. The leg became swollen to "twice its normal size." The next day the entire leg turned black-and-blue. On physical examination 8 days after the onset of symptoms ecchymosis and considerable swelling were still present.

Case Report 11-6

A 60-year-old Caucasian female was sitting on the divan and jumped to her feet on hearing a dog bark. As she did so, she felt a sudden "snapping" pain in her left leg. The leg began to swell and became very sore. Four days later, her ankle and the back of her leg turned black-and-blue. On physical examination 10 days after the acute onset of pain, the left leg was moderately swollen and ecchymosis was present around the ankle and lower third of the leg. Measurements were as follows: right thigh, 39.5 cm; right calf 23.0 cm; right ankle, 21.0 cm; left thigh, 41.0 cm; left calf, 36.0 cm; left ankle, 22.0 cm. Treatment consisted of rubberized bandages on the left leg and rest.

NEURALGIA AND ARTHRALGIA

Some form of neuralgia or arthralgia is by far the most common nonvascular condition observed by the peripheral vascular surgeon. Indeed, at some times, over half of the patients seen in consultation for peripheral vascular diseases are complaining instead of neuritic or arthritic symptoms. As these lie outside the scope of this study, no detailed review of arthralgia and neuralgia is presented. By analyzing patient disorders according to categories, disorders that may or do involve the peripheral arteries or veins are easily recognized; patients with nonvascular conditions are then referred to appropriate specialists.

NEURALGIA OF THE LOWER EXTREMITY

The specific cause of a neuralgia is difficult to determine at times. The pain may be due to a primary disorder of the nerves, to arthritis, to a ruptured intervertebral disc, or to one of the common conditions of the lumbar spine that cause sciatic neuralgia. However, it is a relatively easy matter to recognize these groups and to rule out arterial disease as the etiologic factor. The patient who attributes pain in the lateral aspect of his hip and thigh to "poor circulation" is by far the most typical example. As he runs his hand from his buttocks down the lateral aspect of the thigh towards the knee, demonstrating the course of his pain, he is ruling out a vascular origin. In our experience a vascular condition does not produce this type of pain. Neuralgic pain is present at all times, and although it may be aggravated by walking, it also occurs when the patient is sitting or lying down. Damp weather also may be an aggravating factor, and the patient may be able to predict the onset of discomfort by a change in the weather. At times the pain occurs while he lies in bed or on first arising; as he becomes ambulant, its severity lessens.

Treatment

Heat and aspirin are prescribed for the relief of symptoms.

ASPIRIN

Aspirin sometimes provides an excellent therapeutic test. When a patient denies that aspirin relieves his pain, the physician must make certain that the dose he is taking is adequate. One method is to prescribe 10 grains of aspirin to be taken 3 or 4 times a day for a week as a trial to determine its efficacy in relieving the pain. The physician may enlist the patient's cooperation by explaining that success or failure of aspirin in this dose as an analgesic will be of value in diagnosing the patient's condition.

ARTHRITIS OF THE KNEE

Arthritis of the knee often causes pain in the lateral aspect of the leg 2 or 3 inches below the knee or on the lateral aspect of the thigh above the knee without producing pain in the knee joint itself. The fact that the joint is spared may convince the patient, and quite possibly his physician, that the problem cannot be arthritis. However, the pain of arterial or venous disease differs in character and distribution from that described by the patient with arthritis.

OTHER ARTHROPATHIES OF THE KNEE

Frequently a patient who complains of pain or discomfort in his knee reports that his leg "gives way" without warning, causing him to either come close to falling or actually fall down. Some internal derangement of the knee is invariably the causative factor in this condition.

NEUROGENIC CLAUDICATION

A full description of this type of nerve pain is given in *Vascular Surgery*, Volume I, Chapter 1, pp. 10–11.

NEURALGIA AND ARTHRALGIA WITH ASSOCIATED VASCULAR DISEASES

Some patients with neuritic and arthritic symptoms also have arterial or venous disease. However, it can readily be determined whether the arterial or venous disease is significant enough to cause the symptoms of which the patient complains. Arterial disease can be ruled out as the cause of the pain by the following: the absence of true claudication, which is present only on walking and which is relieved by standing still; the absence of rest pain, specifically pain in the toes or metatarsal heads that occurs when the patient lies down and that is relieved (in the earlier stages) by pendency of the extremity; the absence of atrophy of the muscles; the presence of normal skin color and texture of the limb and normal hair growth; and the presence of peripheral pulses. Venous disease of a degree to cause symptoms of pain and discomfort in the extremity can be detected quite readily. It can be ruled out on inspection by the absence of visible, large varicosities and swelling and by the presence of normal color and texture of the skin of the extremity.

DERMATOLOGIC CONDITIONS

The distinctive cutaneous patterns of chronic venous insufficiency of the lower extremity and obliterative arterial disease make their diagnosis easy in the majority of patients. A rash or skin lesion that does not conform to the characteristic vascular stigmas can be suspected to be of some other origin (Fig. 11-14). Dermatologic conditions frequently present a problem in diagnosis, and these patients are best referred to a dermatologist.

DERMATOLOGIC CONDITIONS IN ASSOCIATION WITH CHRONIC VENOUS INSUFFICIENCY

Treatment

One principle has stood us in good stead over the years in treating the patient with a dermatologic lesion of the lower third of the leg in association with chronic venous insufficiency: correct the faulty hydraulics first by controlling the edema by means of pressure bandages. Otherwise, it will be impossible for the dermatologist to heal the lesion with medicaments of any kind. It is also a good rule to give a therapeutic trial of pressure bandaging to any limb with *normal arterial circulation* in which there is a bizarre or chronic unhealed lesion. Again and again, lesions that appear to be dermatologic rather than vascular in origin respond promptly to the application of pressure bandages despite months and often years of unsuccessful treatment with various medications. In our opinion, the explanation is that normal healing is impeded by gravitational effects on the lower extremity; one has only to observe the slower healing time of even a simple laceration on the lower third of the leg compared with the healing time of a similar lesion on the arm or any portion of the head or torso. Accordingly, it is our policy to apply supportive bandages to any laceration, cut, or ulcerated wound of the lower extremity (except in the presence of arterial disease) in addition to whatever other treatment may be instituted (see Color Plate IV. G and H). As a corollary to the thesis that overcoming the unfavorable effects of gravity accelerates healing, elevation of the foot of the bed is prescribed to aid the elimination of swelling.

Figure 11-14. Bluish purplish blotchy intracutaneous hemorrhages almost invariably indicate that patient is undergoing steroid therapy.

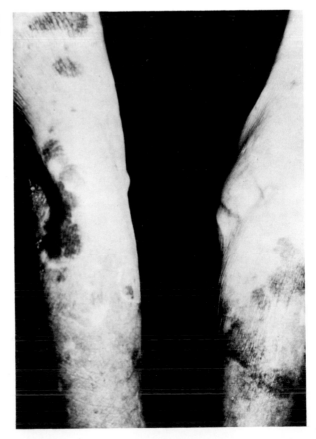

MISCELLANEOUS LESIONS OF THE EXTREMITIES

Figures 11-15 to 11-17 illustrate nonvascular conditions occasionally encountered in practice.

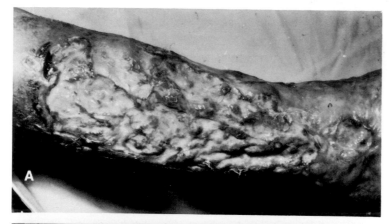

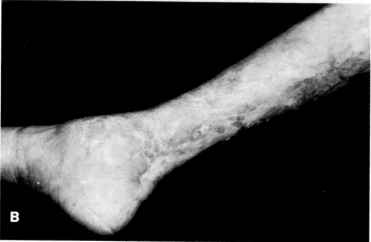

Figure 11-15. A. Such a bizarre atypical lesion suggests a rare disorder. This patient had tertiary lues. **B.** Extraordinarily rapid healing with penicillin therapy.

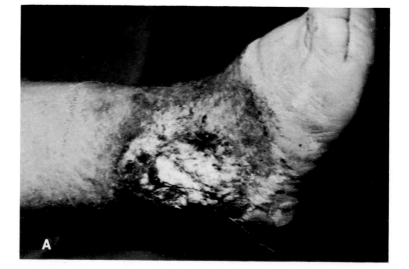

Figure 11-16. A, B, C and **D.** Five patients were encountered with malignant degeneration of an ulcerated leg, or at least associated with ulcer of leg. Four were so bizarre that it was immediately obvious that biopsy should be obtained. One patient was discovered only after biopsy of an ulcer that had failed to respond to therapy.

D. Ulcer of right leg of 70-year-old male; it appeared atypical. Biopsy showed hyperkeratosis. Final diagnosis was verrucous carcinoma (giant papillomatosis). Patient died 3 months after amputation of coronary infarct. Postmortem revealed no evidence of cancer.

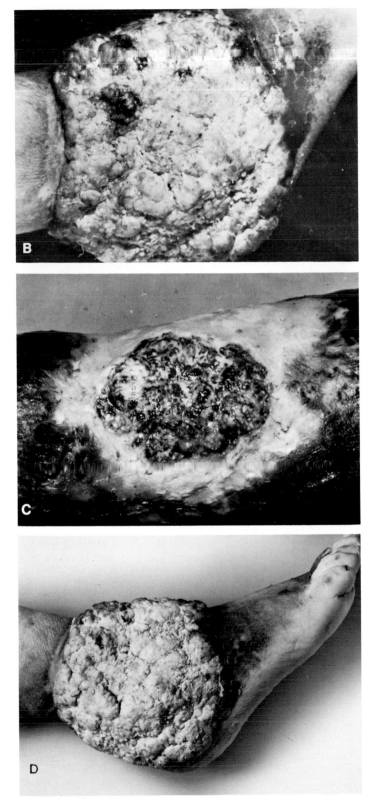

Figure 11-17. Typical picture of "ainhum," formerly believed to be a mysterious disease of the tropics. Dr. Marshall Lee while in the Far East during World War II found that some natives deliberately tied a fine hair around the toe after sustaining a laceration; this was done out of fear of a serious illness recognized to follow infections. (*From teaching collection of late Dr. Louis G. Herrmann.*)

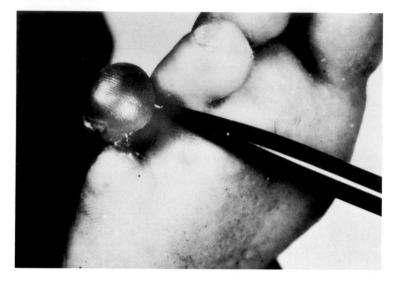

REFERENCES

1. Starling, E. H. On the absorption of fluid from the connective tissue spaces. *J Physiol 19:*312, 1896.
2. Kinmonth, J. B., Rob, C. G., and Simeone, F. A. *Vascular Surgery.* Baltimore, Williams & Wilkins, 1962, pp 342–373.
3. Pappenheimer, J. R. Passage of molecules through capillary walls. *Physiol Rev 33:*387, 1953.
4. Wood, E. H. Physiologic mechanisms for preventing edema of the lower extremities. *Proc Staff Meet Mayo Clin 27:*2, 1952.
5. Landis, E. M., Jones, L., Angevine, M., and Erb, W. The passage of fluid and protein through the human capillary wall during venous congestion. *J Clin Invest 11:*717, 1932.
6. Crockett, D. J. The protein levels of oedema fluids. *Lancet 2:*1179, 1956.
7. Thompson, N. The surgical treatment of chronic lymphoedema of the extremities. *Surg Clin North Am 47:*445, 1967.
8. Malek, P., Belan, A., and Kocandrle, V. L. The superficial and deep lymphatic system of the lower extremities, and their mutual relationship under physiological and pathological conditions. *J Cardiov Surg 5:*686, 1964.
9. Taylor, G. W., Kinmonth, J. B., and Dangerfield, W. G. Protein content of oedema fluid in lymphoedema. *Br M J 1:*1159, 1958.
10. Hudack, S. S., and McMaster, P. D. The lymphatic participation in human cutaneous phenomena. *J Exp Med 57:*751, 1933.
11. Kinmonth, J. B. Lymphangiography in man: A method for outlining lymphatic trunks at operation. *Clin Sci 11:*13, 1952.
12. Kinmonth, J. B., and Taylor, G. W. The lymphatic circulation in lymphedema. *Ann Surg 139:*129, 1954.
13. Kinmonth, J. B., Harper, R. A., and Taylor, G. W. Lymphangiography by radiological methods. *J Fac Radiol 6:*217, 1955.
14. Kinmonth, J. B., Taylor, G. W., Tracy, G. D., and Marsh, J. D. Primary lymphoedema: Clinical and lymphangiographic studies of a series of 107 patients in which the lower limbs were affected. *Br J Surg 45:*1, 1957.
15. Kinmonth, J. B. *The Lymphatics: Diseases, Lymphography and Surgery.* Baltimore, Williams & Wilkins, 1972.
16. Allen, E. V. Lymphedema of the extremities: Classification, etiology and differential diagnosis: A study of three hundred cases. *Arch Int Med 54:*606, 1934.
17. Fairbairn, J. F., Juergens, J. L., and Spittell, J. A., Jr., eds. Allen, E. V., Barker, N. W., Hines, E. A. *Peripheral Vascular Diseases,* ed 4. Philadelphia, Saunders, 1972, p 638.

18. Samman, P. D., and White, W. F. The "yellow nail" syndrome. *Br J Derm 76:*153, 1964.

19. Emerson, P. A. Yellow nails, lymphoedema, and pleural effusions. *Thorax 21:*247, 1966.

20. Dilley, J. J., Kierland, R. R., Randall, R. V., and Shick, R. M. Primary lymphedema associated with yellow nails and pleural effusions. *JAMA 204:*670, 1968.

21. Milroy, W. F. An undescribed variety of hereditary lymphoedema. *NY Med J 56:*205, 1892.

22. Osler, W. *The Principles and Practice of Medicine: Designed for the Use of Practitioners and Students of Medicine.* New York, Appleton, 1892.

23. Meige, H. Dystrophe oedémateuse héréditaire. *Press méd 6:*341, 1898.

24. Milroy, W. E. Chronic hereditary oedema. *JAMA 91:*1172, 1928.

25. Handley, W. S. Lymphangioplasty: A new method for the relief of the brawny arm of breast cancer and for similar conditions of lymphatic oedema: Preliminary note. *Lancet 1:*738, 1908.

26. Gillies, H. D., and Fraser, S. Treatment of lymphoedema by plastic operation. *Br. Med J 1:*96, 1935.

27. Thompson, N. The subcutaneous dermis graft: A clinical and histologic study in man. *Plast Reconstr Surg 26:*1, 1960.

28. Thompson, N. A clinical and histologic investigation into the fate of epithelial elements buried following grafting of "shaved" skin surfaces. *Br J Plastic Surg 13:*219, 1960.

29. Thompson, N. Surgical treatment of chronoc lymphoedema of the lower limb: with preliminary report of new operation. *Br Med J 2:*1566, 1962.

30. Thompson, N. Surgical treatment of chronic obstructive lymphoedema of upper and lower limbs by cutaneous lymphatic transposition. *III Internat Congr Plast Surg,* 1964, p. 849.

31. Thompson, N. Surgical treatment of primary and secondary lymphoedema of the extremities by lymphatic transposition. *Proc Roy Soc Med 58:*1026, 1965.

32. Nielubowicz, J., and Olszewski, W. Surgical relief of lymphoedema, abstracted. *World Med* 90, 1966.

33. Rivero, O. R., Calnan, J. S., Reis, N. D., and Mercurius-Taylor, L. Experimental peripheral lymphovenous communications. *Br J Plastic Surg 20:*124, 1967.

34. Calnan, J. S., Reis, N. D., Rivero, O. R., Copenhagen, H. J., and Mercurius-Taylor, L. The natural history of lymph node-to-vein anastomosis. *Br J Plastic Surg 20:*134, 1967.

35. Goldsmith, H. S., DeLos Santos, R., and Beattie, E. J. Relief of chronic lymphedema by omental transposition. *Ann Surg 166:*573, 1967.

36. Goldsmith, H. S., and DeLos Santos, R. Omental transposition in primary lymphedema. *Surg Gynecol Obstet 125:*607, 1967.

37. Lanzara, A. Surgical treatment of lymphoedema by omental transplantation. *J Cardiovasc. Surg.* Special No. for XVIIth Congress of the European Society of Cardiovascular Surgery, 1968, p 122.

38. Charles, R. H. *A System of Treatment.* London, Churchill, 1912, vol. 3, p 504.

39. Kondoleon, E. Die chirurgische Behandlung der elephantiastischen Oedeme durch eine neue Methode der Lymphableitung. *Münch Med Wchsch 59:*2726, 1912.

40. Sistrunk, W. E. Experiences with the Kondoleon operation for elephantiasis. *JAMA 71:*800, 1918.

41. Auchincloss, H. New operation for elephantiasis. *Puerto Rico J Pub Health Trop Med 6:*149, 1930.

42. Homans, J. Treatment of elephantiasis of the legs: A preliminary report. *N Engl J Med 215:*1099, 1936.

43. Miller, T. A., Harper, J., and Longmire, W. P. The management of lymphedema by staged subcutaneous excision. *Surg Gynecol Obstet 136:*586, 1973.

44. Sabouraud, R. Sur la parasitologie de l'elephantiasis nostras. *Ann Derm Syph 3:*592, 1892.

45. Edwards, E. A. Recurrent febrile episodes and lymphedema. *JAMA 184:*858, 1963.

46. Ochsner, A., Longacre, A. B., and Murray, S. A. Progressive lymphedema associated with recurrent erysipeloid infections. *Surgery 8:*383, 1940.

47. McGlasson, J. L. Recurrent erysipelas of legs with dermatitis of feet. *Arch Derm 14:*679, 1926.

48. Goldberg, M. J. A syndrome that is already a syndrome: "Coup de fouet" is "Tennis leg." *Angiology 21:*230, 1970.

49. Martorell, F. Le syndrome de coup de fouet. *Presse méd 63:*522, 1955.

50. Henzel, J. H. Pories, W. J., Smith, J. L., Burget, D. E., and Plecha, F. R. Pathogenesis and management of abdominal wall hematomas. *Arch Surg 93:*929, 1966.

51. Gilcreest, E. L. Rupture and tears of muscle and tendons of the lower extremities: Report of fifteen cases. *JAMA 100:*153, 1933.

52. Costeas, F. R., Papastavrou, E., and Alexandrides, K. The "coup de fouet" syndrome of lower extremities. *Angiology 16:*252, 1965.

Index

Page numbers in italic indicate illustrations. Page numbers followed by the letter t indicate tabular information.